Assisted Reproductive Technologies

ASSISTED REPRODUCTIVE TECHNOLOGIES

Current Methods and Future Directions

Edited by

Indira Hinduja

Kusum Zaveri

Chander Puri

OXFORD
UNIVERSITY PRESS

OXFORD
UNIVERSITY PRESS

YMCA Library Building, Jai Singh Road, New Delhi 110001

Oxford University Press is a department of the University of Oxford. It furthers the University's objective of excellence in research, scholarship, and education by publishing worldwide in

Oxford New York
Athens Auckland Bangkok Bogota Buenos Aires Cape Town
Chennai Dar es Salaam Delhi Florence Hong Kong Istanbul
Karachi Kolkata Kuala Lumpur Madrid Melbourne Mexico City Mumbai
Nairobi Paris Sao Paolo Singapore Taipei Tokyo Toronto Warsaw

with associated companies in

Berlin Ibadan

Oxford is a registered trade mark of Oxford University Press in the UK and in certain other countries

Published in India
By Oxford University Press, New Delhi

First published 2001

ISBN 0 19 5656067

Typset in Galliard by Eleven Arts, Keshav Puram, New Delhi 110035
Printed in India by Pauls Press, New Delhi 110 020
and published by Manzar Khan, Oxford University Press
YMCA Library Building, Jai Singh Road, New Delhi 110 001

Contents

Foreword

The birth of the first test tube baby, Louise Brown, in 1978 through the use of Assisted Reproductive Technologies (ART) rekindled hopes of parenthood in a large number of infertile couples. This historical milestone achieved by Dr Patrick Steptoe and Dr Robert Edwards demonstrated that human gametes can be fertilized in-vitro and can be grown into a healthy baby when the fertilized egg is placed inside a woman's womb. Significant advancement has been made in ARTs since then and these have succeeded in realizing the dreams of parenthood of azoospermic men, women with tubal blockage or endometriosis, and many others with reproductive anomalies. With the advent of these techniques, now it is feasible to fertilize the egg with one single spermatozoon recovered from the testes or epididymis, or picked up from the ejaculate of men with normal or deficient spermatogenesis. Success of various ART techniques and their acceptance in the society is evident from the fact that more than 6,00,000 babies have been born all over the world using these techniques since 1978.

It is matter of great pride for us that India has been at the forefront of the development and adoption of ART. India's first scientifically documented 'test tube baby' Harsha was born in 1986 due to the concerted efforts of the Institute for Research in Reproduction (IRR), an Institute of the Indian Council of Medical Research (ICMR), and the K.E.M. Hospital in Mumbai.

Today, a number of centres have started extending ART services in remote corners of the country. The take-home-baby rate through the use of these techniques in India is comparable to that of the most reputed centres in the world. While the potential for ARTs in overcoming the barriers to successful fertilization is huge, its use has been limited to some degree because of the high expenses incurred in establishing and sustaining these facilities. Consequently, only the privileged sections of the society can avail benefits of ARTs. However, as research continues, there is no doubt that ARTs will be made available to larger sections of the population by public as well as private sector institutions.

This book provides a comprehensive and detailed overview of the entire gamut of assisted reproduction techniques. Collectively, this book represents the insight gathered by more than 500 years of clinical, scientific and research experience. It captures every nuance of the practice, the methods, the benefits, the pitfalls and the precautions involved in ART technologies. Moreover, it also presents the views and thoughts of the scientists who themselves have contributed to the standardization and refinement of ARTs. This book also offers valuable information for those interested in pursuing research in reproductive biology using ARTs.

I am particularly pleased that this book has been edited by Indian scientists who have pioneered India's foray into this cutting edge area of medicine.

Nirmal K. Ganguly, M.D.
Director General
Indian Council of Medical Research

Preface

The rapid progress in medical technology and molecular medicine during recent years has resulted in a better understanding of the process of human reproduction. Our insight into this complex process of nature has given us the ability not only to assist it, but also to manipulate it. In a lot of cases, greater understanding has helped us develop simpler treatments for conditions that were hitherto difficult to manage. The treatment of male infertility, for instance, has drawn upon the knowledge from other fields such as preimplantation genetic diagnosis.

Today the field of Assisted Reproduction has evolved into a flourishing science with several sub-specialities, each of which have their own significant roles to play in the overall treatment of male and female infertility. In this book, we have tried to provide a detailed discussion on each of the sub-areas in Assisted Reproduction. We are delighted that national and international authorities on each of the subjects agreed to contribute. No doubt, each of the subjects could be dealt with in separate dedicated books, and indeed they have been. This book attempts to collate the state-of-the-art in each of the Assisted Reproductive Technologies (ARTs) under one umbrella, and to provide the reader with an insight into what lies ahead in the area of Assisted Reproduction.

Often it is asked whether ARTs are required in a world that is plagued by hunger, disease, lack of education and various other ailments. There is no doubt a larger social question needs to be addressed. At the very outset, therefore, we have tried to put ARTs in perspective with the social issues as a background. This is followed by the scientific aspects of ARTs, starting with evaluation of female infertility to various techniques of Assisted Reproduction.

We hope that through the flow of chapters in this book, the reader will derive an overview of where ARTs have come from, what are the techniques in use today and where they are likely to go. We begin by discussing the social and scientific impact of ARTs. The next few chapters deal with various aspects of female infertility, its evaluation and treatment, the normal menstrual cycle, ovarian stimulation in Assisted Reproduction, and oocyte maturation both *in vivo* and *in vitro*. These are followed by discussing the recent advances in embryo culture, and Assisted Reproduction in cases with other conditions such as polycystic ovaries and genital tuberculosis. The diagnosis and treatments associated with male infertility are discussed in length in the next few chapters. The role of imaging techniques in cases of Assisted Reproduction is also covered as a separate topic. Finally, several issues around recent advances in ARTs, as also the clinical and medico-legal aspects of ARTs, are explored in the final chapters of this book.

We are deeply grateful to all the contributors who have encapsulated their years of experience and knowledge into individual manuscripts. We also wish to thank Oxford University Press, New Delhi for assistance in preparing this book.

List of Contributors

Anibal Acosta
Scientific Director,
CEGYR
Centro De Estudios En Ginecologia Reproducion
Institucion afiliada a la Facultad de Medicina
de la Universidad de Buenos Aires
Viamonte 1438 (1055)
Buenos Aires, Argentina.

David T. Baird
Clinical Research Professor,
Centre for Reproductive Biology
University of Edinburgh

J.C. Calamera
Investigacion Basica
CEGYR
Centro De Estudios En Ginecologia Reproducion
Institucion afiliada a la Facultad de Medicina
de la Universidad de Buenos Aires
Viamonte 1438 (1055)
Buenos Aires, Argentina.

Alan Decherney
Edito-in-Chief.
Department of Obst & Gynec., UCLA School of Medicines
10833 Le Conte Avenue, 22–132 CHS, Los Angeles,
California, 90095–1740, U.S.A.

Sadhana K. Desai
Director Fertility Clinic
Spring field,
Vatchha Gandhi Road
Mumbai-400007.
India.

Marc Dhont
Professor of Obstetrics & Gynaecology
Chairman of Department and Head of Fertility Centre
University of Ghent, Belgium

Josiane Van der Elst
Head of IVF Laboratory
Infertility Centre
Ghent University Hospital
De Pintelaan 185
9000 Ghent
Belgium

Sozos J. Fasouliotis
Department of Obstetrics and Gynaecology,
Hebrew University-Hadassah Medical Centre
Jerusalem, 911020, Israel.

Anuradha Goud
Centre for Molecular Medicine and Genetics and
Department of Obstetrics and Gynaecology
Wayne State University School of Medicine
Detroit, Michigan, U.S.A.

Pravin Goud
Division of Reproductive Endocrinology and Infertility
Department of Obstetrics and Gynaecology
Wayne State University School of Medicine
Detroit, Michigan, U.S.A.

Jesse J. Hade
Department of Obst & Gynec., UCLA School of Medicines
10833 Le Conte Avenue, 22–132 CHS, Los Angeles,
California, 90095–1740, U.S.A.

Dr Indira Hinduja
Scientific Director
Inkus IVF Centre,
311, Mehta Bhavan,
Charni Road,
Mumbai-400004.
India.

Michelle Hutchison
Department of Obst & Gynec., UCLA School of Medicines
10833 Le Conte Avenue, 22–132 CHS, Los Angeles,
California, 90095–1740, U.S.A.

Semra Kahraman
Associate Professor
Reproductive Endocrinology,
ART and Genetics Unit
Istanbul Memorial Hospital
Talatpasa Bulvari, 80270,
Okmeydani,
Istanbul, Turkey

Iqbal Khan
Scientific Director
IVF Michigan
Rochester Hills,
Michigan, U.S.A.

C.P. Lulla
Sonologist
Ria Clinic
Geeta B,
Huges Road,
Mumbai-400007
India.

Nijs Martine
Clinical Embryologist
Schoysman Infertility Management Foundation
Van Helmont Ziekenhuis
Vaartstraat 42
1800 Vilvoorde-Belgium

M.B. Minbattiwalla
Embryologist
Inkus IVF Centre,
311, Mehta Bhavan,
Charni Road,
Mumbai-40004.
India.

F. Nodar
Directores Asociados
CEGYR
Centro De Estudios En Ginecologia Reproducion
Institucion afiliada a la Facultad de Medicina
de la Universidad de Buenos Aires
Viamonte 1438 (1055)
Buenos Aires, Argentina.

P.L. Oei
Assistant Professor
Dept of Obstetrics & Gynaecology
National University of Singapore
National University Hospital
Lower Kent Ridge Road
Singapore 119074

Pritam P. Phatnani.
Hon. Professor & Head, Dept of Forensic Medicine & Toxicology,
L.T.M. Medical College,
Mumbai.

Vanderzwalmen Pierre
Clinical Embryologist
Schoysman Infertility Management Foundation
SIMAF
Van Helmont Ziekenhuis
Vaartstraat 42, 1800 VILVOORDE
Belium.

Chander Puri
Director
Institute of Research in Reproduction
Parel,
Mumbai-400012
India.

Prof. S.S. Ratnam
Emeritus Professor
Department of Obstetrics & Gynaecology
National University of Singapore
National University Hospital
Lower Kent Ridge Road,
Singapore 119074

V. Rawe
Investigacion Basica
CEGYR
Centro De Estudios En Ginecologia Reproducion
Institucion afiliada a la Facultad de Medicina
de la Universidad de Buenos Aires
Viamonte 1438 (1055)
Buenos Aires, Argentina.

G. Sachdeva
Research Officer
Primate Biology Lab
Institute of Research in Reproduction
Parel,
Mumbai-400012
India.

Josheph G. Schenker
Professor of Obstetrics & Gynaecology
Hebrew University-Hadassah Medical Centre
P.O. Box 12000
Jerusalem, 91120, Israel

Rupin Shah
Consultant Andrologist & Infertility Microsurgeon,
Bhatia General Hospital, Mumbai-400007
India.

K. Joo Thong
Director, Assisted Conception Unit
Simpson Memorial Maternity Pavilion/
Lothian University NHS Trust

Kusum Zaveri
Medical Director
Inkus IVF Centre,
311, Mehta Bhavan,
Charni Road,
Bombay-400004.
India.

1

IVF in the Contemporary World— Its Necessity

Indira Hinduja, Kusum Zaveri and Chander Puri

The desire for children by the normal woman is stronger than self-interest in beauty and figure, stronger than the claims of a career: in the man it is less intense. Childlessness is generally a tragedy to the married woman and can be a cause of mental upset, as well as of personal unhappiness and ill health. The having of children cements a marriage and when a breakdown is threatened, the future welfare of their offspring often deters man and wife from separating.—Sir Norman Jeffcoate

Infertility is a distressing condition. It is a problem affecting couples worldwide, irrespective of geographical location, religion, community, socio-economic status, or education. The overall incidence of infertility as well as the causes remain the same, whereas the prevalence of causes may differ, e.g. incidence of endometriosis in the developed countries over tuberculosis in the developing countries.

Approximately, 10%–15% of the couples within the reproductive age group are infertile. At any given time, there are an estimated 60–80 million infertile couples, of which almost 18 million are in India alone (WHO, 1998). According to The International Federation of Gynaecology and Obstetrics (FIGO manual, 1990), the incidence of male and female factors is as follows.

Causes	Percentage
Female factor	25–37
Male factor	8–22
Both male & female factors	21–38
Unexplained	3–14

The World Health Organization (WHO) in 1989 carried out a multicentric study of over 10,000 infertile couples and documented approximate percentages as follows—male factor infertility in 33% of the cases, female factor in 25%, and both partners responsible in 25%. The remaining cases were due to unexplained factors.

CAUSES OF INFERTILITY

The causes of infertility in females include tubal disease, ovulatory dysfunction, endometriosis, immunological factors or others that are unexplained. Tubal obstruction is the most common cause. Cates et al. (1985) found tubal obstruction in 36% of infertile women in developed countries, 39% in Asia, 44% in Latin America and 85% in Africa. This finding is corroborated by a WHO sponsored multicentric collaborative investigation (WHO, 1987) of the infertile couple between 1979 and 1984, carried out at 33 centres in 25 countries throughout the developed and developing worlds. Bilateral tubal occlusion and other infection-related infertility diagnoses were found to be strongly connected to a previous history of sexually transmitted disease (STD), pelvic inflammatory disease (PID) and post-abortal and postpartum infectious morbidity. The main purpose of this study was to underline the fact that tubal disease becomes the major cause of infertility among women consequent to genital tract infections—either STDs (Chlamydia, gonorrhoea) or post-abortal or postpartum infections, which are preventable. Therefore, there is a necessity for culturally sensitive public education programmes to spread awareness among the general population about the causes, dangers and ways to prevent STDs, and simultaneously, for setting up more STD clinics for proper diagnosis and treatment. Traditional birth attendants practising in developing countries can be trained to use hygienic procedures and asepsis and antisepsis to reduce secondary postpartum infection. There is also a need to intensify the practice of contraceptive methods to prevent unwanted pregnancies and subsequent abortions. Another aetiology for tubal occlusion is abdominal tuberculosis, which often results in irreversible tubal damage. Preventive measures like early diagnosis and timely treatment of tuberculosis are hence very important.

In males, varicocele, primary testicular failure, accessory gland infection, abnormal sperm count, motility and morphology are the main causes. Other less common causes include congenital anomalies, obstructive and endocrine pathologies. Sometimes, however, there is no demonstrable cause. Defective spermatogenesis may be due to pituitary disorders, genetic factors, testicular cancer, germ cell aplasia, varicocele, certain drugs, environmental and therapeutic factors, or toxins. Over the past 50 years, there has been a trend of decline in semen quality (Carlsen et al., 1992). They found a significant decrease in the mean sperm count among proven fertile males from 113 million/ mL in 1940 to 66 million/ mL in 1990, as also a decrease in semen volume from 3.4 mL to 2.75 mL. This could be the effect of increasing environmental pollution on the reproductive ability. Auger et al. (1995) have also proved that the concentration, motility and percentage of morphologically normal spermatozoa have declined over the past 20 years. In other words, given that the same environmental conditions continued, 50 years hence, the sperm count would range between 15 and 20 million. However, both the studies have highlighted the decline in normal sperm parameters. There is no such data available for males having abnormal sperm parameters.

In the past, the medical and surgical lines of treatment, especially for azoospermia, tubal blockage and unexplained infertility, yielded poor results and the childless couple could do little to achieve pregnancy. Childlessness is seldom accepted completely and feelings of grief do emerge from time to time.

With the increase in the knowledge of reproductive physiology and improved diagnostic methods, the management of infertility has improved. The birth of Louise Brown, the world's first successful baby following *in vitro*-fertilization and embryo transfer (IVF-ET) (Steptoe and Edwards, 1978), gave hope to millions of infertile couples. Since then, the many advances in Assisted Reproductive Technology (ART) have improved the pregnancy rates immensely. India's own first scientifically-documented IVF baby (Harsha), born in 1986, and subsequent successes since then have been widely publicized (Hinduja et al., 1988). This has given a ray of hope to even illiterate, poor couples residing in remote villages. They dream of being successful in having their very own baby one day.

The success rates of ART depend on the ovulation stimulation protocols used, technique of retrieval and handling of oocytes, preparation of spermatozoa prior to fertilization, optimal conditions of embryo growth, endometrial preparation, embryo replacement techniques, luteal-phase support, etc. Variations in patient characteristics, like the duration of infertility, maternal age, presumed cause(s) of infertility, previous history of infertility and treatment, also determine the success rate.

In a report by the Society for Assisted Reproductive Technology and the American Society for Reproductive Medicines, 1994, data on 42,509 ART treatment cycles initiated at 249 centres operating in the US and Canada is summarized. The rate of deliveries per retrieval for stimulated IVF cycles in women < 40 years of age with male factor infertility was 20.2%, as compared to 24.5% among women in the same age-group without male factor. The clinical pregnancy rates per retrieval for IVF, Gamete Intra-Fallopian Transfer (GIFT) and Zygote Intra-Fallopian Transfer (ZIFT) were found to be 26.3%, 36.3% and 34.8% respectively, and the delivery rates per retrieval were 21.1% in IVF, 28.5% in GIFT and 29.1% in ZIFT. The rates of pregnancy losses were 19%, 22.5% and 16.2% respectively.

In the United Kingdom (UK), 80% of provision

for IVF is estimated as being private, as compared to the 20% provided for by the National Health Service. Depending on the prevalence of infertility among couples in the reproductive age group, an estimated 40 IVF cycles need to be performed per year for a population of 100,000 (NIAC, 1995). Of these 40 cycles, 8.1 cycles per 100,000 were funded by the state during 1994 to 1995. If the magnitude of the need for infertility management in India is equated to that of the UK, then for a population of one billion, approximately 400,000 IVF cycles will have to be performed per year. This highlights the need for a large number of well-equipped ART centres spread all over the country.

Currently in India, most of the facilities for infertility management, including ART, are available through the private sector in some of the metropolitan cities. It is estimated that the cost per cycle, with a take–home–baby rate of just 20%–30%, is between Rs 50,000 to Rs 75,000(US $1,000–2,000), in addition to the subsequent obstetric costs. These high costs are a consequence of expensive infrastructure, the drugs required for inducing multiple ovulations and maintenance expenses. It is expected that the average cost of having a baby through ART may reduce as we understand more about the reproductive physiology, which may help increase the success rate per cycle as well through indigenous technologies. The question that arises is whether in a developing country like India, where there is a population explosion and there are more basic and pressing health necessities like eradication of polio, nutrition-related blindness, rickets, tuberculosis, malaria, dysentery, etc., is the resource drain towards management of infertility with ART justified?

Pushing for adoption by the infertile couple, who is already under immense pressure from the psycho-social point of view, in order to balance the growing population can neither be justified, nor can it be a satisfactory solution to the problem of infertility. The need for parenting a biological child is very intense and it is a basic right of the couple, and no amount of substitution is satisfactory and fulfilling to them. Adoption is a very noble act and it is the responsibility of the society and the country concerned. The problem of population should be tackled by encouraging couples with at least one biological child to adopt the next one, if desired.

A lot of importance is given to tubal microsurgery, especially in cases where a reversal of sterilization is required due to calamity or the death of a child. The anguish of the bereaved parents is something very palpable. But tubal microsurgery may prove unsuccessful in previously infected tubes, especially in cases with a past history of tuberculosis. Ultimately, the couple finds hope in ART. The importance of IVF is thus underlined. In male factor infertility, even after the medical and surgical lines of treatment have been pursued, there is no marked improvement in the outcome and microfertilization is the only hope.

Infertility is a basic component of reproductive health and its prevention and appropriate treatment is essential. To raise the standards of reproductive health, many aspects have to be taken into consideration and improvement in environmental pollution especially has to be tackled aggressively (cause of decreasing semen parameters). There is a need to increase the awareness in society about the importance of the same. Women need to be educated about contraception and prevention of STDs, and knowledge needs to be augmented among midwives and traditional birth attendants regarding the use of proper aseptic techniques, so as to prevent tubal causes of infertility. But how soon can this utopian situation be achieved is anybody's guess. Today in India, in spite of a growing awareness among the general population and the ongoing attempts to decrease pollution, it is difficult to make any headway. Thus till such time as these parameters are controlled, the need for ART remains acute.

Though there are many arguments that highlight the need for ART, the cost factor is unfortunately inhibitive. Infertility is not a life-threatening condition as such and hence, ART is not a life-saving treatment modality, but at the same time, it helps in building up families. Parallel to the efforts to eliminate the preventable causes of infertility, attempts should be made to reduce the cost of ART and improve the results in terms of take-home-baby rates. This will reduce the number of cycle attempts and also reduce the economic burden on the nation as well as the individual, and also achieve a successful family health programme.

ACKNOWLEDGEMENTS

We wish to express our gratitude to Dr Pradyna Parulekar for helping us in preparing the chapter and Mrs Jyotsina Chhabria for her typing assistance.

REFERENCES

Auger, J. et al. (1995). 'Decline in semen quality among fertile men in Paris during the past 20 years', *N. Engl.J. Med.*, **332**: 281-5.

Carlsen, E. et al. (1992). 'Evidence of decreasing quality of semen during past 50 years', *BMJ*, **305**: 609-12.

Cates, W. et al. (1985). 'Worldwide patterns of infertility: Is Africa different?' *Lancet*, **2**: 596-8.

Fathalla, M.F. et al. (eds.) (1990). 'Reproductive health: Global issues', *Figo Manual of Human Reproduction*, Parthenon Publication Group, Lancaster, vol. 3, pp. 65–77.

Hinduja, I. N. et al. (1988). 'The *in vitro* Fertilization and Embryo Transfer (IVF-ET) and Gamete Intra Fallopian Transfer (GIFT) programme at the Institute for Research in Reproduction (ICMR) and the King Edwards Memorial Hospital, Bombay', *J. In Vitro Fert. and Embryo Transfer*, **5**: 376-7.

National Infertility Awareness Campaign (1995). *Report of the Third and Fourth National Surveys of NHS Funding of Infertility Services*, London College of Health.

Sir Jeffcoate, N. (1975). 'Sterility and Subfertility', *Principles of Gynaecology*-4th ed. Butterworth & Co. Ltd., London and Boston, p. 583.

Society for Assisted Reproductive Technology and The American Society of Reproductive Medicines (1996). 'Assisted reproductive technology in the United States and Canada: 1994 results generated from the American Society for Reproductive Medicine/Society for Assisted Reproductive Technology Registry', *Fertil. Steril.*, **66**: 697–705.

Steptoe, P.C. and R.G. Edwards (1978). 'Birth after the re-implantation of a human embryo (letter)', *Lancet*, **2**: 366.

World Health Organization (1987). 'Infection, pregnancies and infertility: Perspectives in prevention', *Fertil. Steril.*, **47**: 964–8.

———(1989). *Biennial Report 1988-89*, Research in Human Reproduction, W.H.O., Geneva p. 35.

———(1998). *Sexual and reproductive health research: Priorities for WHO for the period 1998-2003*. World Health Organization, Geneva.

2

Recent Trends in Evaluation and Management of Female Infertility

P.L. Oei and S.S. Ratnam

Infertility affects approximately 10%–15% of couples in the reproductive age group (Mosher and Pratt, 1991). However, there appears to be an increase in the number of women with infertility. It was projected that the number of women with infertility in the United States would be 5.1 million in 1995 and 4.8–5.9 million in 2020 (Stephen, 1996). These projections have, however, been revised upwards substantially. It is now estimated that the number of infertile women will range from 5.4–7.7 million in 2025, most likely just under 6.5 million (Stephen and Chandra, 1998). Infertility has thus become an important medical issue with social and economic implications.

AGE AND FEMALE INFERTILITY

There is little change in a woman's fecundity when she is in her twenties, and she is at her most successful in achieving a pregnancy and delivery. However, with ageing, there is a decline in the natural ability to reproduce. It would appear that a state of 'reproductive menopause' exists for about 10 years before the onset of the 'endocrine menopause' (Sauer,1996).

After the age of 37, a woman's fertility is reduced by about 50%, and by the time she is 45 years old, her fertility has dropped by 95% (National Centre for Health Statistics, 1983). This decline in a woman's reproductive potential is due to a decrease in oocyte fertilization, embryo hatching, implantation and embryogenesis, which is related to the ageing process (Sauer,1996). There is also an associated decline in uterine receptivity due to the senescent uterus of the older woman (Levran et al, 1991)

EVALUATION OF FEMALE INFERTILITY

A whole gamut of tests are available and these are used in the investigation of female infertility. They range from the simple, cheap and noninvasive to the most advanced techniques in imaging available today. Regardless of the test used, the ultimate aim in the investigation of the infertile female is to detect ovulation, assess the tubes for any pathology that may interfere with patency and transport of the gametes and fertilized oocyte, and to assess the uterine cavity for abnormalities which could interfere with implantation of the embryo.

In the evaluation and management of female infertility, it is crucial to keep in mind the age-related decline in female infertility. Time is of essence, and the investigation and treatment must be instituted without any delay.

INVESTIGATIONS

HORMONES

A serum hormonal assay is part of the preliminary investigations for female infertility. The basic hormones which are estimated include follicular stimulating hormone (FSH), luteinizing hormone (LH), prolactin and progesterone.

Prolactin

A third of the women with no obvious cause of amenorrhoea have a high prolactin level. Elevated prolactin levels interfere with the normal functioning of the menstrual cycle by suppressing the pulsatile secretion of GnRH. In a subfertile patient with hyperprolactinaemia, treatment is by induction of ovulation. In 80% of patients with galactorrhoea and hyperprolactinaemia, ovulatory menses and pregnancy can be achieved (Speroff, 1994). Serum prolactin should always be assayed in a woman with infertility as there may not be any clinical symptoms to suggest hyperprolactinaemia.

Progesterone

Israel et al. (1972) first described a single luteal-phase serum progesterone assay as an indicator of ovulation. However, progesterone secretion is pulsatile throughout the human luteal phase. Hence, a single measurement of progesterone in the mid-luteal phase is not always a reliable indicator of ovulation (Steele et al., 1985).

Comparing endometrial biopsy and serum progesterone in 55 infertile women, it was shown that a single well-timed serum progesterone level is superior to a single endometrial biopsy as a screening method for confirmation of ovulation (Shepard and Senturia, 1977).

Luteinizing Hormone

When measuring the serum LH levels, the reversal of the FSH / LH ratio is a biochemical indicator of polycystic ovaries. The detection of LH, either in the serum or the urine, is also a reliable evidence of ovulation (Vermesh et al., 1987).

However, because of the pulsatile release of LH from the pituitary gland, the serum peak may be missed in a single daily blood sampling. Hence, comparing the serum and urinary detection of LH, Grinsted et al. (1989) noted that doubling values of serum LH were inferior to the urinary detection of the peak. Urinary determination of LH is also rapid and cheap, and has the advantage of ease, without demands on staff operations.

However, Fedele et al. (1990) found that in spontaneous cycles, as well as in cycles induced with gonadotrophins (because of the fluctuating levels of LH and the possible cross-reactivity of the drugs used), urinary LH was less reliable than serum LH in terms of predictability.

Follicular Stimulating Hormone

Follicular stimulating hormone (FSH) is measured as an indication of the ovarian function. An elevated FSH during the reproductive life is an early manifestation of ovarian ageing. In young regularly menstruating infertile women with an elevated FSH, there is significantly slower follicular growth, smaller follicle diameter and lower luteal-phase salivary progesterone. These are features recorded in older women during their menopause transition (Ebbiary et al., 1994).

However, there are wide variations in FSH concentrations from cycle to cycle (Scott and Hofman, 1995). Hence, if the FSH is raised, indicating ovarian failure, a repeat sample is performed to verify this end-stage diagnosis.

The FSH concentration does not fully indicate the extent of ovarian reserve, and usually by the time that FSH concentrations are elevated, the ovaries have become refractory (Lass et al., 1997). Hence, transvaginal measurement of ovarian volume and ovarian biopsy have been investigated as alternative methods of assessing ovarian function.

Ovarian Biopsy

The number of primordial follicles in the human female decreases from >250,000 at menarche to only a few hundreds or thousands at the end of the reproductive life (Block, 1952). This loss accelerates around the age of 37 years and precedes the menopause by about 10–12 years (Faddy and Gosden, 1995,1996). There is, however, variation in the number and rate of depletion of the follicles. Age and regularity of the menstrual cycles are also not reliable indicators of the ovarian reserve (Lass et al., 1997).

In 60 women who were investigated for infertility, the early follicular-phase FSH was measured, the ovarian volume was assessed by transvaginal ultrasound and an ovarian biopsy was obtained for histological assessment of the number of follicles. It was found that follicular density decreased significantly with increasing age, with women >35 years having only a third of the concentration of follicles of younger women. Those women who had practically no follicles in their biopsies were significantly older than those with follicles. This study also showed that FSH was similar in the older (>35 years) and younger women (<35 years), and that there was no correlation with follicular density (Lass et al.,

1997). In this small study, none of the women experienced any complication from the biopsy. FSH is thus a relatively late sign of ageing; and the basal fertility level of a woman who presents for infertility treatment may be better assessed by ovarian biopsy combined with ovarian volume measurements.

Detection Of Ovulation

The detection of ovulation is one of the basic infertility investigations that is recommended by WHO (Rowe et al., 1993). There are numerous methods to document ovulation, and these include serum progesterone measurements, serum/urinary LH measurements, basal body temperature charts (BBT) and follicle measurement by ultrasound.

Basal Body Temperature (BBT) Charts

It was W.S. Squire who first described, in 1868, the biphasic basal body temperature pattern that occurs throughout the menstrual cycle. Progesterone is thermogenic, and the basal body temperature chart is, therefore, an indirect evidence of ovulation. Morning temperatures are subject to wide inter- and intra-individual variations; and it is the pattern of the basal body temperature throughout the menstrual cycle rather than the absolute temperature value which is considered in the evaluation of ovulation.

A distinctly biphasic basal body temperature with a sustained rise in temperature of approximately 14 days' duration is indicative of ovulation. The nadir which precedes the rise in temperature coincides with the luteinizing hormone peak. Ovulation occurs some time between the nadir and the first day of the rise in temperature. On the other hand, anovulation is suggested by a flat monophasic pattern throughout the whole cycle (Insler and Lunenfield, 1986).

The basal body temperature graph is relatively simple, inexpensive and well tolerated (Martinez et al., 1992). When Ayres-de-Campos et al. (1995) analysed 160 BBTs visually, it was found that the reproducibility of the 'ovulatory' graph feature (i.e. the biphasic pattern and the adequate thermal shifts) was excellent. There are reports on BBT graph analysis by computer-based mathematical algorithms, but a clinical evaluation has not been performed. Moreover, using computer analysis would have the disadvantage of making this simple and basic investigation expensive, complicated and less applicable (McCarthy and Rockette, 1983).

However, there are numerous problems associated with charting the basal body temperature. Incorrect measurement and registration of temperature by patients is an important limiting factor (Ayres-de-Campos et al., 1995). The BBT also does not necessarily show evidence of ovulation, and is of limited value in the timing of intercourse. Vermesh et al. (1987), in an evaluation of the accuracy of various methods in the detection of ovulation, reported that the BBT nadir predicted the day of ovulation in only 10% of cycles. Moreover, couples often become anxious and worried when their temperature charts do not follow the expected pattern. The pressure to have sexual intercourse as dictated by the BBT can also lead to anxiety-related sexual dysfunction in both partners. Temperature charts are, therefore, of limited practical use, and the woman should be discouraged from charting her daily temperature to monitor for the day of ovulation. What would be more useful would be a menstrual calendar which, at a glance, would be able to indicate any menstrual irregularities (RCOG, 1992).

Postcoital Test (PCT)

The postcoital test involves assessing the cervical mucus for the presence of progressively motile sperms. It is a measure of how well the sperms can penetrate and survive in the cervical mucus. This test was introduced in 1866 by James Marion Sims (Sims,1866), and was rediscovered in 1913 by Max Huhner (Huhner,1913). It is a mainstay of infertility investigations, and is used in nearly half the fertility clinics in Britain, and in two-thirds of the fertility clinics across Europe (Oei et al., 1995). Despite this immense clinical experience, there are many questions which are unresolved regarding the postcoital test, and its clinical relevance remains debatable.

A point of contention concerns the cut-off point between the normal and abnormal results, with different definitions being used by various authors.

The definition of an abnormal postcoital test varies; less than one motile spermatozoa per high power (X400) field (Harrison, 1981; Glazener et al., 1987), less than five (Collins et al., 1984), seven (Samberg et al., 1985), and even twenty (Jette and Glass, 1972).

When there are no sperms seen on the PCT, a sample must be obtained from the posterior vaginal fornix. If this is also negative, and it has been ascertained that intravaginal intercourse has taken place, it is crucial to exclude azoospermia, or retrograde or anejaculation, as a cause of the infertility.

In a review of 11 published studies with a total of 3,093 women, Oei et al. (1995) related PCT results to pregnancy, and found that the discriminating ability of the PCT is poor, and changing the definitions of normality hardly enhanced the predictive power. However, Eimers et al. (1994) in a retrospective analysis of 956 couples, found that the PCT result was a strong predictor of the fertility within the following year.

Beltsos et al. (1966), in a prospective one-year evaluation of 200 couples who were without risk of infertility, found that the mean sperm count per high power field, and the mean number of highly motile sperm were higher among women in whom pregnancy occurred. Additionally, a high number of sperms in the PCT correlated with a high number of motile sperms in the semen analysis.

In the first randomized controlled study comparing infertility investigations, with and without PCT, a total of 736 consecutive new couples who presented for infertility treatment were followed up for 24 months. It was found that the routine use of the PCT led to more tests and treatment, without a significant effect on the pregnancy rate, the cumulative pregnancy rate at the end of 24 months being similar (Oei et al., 1998).

In addition, due to the circumstances that have to be met to obtain the PCT results, there can be stress in the relationship of the infertile couple (Drale and Grunert,1979; De Vires et al., 1984). However, in a randomized controlled trial of 500 new patients, it was found that the PCT had a positive influence on the sexual relationships of the infertile couple (Oei et al., 1996).

The PCT, though widely used, has limited diagnostic potential and is poorly predictive of the chance of pregnancy. Hence, it should not be included in the routine investigations for infertility.

ULTRASOUND

With the introduction of transvaginal ultrasonography, the screening for pelvic pathologies has improved. With transabdominal ultrasonography, 80% of endometriomas can be picked up (Cochrane and Thomas, 1974). With the use of transvaginal ultrasonography, the efficacy of screening for endometriomas has increased to 97% (Mais et al., 1993).

Transvaginal ultrasonography has also been used in an attempt to assess the ovarian reserve. It has been shown that the ovarian volume is a sign of the ovarian reserve, and that a decrease in the ovarian volume measured on transvaginal ultrasound is a sign of ovarian depletion and is associated with a poor response to ovulation induction (Syrop et al., 1995; Lass et al., 1997). In a woman with an ovarian volume ≤ 3 cm^3, there is a poor chance of adequate ovarian function (Lass et al., 1997).

In polycystic ovaries, the transvaginal colour Doppler ultrasound can assess the vascularization within the stroma. Significant differences have been noted in the ovarian stromal blood flow when polycystic ovaries are compared with normal ovaries. This could perhaps be an additional feature in the ultrasound diagnosis of polycystic ovaries (Zaidi and Tan, 1996).

Ultrasonography is now regarded as an essential element of the fertility practice. It is the role of ultrasonography in the initial infertility work-up which is less clear. Preutthipan and Hesla (1995) compared transabdominal pelvic ultrasonography with laparoscopy in the detection of pelvic pathologies in infertile women. Ultrasonography had an accuracy of 76%, with a sensitivity of 57% and a specificity of 92%; and the authors concluded that transabdominal ultrasonography for the detection of pelvic pathologies should not be used as a routine screening test for the initial infertility work-up.

A prospective study of transvaginal ultrasonography by Ubaldi et al. (1998) showed more promising results. When compared with laparoscopy and pathological findings, transvaginal ultrasonography was accurate in the diagnosis of pelvic pathologies, with the exception of filmy pelvic adhesions. This study demonstrated a sensitivity of 86.2% and a specificity of 97.8% in the detection of pelvic pathologies. Thus, in trained hands, a transvaginal ultrasonography may offer valuable information in the initial infertility investigations.

The introduction of three-dimensional (3D) ultrasound has enabled excellent spatial evaluation of the pelvic organs, volume calculations and three-dimensional reconstruction (Zaidi and Tan, 1996).

In a prospective trial by Wu et al. (1998), it was found that three-dimensional ultrasound was more accurate in assessing the stroma and volume of polycystic ovaries than the traditional two-dimensional ultrasonography. The time taken was short and did not increase patient discomfort. The technique was also simple and did not require the use of other computer-assisted devices to perform the calculations.

Brunner et al. (1995) demonstrated that 3D ultrasound can accurately measure the follicular volumes of patients undergoing ovarian stimulation for *in vitro* fertilization.

Jurkovic et al. (1995) described an innovative technique in which three-dimensional ultrasonography was able to diagnose all uterine abnormalities, especially differentiating between a bicornuate and subseptate uterus in a single 3D examination, without the need for a HSG or laparoscopy or both. This technique may replace traditional methods of assessment of uterine morphology.

Transvaginal ultrasound is an excellent tool for detecting ovulation. It can pinpoint the day of ovulation and also differentiates between ovulation and the luteinized unruptured follicle syndrome. In addition, serial ultrasounds can provide important information about the progressive growth and development of the follicles (Vermesh et al., 1987).

Besides measurements of follicular size and volume in the monitoring of ovulation, ultrasonography is employed in many other aspects of the treatment of the infertile patient. Most centres perform oocyte recovery under ultrasound guidance. In patients going for assisted reproduction cycles, Doppler ultrasonography has been used to assess uterine and endometrial vascularity in an attempt to improve the implantation rates (Zaidi and Tan, 1996).

LAPAROSCOPY

Diagnostic laparoscopy is considered the gold standard in the infertility work-up to assess the presence of pelvic pathologies that might be a cause of the infertility.

Laparoscopy is, however, not innocuous and should be considered as a major surgical procedure (Querleu et al., 1993). There are associated complications of the surgery and general anaesthesia. It is also frequently performed in healthy women without obvious pelvic pathology, thus resulting in normal findings or pathology of doubtful clinical significance. Forman et al. (1993) found that 38% of infertile women who underwent laparoscopy had an entirely normal pelvis, while another 33% had minimal to mild endometriosis. As such, various alternative out-patient procedures, such as minilaparoscopy and transvaginal hydrolaparoscopy, have been employed.

Minilaparoscopy

This procedure has the advantage that it avoids general anaesthesia, and can be performed as an out-patient procedure. However, due to the smaller diameter optic which is used, it does not offer the panoramic view of the pelvis given by laparoscopy. In addition, this is mainly a diagnostic procedure, and in the event that a pelvic pathology is discovered, an operative procedure is out of the question.

Transvaginal Hydrolaparoscopy

This technique is described by Gordts et al. (1998) as an alternative procedure to a diagnostic laparoscopy in infertile patients without obvious pelvic pathology. Transvaginal introduction of an endoscope is performed, with hydroflotation, using saline as the irrigation media.

It is performed under a local anaesthetic and avoids the surgical and general anaesthetic complications associated with a laparoscopy. In addition, there is no transabdominal insertion of the Veress needle and trocars, manipulation of organs, and drying and acidosis of the tissues. It may also be utilized for conscious pelvic pain mapping.

However, as a consequence of the smaller optic diameter, this procedure has the same limitation with regard to the angle of view as a minilaparoscopy. Furthermore, because of the transvaginal access, endometriosis of the uterovesical fold may be missed.

Minilaparoscopy and transvaginal hydrolaparoscopy are not substitutes for a diagnostic laparoscopy. However, in the appropriate circumstances, these procedures may be a first-line outpatient investigation in a patient without any obvious pelvic pathology, with recourse to a laparoscopy in the event that any abnormality is suspected or detected.

Evaluation Of The Tubes

Tubal disease is a major cause of female infertility, accounting for approximately 25% of infertility in the United States (Seibel, 1990). Hence, evaluation of the tubes should be performed at an early stage of the investigations. Laparoscopy and dye insufflation, with or without hysteroscopy, is generally accepted as the basic tubal investigation, with the hysterosalpingography as an initial screening investigation (RCOG,1992).

Hysterosalpingography (HSG)

The HSG is the most commonly used screening test for evaluation of the female pelvic anatomy. Glatstein et al. (1997), in a survey of board-certified reproductive endocrinologists in the United States, found that 96% of practitioners routinely rely on the HSG in the initial infertility evaluation of the uterine and tubal status. The HSG is thus an important investigative tool, as the results will often determine the subsequent course of the patient's management. But is the HSG a reliable tool for the assessment of tubal pathology?

In a meta-analysis of 20 studies involving 4,179 patients, in which HSG is compared to laparoscopy (the gold standard) in the diagnosis of tubal patency and peritubal adhesions, Swart et al. (1995) noted that HSG has a low sensitivity and is, therefore, of limited value in the detection of tubal patency. The tubal patency that is demonstrated on HSG is not reliable and would, therefore, require a laparoscopy. HSG was also unreliable in the diagnosis of peritubal adhesions. The high specificity of HSG, however, made it a useful test for ruling out tubal obstruction.

HSG is often used as a screening test before proceeding to laparoscopy, which is a more invasive procedure requiring general anaesthesia. An important criterion of a screening test would be the inter-observer reproducibility. This was assessed by Glatstein et al. (1997) in a prospective study in which 50 HSG films, selected randomly from the medical records, were evaluated by 5 experienced fertility practitioners with a mean experience of 20 years. The results showed that there was considerable variability in the interpretation and clinical management of the HSG.

An advantage that has been frequently noted is the presumed ability of HSG to induce pregnancies (Rice et al., 1986). A meta-analysis by Watson et al. (1994) which included 10 studies in which the therapeutic role of the media was compared, found that the oil-soluble contrast media had a greater pregnancy-inducing effect compared with the water-soluble contrast media, with an odds ratio of 1:9.

Besides tubal patency, HSG is widely used to evaluate the uterine cavity. However, Alatas C. et al. (1997) found that HSG was able to detect only 72.7% of uterine pathologies. There is also a risk of infection with HSG. This risk is said to be less than 1%; however, in a high-risk population, it can be 3% (Stumpf and March, 1978).

The increasing awareness among practitioners of the potential limitations and pitfalls of the HSG has led to newer and potentially more accurate modalities for evaluating the uterine cavity and fallopian tubes. These include on-line digitally enhanced HSG, saline and contrast sonohysterography.

Digitally Enhanced HSG

The use of an on-line digitally enhanced HSG, combined with the measurement of tubal perfusion pressures, can substantially improve the evaluation of the HSG (Karande et al., 1995).

Saline Sonohysterography

This technique was first described by Beresford Buttery in 1973. Saline sonohysterography is an important complementary technique to hysteroscopy. It gives an accurate assessment of intra- and periendometrial pathology. Thus, it may eliminate the need for a diagnostic hysteroscopy and may optimize hysteroscopic surgery (de Crespigney et al., 1997).

Using transvaginal ultrasonography, Alatas C. et al. (1997) found that saline sonohysterography was able to detect all uterine anomalies, except for a single endometrial polyp (90.3%) in 62 patients. This compared favourably with HSG, which could detect only 72.7% of the uterine pathologies.

Compared to HSG, sonohysterography is better tolerated, does not require the use of radiation and provides better diagnostic accuracy. When compared to hysteroscopy, sonohysterography is less invasive and costs less. Hysteroscopy only evaluates the uterine cavity; in contrast, sonohysterography evaluates both the uterus as well as the adnexae. Sonohysterography is also performed easily in the out-patient setting, with minimal discomfort and risk of infection (Kim et al., 1998). As there is a very high correlation between hysteroscopy and sonohysterography, Goldberg et al. (1997) proposed that if the sonohysterogram is normal, a diagnostic hysteroscopy can be avoided.

Contrast Sonohysterography

In an attempt to avoid the ionizing radiation associated with hysterosalpingograpy, hysterosalpingo-contrast sonography (HyCoSy) and transvaginal ultrasonography with an echocontrast agent has been used in the evaluation of tubal status. HyCoSy is an ultrasound-based technique that uses fluid as a contrast agent injected into the fallopian tubes via the uterine cavity (Guerriero et al., 1996).

Tubal disease is largely due to pelvic inflammatory disease, with *Chlamydia trachomatis* as the main cause of the infection (Mol et al., 1997). *Chlamydia trachomatis* is, however, asymptomatic in the majority of cases, and is often not diagnosed, especially in patients with a low-level infection, or persistence of the *C. trachomatis* in a nonculturable state (Lin et al., 1992, Patton et al., 1994).

To establish an unequivocal diagnosis of salpingitis, fallopian tissue sampling with pathogen analysis by polymerase chain reaction (PCR) or cell culture have been employed. Cianci et al. (1989) have described a sampling technique in which fallopian tissue is obtained by laparoscopy. A small study of twenty women by Haeusler et al. (1997) suggests that transcervical fallopian tissue sampling with a cytobrush during hysteroscopy is a reliable and safe technique for detecting Chlamydia tubal infection.

Chlamydial Antibodies

Mol et al. (1997) performed a meta-analysis of 23 studies, with a total of 2,729 patients with subfertility, comparing Chlamydia antibody titres and laparoscopy for tubal patency and peritubal adhesions. The results of this meta-analysis suggested that the discriminative power of Chlamydia antibody testing depended on the assay which was employed, with the ELISA and microimmunofluorescence showing a better discrimination than the immunoperoxidase assay. This meta-analysis of Chlamydia antibody testing was then compared to a meta-analysis of the performance of hysterosalpingography (Swart et al., 1995); and Chlamydia antibody testing was shown to be comparable to the use of hysterosalpingography in the diagnosis of tubal pathology as defined at laparoscopy.

Chlamydia antibody testing is cheaper than performing a hysterosalpingography, and having a sample of blood taken is usually much easier for the patient than a hysterosalpingography, which may be painful. It, however, fails to provide an idea of the architecture of the uterus and cervix. It also detects a past infection and, therefore, gives no information as to the severity of the disease, and is unlikely to be helpful in the prognosis of future fertility.

Hysterosalpingography, despite being more invasive, gives additional information regarding the architecture of the uterus and cervix. It has also been reported to improve the chances of fertility by unblocking the occluded tubes (Watson et al., 1994).

The value of various investigations for the diagnosis of tubal pathology as a cause of infertility is debatable. Generally, most studies have used laparoscopy as the gold standard to verify the tubal pathology. However, laparoscopy is not a perfect gold standard. Occasionally, obstruction at laparoscopy is due to artefacts, because of technical difficulties and differences in resistance between the two tubes (Swart, 1995). Despite these inadequacies, laparoscopy is still the best standard available to date. From that perspective, it could be concluded that laparoscopy is generally regarded as the best method of assessment for tubal disease.

Hysterosalpingography is widely regarded as a basic test which can be done before a diagnostic laparoscopy with dye insufflation. Contrast hysterosonography has demonstrated potential in detecting tubal patency, and in the future, could perhaps be employed as a screening test. Chlamydial antibody testing and fallopian tube tissue sampling are subsidiary methods which are generally used to obtain additional information in the diagnostic work-up for female infertility.

Evaluation Of The Uterine Cavity

The evaluation of the uterus for any abnormality that may interfere with the implantation of the embryo is an essential part of the infertility investigation. HSG is a basic infertility investigation which is often the initial method used to assess the uterine cavity. This is because it also offers information regarding the patency and the architecture of the fallopian tubes, and it may even have a therapeutic effect. When any abnormality is detected on HSG, diagnostic hysteroscopy and laparoscopy are then undertaken.

Hysteroscopy

A diagnostic hysteroscopy is performed to confirm the existence of an uterine pathology. However, this is an invasive procedure and may require anaesthesia in an operating theatre. Out-patient hysteroscopy can be performed as an office procedure. However, there may be problems with asepsis, vasovagal attacks and failure of the procedure (de Crespigney et al., 1997). Despite these limitations, hysteroscopy provides a clear view of the uterine cavity and the cervical canal, and is the gold standard for the diagnosis of uterine pathologies (Gillespie and Nicholas, 1994).

Magnetic Resonance Imaging (MRI)

The pelvis is an ideal site for utilizing MRI. High-quality multiplaner images can be obtained as there is minimal motion artefact from respiration or large blood vessels (Ayida et al., 1997). It provides more information than an ultrasound, and has been shown to reduce the total health care expenditure in gynaecology by reducing the number of invasive procedures (Schwartz et al., 1994). MRI is, however, time-consuming and expensive, and may not be available in certain health care settings. It, therefore, has limited value in the assessment of an uterine abnormality (Haynor et al., 1988).

STANDARD INFERTILITY EVALUATION

The Practice Committee of the American Fertility Society published its guidelines for the evaluation of the infertile couple in 1992. The standard infertility evaluation recommended included semen analysis, HSG, PCT, endometrial biopsy and laparoscopy (Guzick et al., 1995).

There exists, however, a controversy over which tests should be regarded as part of the standard infertility work-up. It has been shown in the United States that the board-certified reproductive endocrinologists, in their practice, relied on five 'traditional' infertility tests: semen analysis, an assessment of ovulation, HSG, laparoscopy and PCT. With regard to other investigations, there was marked variability by physician sex, age, type of practice and geographic location. Over half of the respondents routinely ordered TSH, early follicular FSH and prolactin. Over half also routinely ordered pelvic ultrasound, hysteroscopy and cervical chlamydia cultures (Glatstein et al., 1997)

In the WHO's recommendations for investigation of the infertile couple, the minimal requirements in the female include a general physical examination, gynaecological examination, ovulation detection and laparoscopy with a dye test. However, in western Europe, there is only a weak adherence to the WHO guidelines. The detection of ovulation was standard in practically all departments, but the method used varied greatly across departments and countries. Although laparoscopy with a dye test is recommended by WHO as part of the routine investigation, only 57% of the departments reported this as a standard investigation. The data suggest that fertility investigations are based on personal preference and tradition (Helmerhorst et al., 1995).

Guzick et al. (1994) reported a study in which standard infertility tests were conducted in both fertile and infertile couples. Surprisingly, over two-thirds of the fertile couples had at least one abnormal infertility test. This was comparable to the 84% of infertile couples with at least one abnormal test. With the exception of tubal damage and endometriosis, which were expected to be more common in the infertile couple, there was no significant difference in the other infertility tests.

This study is an important reminder to be cautious when selecting the type of test to perform in an infertile patient. Only tests which are grounded in research and of proven prognostic value should be selected. Other investigations that have an intuitive appeal because of historical roots, but do not offer any diagnostic or therapeutic advantage to the patient, should be discarded. Any 'abnormal' result must be interpreted with respect to the degree of departure from 'normality' (Guzick, 1995).

It is impossible to define a 'standard' infertility evaluation that would apply across the board. Economic, social and cultural factors would influence the type of investigations that would be applicable or affordable in different clinical practices across the world. However, where possible, the basic investigation for infertility in the female partner should include an analysis of hormones (FSH, LH, prolactin), detection of ovulation and assessment of tubal patency, at least with a HSG, but preferably by laparoscopy with a dye test.

REFERENCES

Alatas, C., E. Aksoy, C. Akarsw et al. (1997). 'Evaluation of intrauterine abnormalities in infertile patients by sonohysterography', *Human Reproduction*, **12** (3): 487–90.

American Fertility Society (1992). 'Investigation of the infertile couple', American Fertility Society, Birmingham, AL, USA.

Ayida, G., P. Chamberlain, D. Barlow et al. (1997). 'Is routine diagnostic laparoscopy for infertility still justified? A pilot study assessing the use of hysterosalpingo-contrast sonography and magnetic resonance imaging', *Hum. Reprod.*, **12** (7): 1436–9.

Ayres-de-Campos, D., J.L. Silva-Carvalho, C. Oliveira et al. (1995). 'Inter-observer agreement in analysis of basal body temperature graphs from infertile women', *Hum. Reprod.*, **10**: 2010–16.

Beltsos, A.N., S. Fisher, M.L. Uhler et al. (1996). 'The relationship of the postcoital test and semen characteristics to pregnancy rates in 200 presumed fertile couples', *Int. J. Fertil. Menopausal Stud.*, **41**(4): 405–11.

Block, E. (1952). 'Quantitative morphological investigations of the follicular system in women: Variation at different ages', *Acta. Anat.*, **14**: 108–123.

Bonilla-Musoles, F., C. Simon, V. Serra et al. (1992). 'An assessment of hysterosalpingo-sonography (HSSG) as a diagnostic tool for uterine cavity defects and tubal patency', *J. Clin. Ultrasound*, **20**: 175–8.

Brunner, M., A. Obruca, P. Bauer et al. (1995). 'Clinical application of volume estimation based on three-dimensional ultrasonography', **6**: 358–61.

Buttery, B. (1973). 'Ultrasonic hysterography: A new technique', *Lancet*, **2**: 595–6.

Cianci, A., G. Palumbo et al. (1989). 'Chlamydia trachomatis detection in infertile women by using a tubal cytobrush during laparoscopy', *Acta. Eur. Fertl*, **20**: 363–5.

Cochrane, W.J. and M.A. Thomas (1974). 'Ultrasound diagnosis of gynecological pelvic mass', *Radiology*, **110**: 649–54.

Collins, J.A., Y. So, E.H. Wilson et al. (1984). 'The postcoital test as a predictor of pregnancy among 355 infertile couples', *Fertil. Steril.*, **41**: 703–8.

Dechaud, H., J.P. Daures, B. Hedon et al. (1998). 'Prospective evaluation of falloposcopy', *Hum. Reprod.*, **13** (7): 1815–8.

de Crespigney, L., R. Kuhu, D. Mc Ginnes et al. (1997). 'Saline infusion sonohysterosalpingography: An underutilized technique', *Aust. N.Z.J. Obstet. Gynaecol.*, **37** (2): 206–9.

De Vries, K., S. Degani, I. Eib Schitz et al. (1984). 'The influence of the post-coital test on the sexual function of infertile women', *J. Psychosom. Obstet. Gynaecol.*, **3**: 101–6.

Drale, T.S. and G.M. Grunert (1979). 'A cyclic pattern of sexual dysfunction in the infertility investigation', *Fertil. Steril.*, **32**: 542–5.

Ebbiary, N.A.A., E.A. Leuton, C. Sait et al. (1994).

'The significance of elevated basal follicular stimulating hormone in regularly menstruating infertile women', *Hum. Reprod.*, 9 (2): 245–52.

Eimers, J.M., E.R. te Velde, R. Gerritse et al. (1994). 'The validity of the postcoital test for estimating the probability of conceiving', *A.M.J. Obstet. Gynecol.*, 171: 65–70.

Faddy, M.J. and R.G. Gosden (1995). 'A mathematical model of follicle dynamics in the human ovary', *Hum. Reprod.*, 10: 770–75.

______(1996). 'A model confirming the decline in follicle numbers to the age of menopause in women', *Hum. Reprod.*, 11: 1484–6.

Fedele, L., M. Brioschi, F. Dorta et al. (1990). 'Timing of ovulation in spontaneous and induced cycles', *Int. J. Gynecol. Obstet.*, 32: 369–75.

Forman, R., J. Robinson, Z. Mehta et al. (1993). 'Patient history as a simple predictor of pelvic pathology in subfertile women', *Hum. Reprod.*, 8: 53–5.

Gillespie, A. and A. Nicholas (1994). 'The value of the hysteroscopy', *Aust. N.Z.J. Obstet. Gynaecol.*, 34: 85–7.

Glatstein, I.Z., B.L. Harlow and M.D. Hornstein (1997). 'Practice patterns among reproductive endocrinologists: the infertility evaluation', *Fertil. Steril.*, 67 (3): 443–51.

______(1998). 'Practice patterns among reproductive endocrinologists: Further aspects of the infertility evaluation', *Fertil. Steril.*, 70 (2): 263–9.

Glatstein, I.Z., L.A. Sleeper, Y. Lavy et al. (1997). 'Observer variability in the diagnosis and management of the hysterosalpingogram', *Fertil. Steril.*, 67 (2): 233–7.

Glazener, C.M.A., N.J. Kelly, M.J. Weir et al. (1987). 'The diagnosis of male infertility—prospective time-specific study of conception rates related to seminal analysis and post-coital sperm-mucus penetration and survival in otherwise unexplained infertility', *Hum. Reprod.*, 2: 665–71.

Goldberg, J.M., T. Falcone, M. Attaran et al. (1997). 'Sonohysterographic evaluation of uterine abnormalities noted on hysterosalpingography', *Hum. Reprod.*, 12 (10): 2151–3.

Gordts, S., R. Campos, L. Rombauts et al. (1998). 'Transvaginal hydrolaparoscopy as an outpatient procedure for fertility investigation', *Hum. Reprod.*, 13(1): 99–103.

Grinsted, J., J.D. Jacobson, L. Grinsted et al. (1989). 'Prediction of ovulation', *Fertil. Steril.*, 52 (3): 388–93.

Guerriero, S., S. Ajossa, V. Mais et al. (1996). 'The screening of tubal abnormalities in the infertile couple', *J. Assist. Reprod. Genet.*, 13 (5): 407–12.

Guzick, D.S., L. Grefenstette, K. Baffone (1995). 'Do infertility tests discriminate between fertile and infertile populations?' *Hum. Reprod.*, 10 (8): 2008–9.

Guzick, D.S., L. Grefenstette, K. Baffone et al. (1994). 'Infertility evaluation in fertile women: A model for assessing the efficacy of infertility testing', *Hum. Reprod.*, 9: 2306–23.

Haeusler, G., C. Tempfer, R. Lehuer et al. (1997). 'Fallopian tube sampling with a cytobrush during hysteroscopy: A new approach for detecting tubal infection', *Fertil. Steril.*, 67: 580–82.

Harrison R.F. (1981). 'The diagnostic and therapeutic potential of the post-coital test', *Fertil. Steril.*, 36: 71–5.

Haynor, D.R., L.A. Mack, M.R. Shouldes et al. (1988). 'Changing appearance of the normal uterus during the menstrual cycle: MR studies', *Radiology*, 161: 459–62.

Helmerhorst, F.M., S.G. Oei, K.W.M. Bloemenkamp et al. (1995). 'Consistency and variation in fertility investigations in Europe', *Hum. Reprod.*, 10 (8): 2027–30.

Huhner, M. (1913). *Sterility in the male and female and its treatment.*, Rebman, New York.

Insler, V. and B. Lunenfield (eds.) (1986). *Infertility: male and female,* Churchill Livingstone.

Israel, R., D.R. Mishell, S.C. Stone et al. (1972). 'Single luteal phase serum progesterone assay as an indicator of ovulation', *Am. J. Obstet. Gynecol.*

Jette, N.T. and R.H. Glass (1972). 'Prognostic value of the post-coital test', *Fertil. Steril.*, 23: 29–32.

Jurkovic, D., A. Geipel, K. Grubeck et al. (1995). 'Three-dimensional ultrasound for the assessment of uterine anatomy and detection of congenital uterine anomalies: A comparison with hysterosalpingography and two-dimensional ultrasonography', *Ultrasound Obstet. Gynecol.*, 5: 228–32.

Karande, V.C., D.E. Pratt, D.S. Rabin et al. (1995). 'The limited value of hysterosalpingography in assessing tubal status and fertility potential', *Fertil. Steril.*, 63: 1167–71.

Kim, A.H., H. McKay, M.D. Keltz et al. (1998). 'Sonohysterographic screening before *in vitro* fertilization', *Fertil. Steril.*, **69** (5): 841–4.

Lass, A., R. Silye, D.C. Abrams, et al. (1997). 'Follicular density in ovarian biopsy of infertile women: a novel method to assess ovarian reserve', *Hum. Reprod.*, **12** (5): 1028–31.

Lass, A., J. Skull, E. Mc Veigh et al. (1997). 'Measurement of ovarian volume by transvaginal sonography before human menopausal gonadotrophin superovulation for *in vitro* fertilization can predict poor response', *Hum. Reprod.*, **12**: 294–7.

Lin, J.S., W.E. Jones, L. Yan et al. (1992). 'Underdiagnosis of Chlamydia trachomatis infection. Diagnostic implications in patients with low-level infection', *Sex Transm. Dis.*, **19**: 259–65.

Levran, D., I. Ben Shlomo, J. Dor et al. (1991). 'Ageing of endometrium and oocytes: Observation on conception and abortion rates in an egg donation model', *Fertil. Steril.*, **56**: 1091–4.

Lundberg, S., C. Rasmussen, A.A. Berg et al. (1998). 'Falloposcopy in conjunction with laparascopy: Possibilities and limitations', *Hum. Reprod.*, **13** (6): 1490–2.

Mais, V., S. Guerriero, S. Ajassa et al. (1993). 'The efficiency of transvaginal ultrasonography in the diagnosis of endometrioma', *Fertil. Steril.*, **60**: 776–80.

Martinez, A.R., M.H.A. van Hooff, E. Schoute et al. (1992). 'The reliability, acceptability and applications of basal body temperature (BBT) records in the diagnosis and treatment of infertility', *Eur. J. Obstet. Gynecol. Reprod. Biol.*, **47**: 121–7.

McCarthy, J.J.Jr. and H.E. Rockette (1983). 'A comparison of methods to interpret the basal body temperature graph', *Fertil. Steril.*, **39**: 640–6.

Mol, B.W.J., B. Dijkman, P. Nertheim et al. (1997). 'The accuracy of serum chlamydial antibodies in the diagnosis of tubal pathology: A meta-analysis', *Fertil. Steril.*, **67**: 1031–7.

Mosher, W.D. and W.F. Pratt (1991). 'Fecundity and infertility in the United States: Incidence and trends', *Fertil. Steril.*, **56**: 192.

National Center for Health Statistics (1983). 'Advances report of final natality statistics, 1981', *Monthly Vital Stat. Rep.*, **32**: 1–12.

Oei, S.G., M.J.N.C. Keirse, K.W. Bloemenkamp et al. (1995). 'European postcoital tests: opinions and practice', *Br. J. Obstet. Gynecol.*, **102**: 621–4.

Helmerhorst, F.M. and K.W. Bloemenkamp (1996). 'Effect of the postcoital test on the sexual relationship of the infertile couples: A randomized controlled trial', *Fertil. Steril.*, **65**(4): 771–5.

——(1998). 'Effectiveness of the postcoital test: Randomized controlled trial', *BMJ*, **317** (7157): 502–5.

Oei, S.G., F.M. Helmerhorst and M.J.N.C. Keirse (1995). 'When is the postcoital test normal? A critical appraisal', *Hum. Reprod.*, **10**(7): 1711–4.

Patton, D.L. et al. (1994). 'Detection of chlamydia trachomatis in fallopian tube tissue in women with postinfection tubal infertility', *Am. J. Obstet. Gynecol.*, **171**: 95–101.

Preutthipan, S. and J. Hesla (1995). 'A comparative study between pelvic ultrasonography and laparoscopy in the detection of pelvic pathology in the initial work-up of subfertile women', *J. Med. Assoc. Thai.*, **78**: 596–9

Querleu, D., L. Chevalier, C. Chapron et al. (1993). 'Complications of gynaecological laparoscopic surgery: A French multicentre collaborative study', *Gynaecol. Endosc.*, **2**: 3–6.

Rice, J.P., S.N. London, D.L. Olive et al. (1986). 'Revaluation of hysterosalpingography in infertility investigations', *Obstet. Gynecol.*, **67**: 718–21.

Rowe, P., F. Comhaire, T. Hargreave et al. (1993). *WHO manual for the standardized investigation and diagnosis of the infertile couple,* Cambridge University Press, Cambridge.

Royal College of Obstetricians and Gynaecologists (1992). *Infertility Guidelines for practice,* RCOG Press.

Samberg, I., M. Du Pan, B. Bourrit et al. (1985). 'The value of the postcoital test according to etiology and outcome on infertility', *Acta. Eur. Fertil.*, **16**: 147–9.

Sauer, M.V. (1996). 'Pregnancy wastage and reproductive ageing: The oocyte donation model', *Current Opinion in Obstetrics and Gynecology*, **8**: 226–9.

Seibel, M. (1990). *Infertility: A comprehensive textbook,* Appleton and Lange, Norwalk, CT.

Schwartz, K., E. Panageas, R. Lange et al. (1994). 'Female pelvis: Impact of MR imaging on treatment decisions and net cost analysis', *Radiology*, **192**: 55–60.

Scott, R.T. and G.E. Hofman (1995). 'Prognostic assessment of ovarian reserve', *Fertil. Steril.*, **63**: 1–11.

Sims, J.M. (1866). Clinical Notes on Uterine Surgery (with special reference to the management of the sterile condition). Robert Hardwicke, London.

Speroff, L., R.H. Glass, N.G. Kase et al. (eds.) (1994). *Clinical Gynecologic Endocrinology and Infertility*, 5th ed., Williams and Wilkins, Baltimore, USA.

Steele, P.A., G.H. White, S.J. Judd et al. (1985). 'Reliability of a single progesterone determination as an indicator of ovulation', *Clin. Reprod. Fertil.*, Jun **3**(2): 25–30.

Stephen, E.H. (1996). 'Projections of impaired fecundity among women in the United States: 1995–2025', *Fertil. Steril.*, **66**: 205–9.

Stephen, E.H. and A. Chandra (1998). 'Updated projections of infertility in the United States: 1995–2025', *Fertil. Steril.* July **70** (1), 30–34.

Stumpf, P.G. and C.M. March (1978). 'Febrile morbidity following hysterosalpingography', *Fertil. Steril.*, **30**: 733–8.

Squire, W.S. (1868). 'Puerperal temperatures', *Trans. Obstet. Soc.* (London), **9**: 129–144.

Swart, P., B.W. Mol, F. Vander Veen et al. (1995). 'The accuracy of hysterosalpingography in the diagnosis of tubal pathology, a meta-analysis', *Fertil. Steril.*, **64**: 486–91.

Syrop. C.H., A. Wilhoite, B.J. Van Voorhis et al. (1995). 'Ovarian volume: a novel outcome predictor for assisted reproduction', *Fertil. Steril.*, **64**: 1167–71.

Ubaldi, F., A.Wisanto, M. Camus et al. (1998). 'The role of transvaginal ultrasonography in the detection of pelvic pathologies in the infertility work-up', *Hum. Reprod.*, **13**(2): 330–3.

Vermesh, M., O.A. Klitzky, V. Davajan et al. (1987). 'Monitoring techniques to predict and detect ovulation', *Fertil. Steril.*, **47** (2): 259–64.

Watson, A., P. Vandekerckhove, R. Lilford et al. (1994). 'A meta-analysis of the therapeutic role of oil solution contrast media at hysterosalpingography: A surprising result?' *Fertil. Steril.* **61**: 470–7.

Wu, M.H., H.H. Tang, C.C. Hsu et al. (1998). 'The role of three-dimensional ultrasonographic images in ovarian measurement', *Fertil. Steril.*, **69** (6): 1152–5.

Yarali, H., T. Gurgan, A. Erden et al. (1994). 'Colour Doppler hysterosalgingosonography: A simple and potentially useful method to evaluate fallopian tube patency', *Hum. Reprod.*, **9**: 64–66.

Zaidi, J. and S.L. Tan (1996). 'Advances in the use of ultrasound in infertility management', *Current Opinion in Obstetrics and Gynecology.*, **8**: 161–5.

3

Normal Menstrual Cycle

Geetanjali Sachdeva and Chander Puri

Biological clocks are one of the most intriguing and beautiful instances of nature's ways to make us ponder over its enigmas. One of these periodic events is the maturation and discharge of a fertilizable egg at a regularly spaced interval in a fertile female. This cycle of female reproductive activity is popularly known as the menstrual cycle. The ovary, oviducts and uterus (Fig. 3.1) undergo remarkable structural and functional changes in a normal menstrual cycle in the sexually mature female. In

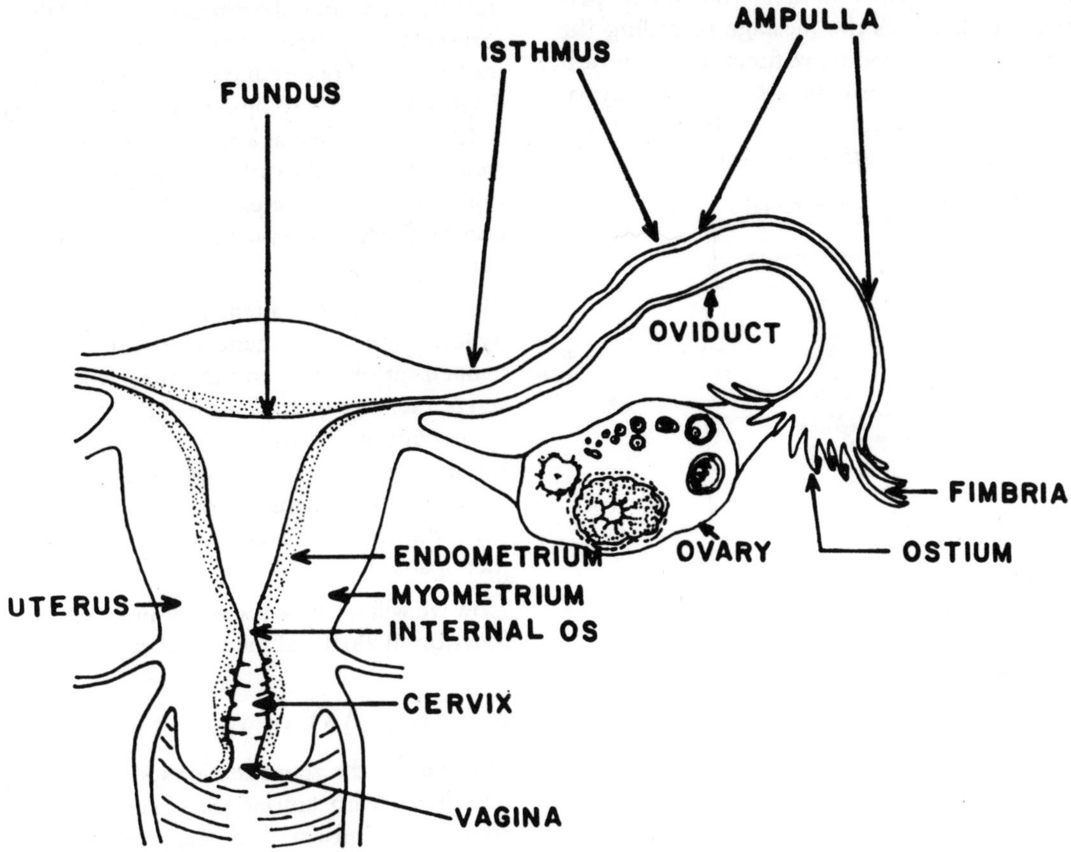

Fig. 3.1. Schematic diagram showing major reproductive organs in a sexually mature woman

this chapter, the authors will review the existing information on the structures and functions of ovary and endometrium during the menstrual cycle as these two occupy very significant places in the whole cascade of female reproductive physiology. The ovary contributes to the process by providing potential candidates for fertilization (i.e., oocytes or eggs), while the endometrium, an inner lining of the uterus, provides shelter to the fertilized entity. However, the ovary and endometrium do not function independently.

1. REGULATION OF MENSTRUAL CYCLE

The physiological regulation of the menstrual cycle involves precisely controlled and timed interaction between the hypothalamus-pituitary, ovary and uterus (Fig. 3.2). The central nervous system perceives and integrates the message regarding the status of female reproductive functions from various sources. This information is sent to the hypothalamus via neural transmission. It leads to the secretion of the gonadotrophin-releasing hormones

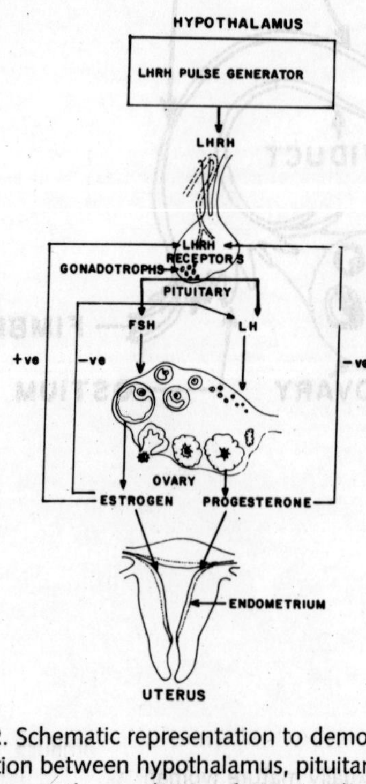

Fig. 3.2. Schematic representation to demonstrate interaction between hypothalamus, pituitary, ovary and uterus in the regulation of menstrual cycle

(GnRH or LHRH) by highly specialized neurons termed the hypothalamic pulse generator or LHRH pulse generator. LHRH released into hypothalamic-hypophyseal portal blood vessels act on the anterior pituitary to stimulate the synthesis and release of gonadotrophins—follicle stimulating hormone (FSH) and luteinizing hormone (LH).

FSH and LH bind to specific receptors on the ovarian cells to stimulate the release of oestrogen, progesterone, inhibin and other factors. These factors exert feedback effects on the hypothalamus and pituitary. Oestrogen increases the concentrations of LHRH receptors on gonadotrophs, while progesterone decreases the levels of these receptors. The regulation of LH pulses is also affected by some neurotransmitters, such as endogenous opiods, including methionine and leucine encephalins, endorphins and dynorphins. Probably, these opiods mediate the actions of oestrogens on LHRH neurons (Shivers et al., 1983). These hypothalamic opiods inhibit LHRH release and gonadotrophin secretion. High levels of these opiods reduce the frequency of LH pulses, whereas low levels are associated with frequent LH pulses of high amplitude. Thus, a regulatory network exists which is essential to prevent the female reproductive system from going berserk.

Menstrual cycles in a female begin only when the hypothalamic pulse generator is activated. This happens at puberty, and the time when a female starts menstruating is called menarche. These cycles continue till the age of menopause, the time when no more menstrual cycles occur. However, in some women, menstrual cycles are never initiated, either due to lack of ovaries or because of premature menopause.

Now we will see how the ovary and endometrium function in a natural menstrual cycle.

2. THE OVARY

This part of the reproductive system is intensely innervated with autonomic nerve fibres, which convey the information regarding the ovarian function to the central nervous system. A continuous sheet of squamous or cuboidal epithelium made of polygonal cells, known as the germinal epithe-

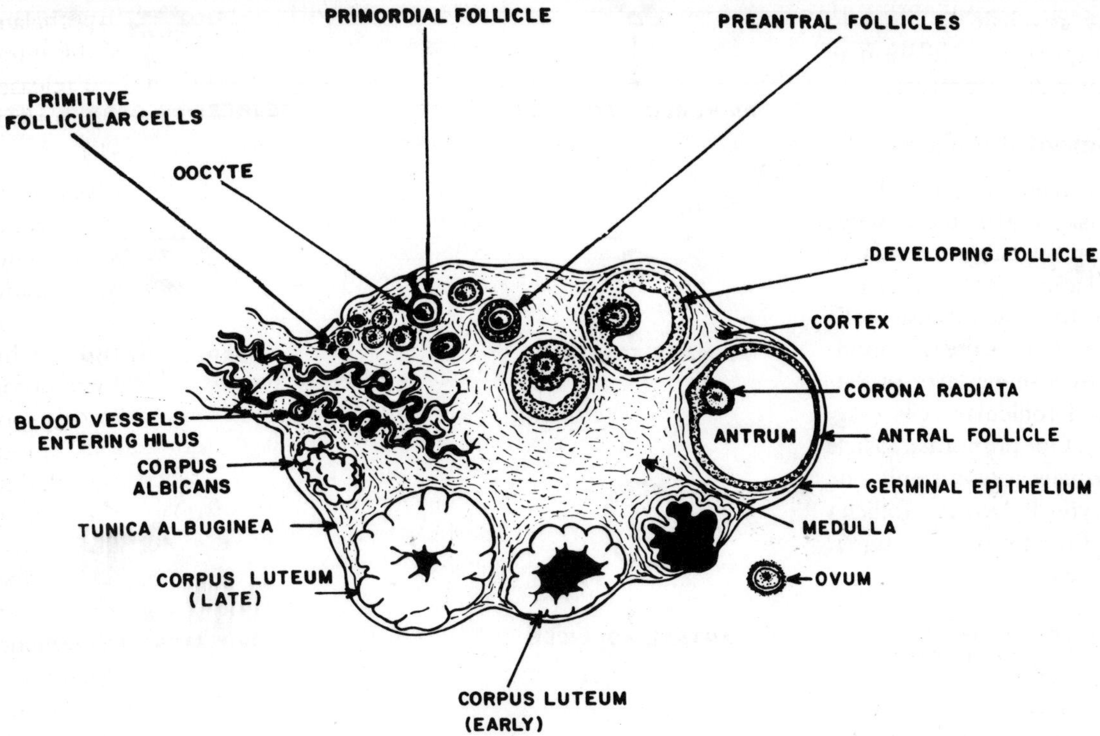

Fig. 3.3. Ovary from a sexually mature woman showing organization of various cellular components

lium, encovers the ovary. Beneath the germinal epithelium lies a layer of dense connective tissue, the tunica albuginea (Fig. 3.3). The ovary has a thick peripheral zone, called the cortex, which surrounds the medulla or zona vasculosa. The ovarian cortex consists of the stroma and the follicles at various stages of maturation and degeneration. The medulla consists mainly of loose connective tissue and a mass of large contorted blood vessels. The boundary between the cortex and medulla is not distinct.

The germ cells, precursors of the female gametes in the ovary, pass through a certain sequence of differentiation. During fetal life, germ cells continue to divide mitotically as oogonia. When the oogonium is triggered to enter into the meiotic prophase, it is called an oocyte. The oocyte then becomes arrested at the diplotene stage and is enclosed within a follicle. Follicles are the lifeboats of the ovary as they nourish and regulate the development of oocytes. Oocytes which are not encapsulated by follicles are doomed to die. The follicles containing oocytes remain embedded in the connective tissue of the cortex. However, all the follicles are not of uniform size as they represent various stages of development.

2.1. Development Of Follicles

Primitive Follicular Cells

Primitive follicular cells or pregranulosa cells are smaller than oocytes and differ from them in the structure of both the nucleus and cytoplasm. The nucleus is ovoid. Chromatin condensation is seen at the nuclear envelope. Occurrence of reticular type nucleoli is rather rare. Mitochondria, smooth endoplasmic reticulum, Golgi complex, secondary lysosome and lipid droplets are distributed in the cytoplasm. There also exist junctional apparati between the oocyte and the follicular cells. However, it is not known whether they play any role in nutrient transport or regulation of follicle development.

Primordial Follicles

The majority of follicles in females of the reproductive age-group are primordial or unilaminar follicles. A primordial follicle consists of a quiescent oocyte surrounded by a single layer of flattened follicular cells (Fig. 3.4). One primordial follicle normally contains only one oocyte. Polyovular follicles are found mostly in immature girls.

Primary Follicle or Preantral Follicle

An inactive primordial follicle develops into a primary follicle. This process is accompanied by cytological changes in the oocyte, the follicular cells and the adjacent connective tissue. With enlargement of the oocyte, the flattened follicular cells first become cuboidal or low columnar, and then undergo mitotic divisions to give rise to granulosa cells that form a stratified epithelium as called the stratum granulosum.

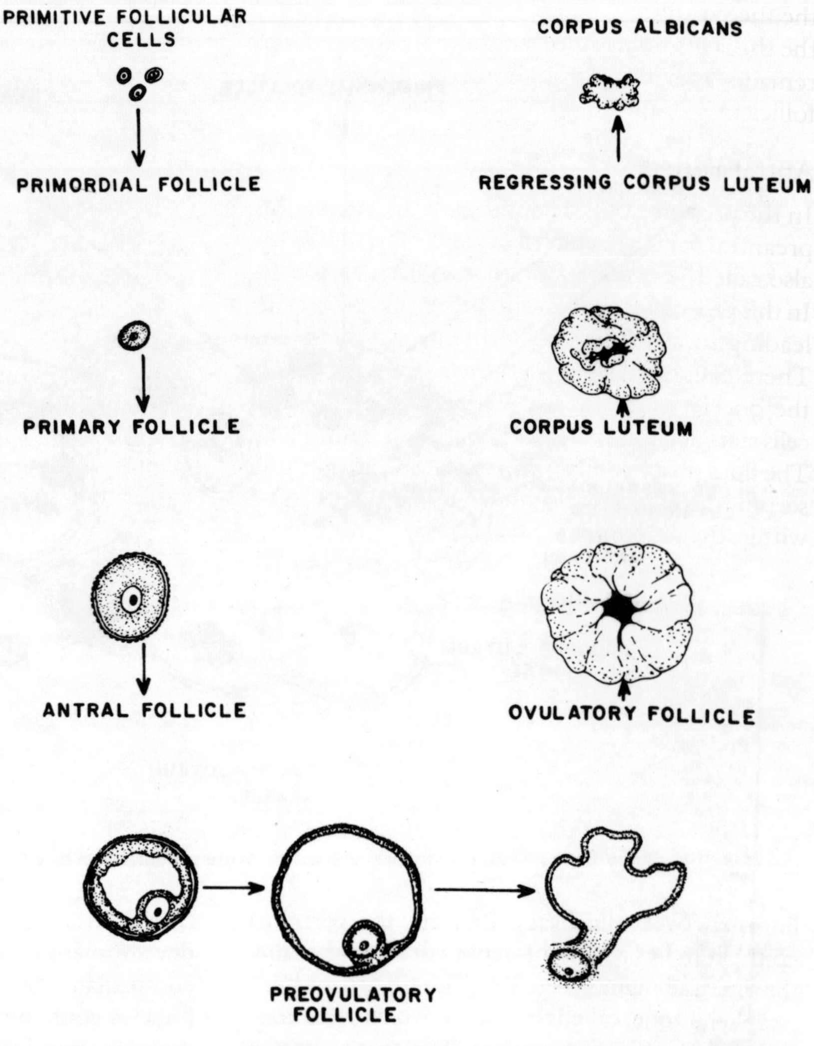

Fig. 3.4. Diagrammatic illustration to demonstrate different stages of follicular development

Interposed between the oocyte and the granulosa cells is a refractile, deeply staining, acellular layer of uniform thickness known as the zona pellucida. This glycoprotein coat is secreted by granulosa cells during oogenesis. The various functions attributed to the zona pellucida include presentation of receptors to the sperm, induction of acrosome reaction, polyspermy block and physical protection of the embryo afterwards.

A sheath of ovarian stroma cells—the theca folliculi—develops around the follicle as the growing follicles increase in size. Theca folliculi subsequently differentiate into a highly vascular, inner layer of oestrogen-secreting cells—the theca interna, and an outer layer composed largely of connective tissue—the theca externa. A basement membrane distinguishes the theca interna from the stratum granulosum. No blood vessel penetrates this basement membrane. As a result, the oocyte and its supporting cells are devoid of any vascular support. In contrast, numerous small blood vessels penetrate the theca externa to supply a rich capillary plexus in the theca interna. However, the granulosa cell layer remains avascular throughout the growth of the follicle.

Antral Follicles

In the presence of FSH and LH in the circulation, preantral follicles are converted to antral follicles, also called Vesicular or Graffian follicles (Fig. 3.5). In this process, granulosa and thecal cells proliferate, leading to a further enlargement of the follicles. There occurs no significant increase in the size of the oocyte itself, though. The dividing granulosa cells start accumulating fluid between themselves. The fluid drops comprise mucopolysaccharides and serum transudates, and coalesce to follicular fluid within the antrum.

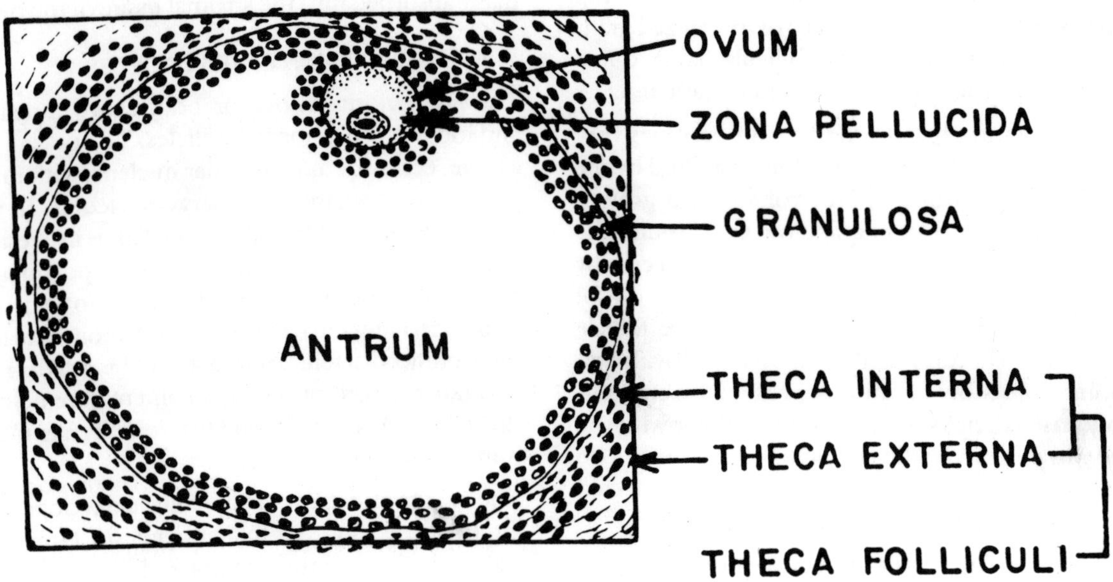

Fig. 3.5 An antral follicle containing fully grown oocyte surrounded by zona pellucida and layers of granulosa cells

Antral follicles synthesize androgens (e.g., androstenedione and testosterone) and oestrogens (e.g., oestradiol). This process of steroidogenesis by the follicles is controlled by the gonadotrophins. FSH binds to the granulosa cells, while LH binds to the theca interna. The theca interna cells synthesize androgens and this process is stimulated by LH. The granulosa cells do not synthesize androgens; however, the enzymes present in these cells aromatize androgens to oestrogens. With the increase in follicular size, there is, concomitant rise in oestrogen synthesis. These steroids are released into the circulation, resulting in an oestrogen surge.

Oestrogens, besides exerting the systemic effects, also have a local intrafollicular role. They bind to the granulosa and stimulate them to proliferate and synthesize more oestrogen. Thus, a system of positive feedback operates in which oestrogen stimulates further oestrogen output. At the end of antral phase, oestrogen, in conjunction with FSH, stimulates the appearance of LH-binding sites on the outer layers of granulosa cells.

Preovulatory Follicle

Only those antral follicles which express LH receptors on the outer granulosa cells enter into the preovulatory phase of follicular growth. LH induces terminal growth changes in the follicle as well as the oocyte. The changes in the oocyte following the LH surge include the breaking of the nuclear membrane and resumption of the meiotic prophase. This results in a division of the oocyte into a secondary oocyte, which contains half the chromosomes but almost all the cytoplasm; and the polar body containing the remaining chromosomes, with little cytoplasm. This is followed by another arrest of meiosis, now at the metaphase stage.

The LH surge is followed by a transient rise and subsequent decline to significant levels of the follicular oestrogens and androgens. Granulosa cells start synthesizing progesterone under the influence of LH. Progesterone levels in the circulation become significant several hours prior to ovulation.

Ovulatory Follicle

After the ovulatory surge of LH, the follicular cells in the vicinity of the oocyte become detached from the follicular wall and become highly dispersed (Greep, 1963). The oocyte, with its surrounding corona radiata and a dense mass of specialized granulosa cells in the innermost follicular layer, called cumulus oophorous, floats free in the antrum.

As the follicle expands, the antrum becomes very large. This rapid expansion of follicular fluid by the end of the preovulatory phase of follicular growth results in a thin layer of granulosa cells around the oocyte. The oocyte is attached to the thecal cells by a thin stalk of cells. This leads to a bulging out of the follicle from the ovarian surface. The follicle ultimately ruptures at the 'stigma' or 'ovulation point', probably because of proteolytic and collagenase activities. Follicular fluid, along with the oocyte and surrounding cumulus cells, flows out on to the ovarian surface. The oocyte is then collected by the cilia on the fimbriae of the oviduct.

The remaining parts of the follicle within the ovary collapse into the space left by the follicular fluid, oocyte and the cumulus mass. Thus the post-ovulatory follicle consists of a fibrin core and several collapsed layers of granulosa cells enclosed within a fibrous theca. The collapsed follicle undergoes luteinization to form a corpus luteum, which assumes an endocrine function. The process of luteinization involves various steps, such as fibrosis of the granulosa cell layer, breakdown of the membrane between the granulosa and thecal layers, and vascularization of granulosa. The granulosa cells become rich in mitochondria, smooth endoplasmic reticulum, lipid droplets, Golgi bodies and lutein, a carotenoid pigment.

Luteinization is associated with high levels of progesterone secretion and an insignificant amount of oestradiol from the corpus luteum. In a non-pregnant female, the corpus luteum persists for 2–14 days. Prolactin, an important component of the luteotrophic complex, and low levels of LH levels are required for the maintenance of the corpus luteum. Withdrawal of the luteotrophic complex or activation of luteolytic factors leads to corpus luteum regression or luteolysis. This involves a collapse of the lutein cells, ischaemia and progressive cell death, which results in declining progesterone levels. Degeneration of the corpus luteum leads to the formation of a whitish scar tissue called the corpus albicans. This tissue is eventually absorbed into the stromal tissue of the ovary.

2.2. Development Of Oocytes

The vast majority of ovarian oocytes are immature and lodged in primordial follicles. The oocyte has a large, eccentric and vesicular nucleus, with finely dispersed chromatin and a large nucleolus. In primordial follicles, although the nucleus is in a resting state, the presence of nucleoli, RNA polymerase activity and continuous uptake of amino acids and ribonucleosides into small oocytes demonstrate that these primordial follicles are active. This activity may facilitate the continuous repair and replacement of the damaged organelles and macromolecules in the primordial follicles.

The oocyte also grows as the follicle develops during the early stages of folliculogenesis. However, the oocyte's growth is complete by the time the surrounding follicular layer is 20- to 30-cells-thick. There occur changes in the ooplasm throughout the period of follicular development. Lipid and proteins, which form a major part of the ooplasm, are deposited in the oocyte during the growth-period. Oocytes expand remarkably, without undergoing mitosis or cleavage of the cytoplasm. However, nuclear maturation remains arrested at the diplotene stage of meiosis. The oocyte nucleus which is arrested at diplotene is called a germinal vesicle. The large size and absence of heterochromatic material are the major characteristics of the germinal vesicle.

With the growth of the oocyte, there occur prominent changes in its organelle distribution. The germinal vesicle increases in size during oocyte growth. The Golgi complex, initially existing as a single mass in the juxtanuclear region of the early oocyte layer, gives rise to multiple Golgi complexes widely dispersed in the ooplasm. The endoplasmic reticulum gradually becomes more extensive and the number of free ribosomes in the ooplasm increases. The spherical or short plump mitochondria initially clustered around the cell centre tend to disperse throughout the ooplasm. The cytoplasm of growing oocytes contains numerous membrane-bound vesicles, as well as multivesicular bodies. These organelles are believed to be involved in moving materials across the cell membrane. Some of these vesicles in the cortex contain products for export, while others contain products of granulosa cell secretions and serum transudates from follicular fluid. There are a few lipid droplets and occasional heterogeneous masses, identified as lipochrome pigment. Centrioles, which are involved in assembling the spindle apparatus required for segregating the chromosomes during cell division, are present in primordial oocytes but disappear by the mid-growth stage.

In contrast to primordial follicles, mature oocytes have the potential to undergo fertilization. This ability to fertilize is achieved due to resumption of meiosis after the LH surge, expression of new gene products, and the organization and redistribution of cytoplasmic organelles.

2.3. Follicle Recruitment

This is the process by which a primordial follicle is initiated into the process of growth. The first signs of a follicle being recruited are a slow increase in the number of pregranulosa cells, the secretion of zona proteins and enlargement of the oocyte. Once the growth of a follicle starts, it continues without a pause until ovulation, or in the majority of cases, till atresia (follicular death).

The first follicles begin growing in the human ovary soon after their formation and by the time of birth, a few multilaminar follicles are usually present. Follicles are recruited continuously until the original store is exhausted after menopause in mid-life. Far more than one follicle is recruited for growth, although only one ovulates each month. All others which are recruited undergo atresia, a process probably initiated by the programmed cell death (apoptosis) of the granulosa and theca cells (Tilly et al., 1992).

Primordial follicles in the ovarian cortex give rise to successive growing stages, which are found at progressively deeper levels towards the medulla in the ovary. The apparent orderliness of oogenesis and follicle utilization is suggestive of the possibility that there exists some sort of production line. According to this hypothesis, the first formed oocytes are the first to be recruited for the growth and the last formed are the last to be ovulated.

Follicle growth can be classified into two stages according to the stage of oocyte development. The first stage involves the growth of the oocyte to almost full size (120 μm), and this is reached when several layers of granulosa cells are present and the fluid-filled antrum is appearing. The second stage is the formation and expansion of the antrum in the Graffian follicle, which grows to more than 2 cm in diameter with a fertile oocyte and achieves maximal steroidogenic activity.

Early Follicular Phase

The oocyte lies within its primordial follicle with its chromosomal development arrested at the diplotene stage of the first meiotic division (Baker, 1982). The development of follicles is resumed without any gonadotrophin stimulation. This process occurs continuously throughout childhood and the reproductive years, until menopause. The origin of the dominant follicle destined to undergo ovulation is termed 'selection'. However, till now, this is believed to be a 'random' process as there is no evidence otherwise. To explain this, it has been hypothesized that there occurs a constant flux of dynamic events within the ovary, with individual primordial follicles having the potential to mature at different times during the reproductive life. Baird hypothesized that the 'gate' mechanism may select a cohort of potential dominant follicles. This gate opens transiently in the early follicular phase of the cycle, when FSH levels are high. Only those follicles which have the capability to mature at an appropriate time are allowed to move past this gate and permitted to join a cohort of potential dominant follicles. Those follicles which acquire the ability to mature at other times in the cycle are exposed to low levels of FSH and thus encounter a 'gate' which remains shut. This leads to their atresia.

Mid-Follicular Phase

All follicles recruited into a cohort of primary follicles during the early follicular phase have the potential to form the final dominant follicle (di Zerega and Hodgen, 1981). The size of this cohort depends on the primordial follicle turnover and the time period for which the FSH level remains elevated. The early follicular phase ends with the emergence of a single dominant follicle among the recruited follicles. Selection of the dominant follicle occurs as a result of a decline in the FSH levels, under the influence of increasing amounts of oestrogen secreted into the circulation by the dominant follicle. Once a dominant follicle has emerged, the remainder of the cohort undergoes atresia. It is interesting to note that the contralateral ovary remains quiescent throughout the succeeding events of the cycle. The selection of the ovary which is to be the source of the dominant follicle of the month, is suggested to be a random process (Sallam et al., 1983). Unilateral ovariectomy has been shown to result in incessant ovulation from the remaining ovary, thus indicating that the selection of the site of the dominant follicle of the month is controlled by intraovarian factors rather than by some central control. In one study, surgical removal of the dominant follicle has been shown to cause postponement of ovulation for approximately 14 days, the length of one follicular phase. This experiment clearly demonstrated the irreversible inhibitory effect of the dominant follicle on the development of other members of the mature follicle cohort (Nilsson et al., 1982).

As the follicle grows and develops, the antrum is enlarged and the granulosa and theca interna layers are distinguishable. The rising levels of oestradiol during the mid-proliferative phase of the cycle stimulate endometrial proliferation, as well as priming of the hypothalamus and pituitary in preparation for the mid-cycle gonadotrophin surge. The dominant follicle is thus responsible for the synchronized preparation of the female reproductive tract for ovulation, fertilization and implantation.

2.4. Endocrine Control Of Ovulation

The anterior pituitary perceives and integrates the signals from the ovary and central nervous system, and then triggers a massive release of LH, the ovulatory hormone (Knobil,1980). At the time of the LH surge, the follicle undergoes the following physiological events.

(i) The oocyte attains a capability of fertilization as meiosis I is resumed. The oocyte matures with the transition from prophase I through metaphase I, and the first polar body is extruded at metaphase II. Nuclear maturation is synchronized with the maturation of the cytoplasm and zona pellucida.

(ii) Luteinization is initiated as the follicular granulosa cells start synthesizing and secreting progesterone rather than oestrogen. Although administration of oestrogen alone can lead to an increase in the circulating levels of gonadotrophins—both LH and FSH (Monroe et al., 1972; Liu and Yen, 1983), there is evidence to suggest that progesterone may also play a role in the events leading to the onset of a gonadotrophin surge in women with normal menstrual cycles. A rise in the peripheral levels of progesterone was observed some hours before the onset of the surge (Aono et al., 1976). This was supported by an observation demonstrating the advancement of the time of the surge, and amplification of its magnitude and duration following progesterone administration after oestrogen priming (Permezel et al., 1989). These reports substantiate that progesterone may participate in the initiation of the midcycle surge. Further, it has been shown that the administration of even low doses of antiprogestins in the late follicular phase retards the onset of the LH surge without reducing the preovulatory rise of oestradiol (Ledger et al., 1992; Batista et al., 1992a,b).

(iii) Third in the sequence of events initiated at the time of the LH surge is ovulation itself. The breakdown of the ovarian epithelial surface at ovulation is possibly induced by local synthesis of prostaglandins (Ackermann and Murdoch, 1993). The LH surge is also associated with an increase in the amount of plasminogen activator in the follicular fluid and granulosa cells, with an eventual enzymatic breakdown of the follicle wall, which leads to the subsequent release of the follicular fluid and the oocyte-cumulus complex (Deutinger et al., 1988).

Data regarding the mechanism of regulation of the gonadotrophin surge has mainly originated from studies on rodents, ungulates and primates. It is proposed that the LH surge is initiated by positive feedback from rising levels of oestrogens secreted by the maturing follicles. Oestrogen acts on the hypothalamus and pituitary to stimulate LHRH. Studies on the rat and sheep suggested that oestradiol increases both the number of receptors for LHRH, as well as the responsiveness of the gonadotrophs to LHRH by increasing intracellular synthesis of LH (Naftolin et al., 1972; Fink, 1979; Menon et al., 1985; Gregg et al., 1990).

The positive feedback effects of oestradiol on the hypothalamo-pituitary axis before the LH surge are mediated by various pathways, which combine to produce the dramatic abrupt increase in peripheral levels of LH seen at the time of the surge. The most obvious marker to predict the time of ovulation is, indeed, the LH surge. However, it can occur only if follicular maturation proceeds normally.

Role of Inhibin: Inhibin, the glycoprotein hormone secreted by the corpus luteum, is known to play a role in the regulation of FSH secretion by the pituitary (Franchimont et al., 1979). Circulating levels of inhibin remain low prior to ovulation and rise during the luteal phase of the human cycle (McLachlan et al., 1987; Reddi et al., 1990). It is also known to act as a paracrine regulator within the ovary (Ying, 1988). Inhibin is secreted from both ovaries in similar amounts, thus ruling out the possibility of the dominant follicle being the major source of inhibin (Illingworth et al., 1991). Further, it has been shown by Illingworth that inhibin is secreted by non-dominant follicles during the late follicular phase. Therefore, inhibin does not seem to have any major endocrine role in the initiation of the LH surge, or in the control of ovulation.

It is well established that fertility declines with age, even before ovulation ceases at menopause. The advent of assisted conception, using *in vitro* fertilization and associated technologies, has allowed an unbiased assessment of the effects of age on fertility by excluding the other variables, such as the frequency of intercourse and sperm quality. It has been found that in women over 40 years of age, even in those with regular menstrual cycles, the prognosis for the success of *in vitro* fertilization is poor (Romern et al., 1986). This decline in fertility was found to be associated with a rise in the basal levels of FSH (Pearlstone et al., 1992). The rise of FSH with age is the first detectable endocrine marker of the onset of the perimenopausal period. The FSH rise commonly occurs while the menstrual cyclicity is maintained. Thus, dissociation of FSH and LH has been attributed to the effect of the decrease in the amount of inhibin released from follicles with ageing (Van Look et al., 1977). Although oestradiol levels do not differ between two groups of regularly cycling women aged 20-29 and 40-44 in the follicular phase, high FSH levels and low inhibin levels are reported in the older age-group (MacNaughton et al., 1992). The fall in the circulating levels of inhibin with age might be caused by the decrease in the number of primordial follicles in the ovaries, and a reduction in the ability of the granulosa cells to synthesize inhibin and possibly other peptides.

2.5. Paracrine Regulation And Ovarian Function

The intraovarian regulatory mechanisms involve interaction between the oocyte and two somatic cell types—granulosa and theca cells. This interaction is mediated via steroids, i.e. androgens and oestrogen, growth factors, cytokines and other proteins (Fig. 3.6).

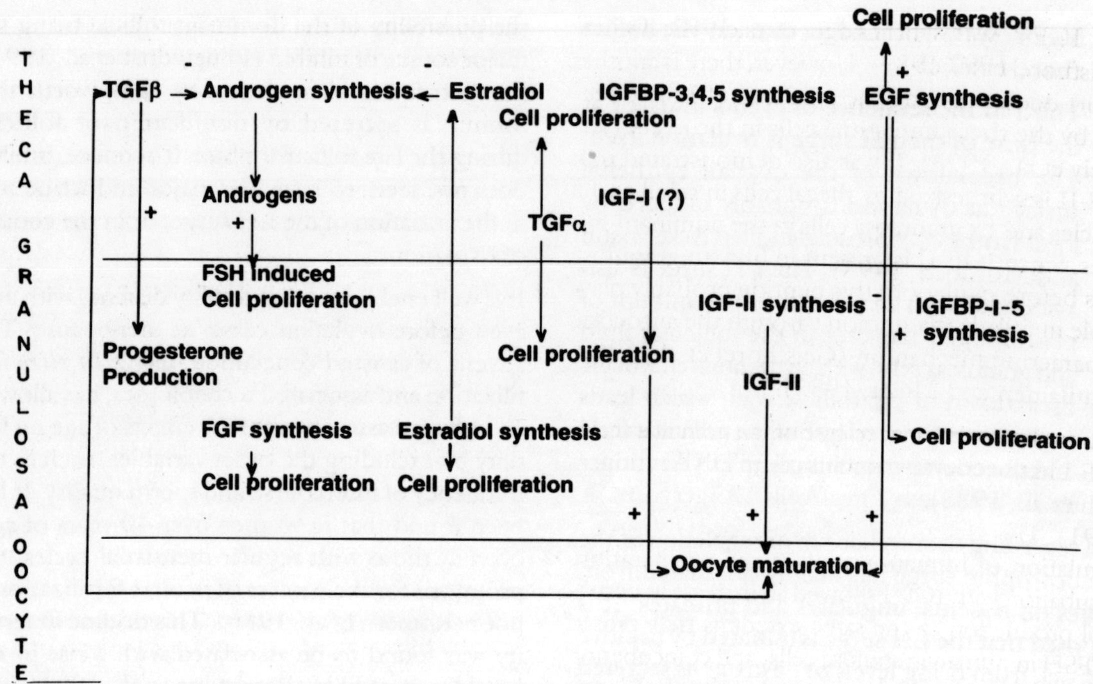

Fig. 3.6. Various factors involved in the regulation of ovarian functions

Steroids

Oestrogen: The theca interna is the principal cellular site of androgen synthesis. Granulosa cells contain androgen receptors, which mediate the effects of thecal androgens to augment FSH-induced granulosa cell differentiation and to control the follicular atresia (Louvet et al., 1975; Hillier et al., 1977).

Oestradiol produced by granulosa cells may regulate theca cell function by suppressing thecal androgen synthesis in response to the midcycle LH surge (Erickson et al., 1985). It potentiates the synthesis of the FSH-induced steroidogenic enzymes, P450aro and P450scc, and stimulates the expression of inhibin and its subunits (Richards et al., 1987; Turner et al., 1989). Oestrogen also acts as an intrafollicular autocrine regulator within the granulosa cells as it stimulates the proliferation of these cells.

Progesterone: The preovulatory rise in follicular progesterone synthesis is suggestive of progesterone playing a role in ovulation. Inhibition of ovulation by systemic administration of anti-progesterone antibodies, or inhibitors of the enzymes involved in progesterone synthesis or blockers of progesterone receptors, supports this idea (Mori et al., 1977; Snyder et al., 1984; Loutradis et al., 1991).

Growth Factors

Insulin-like Growth Factors (IGFs): IGF-I and IGF-II peptides, which show structural homology with proinsulin and insulin, respectively, are suspected to be involved in the intraovarian regulation system through endocrine, paracrine and autocrine mechanisms. Human follicular fluid has been shown to contain both IGF-I and IGF-II (Geisthorel et al., 1989; Ramasharma et al., 1986).

The concentrations of IGF-I and IGF-II in ovarian blood samples from females undergoing abdominal hysterectomy demonstrated a decreased ovarian gradient for IGF-II, but not for IGF-I. This was suggestive of the possibility that IGF-II, but not IGF-I, may be locally regulated by the ovary (Jesionowska et al., 1990). This was supported by a report indicating the presence of IGF-II but not IGF-I mRNA in human granulosa cells (Voutilainen and Miller, 1987). It was presumed that IGF-I was synthesized outside the follicle (Geisthorel et al., 1989). However, there is another report demonstrating the synthesis of IGF-I peptide by the theca interstitial cells in the ovary (El-Roeiy et al., 1993). It was also demonstrated that IGF-II is synthesized by thecal cells in small antral follicles and by granulosa cells in the dominant follicles. Since IGF-II is present in human granulosa cells before ovulation, this peptide probably plays a role in follicle maturation through the autocrine or paracrine mechanism (Geisthorel et al., 1989; Voutilainen and Miller, 1987).

Although not synthesized by human granulosa cells, IGF-I has been shown to stimulate DNA synthesis in human granulosa luteal cells (Angervo et al., 1991). This is indicative of a role for IGF-I in the regulation of human granulosa cell proliferation. Incubation with IGF-I showed an increase in oestradiol production to the same extent as that caused by FSH in human granulosa cells, and coincubation with FSH and IGF-I increased oestradiol levels to more than FSH alone (Erickson et al., 1989; Mason et al., 1992). IGF-I was found to increase the synthesis of P–450 aromatase in granulosa-luteal cells from women undergoing *in vitro* fertilization (Steinkampf et al., 1988). Further, IGF-I and IGF-II have been shown to stimulate human oocyte maturation (Gomez et al., 1993).

IGF-Binding Proteins (IGFBPs): El-Roeiy and his group studied the expression of IGFBPs 1–6 in the normal ovary. They reported the synthesis of IGFBP-1 by the granulosa cells of dominant follicles; IGFBP-3 by the theca cells of all follicles and by the granulosa cells of dominant follicles; and IGFBPs -2, -4 and -5 by the granulosa cells of atretic follicles, IGFBP-4 and -5 also by thecal and stromal tissues. No IGFBP-6 could be detected in the human ovary (El-Roeiy et al.,1992).

IGFBP-1 is also known as PP12 (placental protein-12), α1-PEG (α1-pregnancy associated endometrial globulin), BP28 (Koistinen et al., 1987; Bell and Keyte, 1988; Lee et al., 1988). IGFBP-1 binds to IGF-I with high affinity (Julkunen et al., 1988).

Human follicular fluid and luteinized granulosa cells have been shown to express IGFBP-1 and its mRNA (Seppala et al., 1984; Koistinen et al.,1990). *In vitro* studies have also demonstrated prostaglandin E2-stimulated secretion of IGFBP-1 from human granulosa luteal cells (Julkunen et al., 1988). Further, a positive correlation was observed between follicular fluid oestradiol and IGFBP levels, and also between progesterone and IGFBP levels (Seppala et al., 1984). It has been demonstrated that IGF-I inhibits IGFBP-I secretion in unstimulated human granulosa cells (Mason et al., 1993). Interestingly, according to another report, IGFBP-1 produced by granulosa cells inhibits IGF-stimulated DNA synthesis of the same cells (Angervo et al., 1991). It also inhibits IGF-I-stimulated progesterone secretion from granulosa cells (Adashi et al., 1992).

IGFBP-2 and IGFBP-3 transcripts have also been detected in human granulosa cells (Guidice et al., 1991). IGFBP-3 seems to be the most abundant IGFBP in follicular fluid (Holly et al.,1990). IGFBP-3 is reported to inhibit FSH- and IGF-I-induced oestradiol and progesterone secretion in granulosa cells (Mason et al., 1993).

As the follicle grows, the concentration of IGFBP-3 decreases, while in atretic follicles, IGFBPs-2 and -4 are expressed (San Roman and Magoffin, 1993). These studies indicate that the IGF system plays a role in the local regulation of follicular maturation and steroidogenesis.

Epidermal Growth Factor (EGF): EGF is a polypeptide growth factor, and acts as a mitogen and differentiation-inducing factor. Granulosa and thecal cells both express EGF receptors (EGFR) (Feng et al., 1987; Skinner and Coffey,1988).

Immunohistochemical staining to localize EGF and EGFR in the ovary failed to detect any signal for EGF and EFGR in primordial follicles, while positive staining was observed on the oocyte in the preantral follicles (Maruo et al., 1993). EGF and EGFR were localized in antral follicles on the granulosa and theca interna, without appreciable staining in the surrounding stroma. A similar pattern with intensified staining was observed in the mid-luteal phase on the corpus luteum, whereas no staining was observed for both EGF and EGFR in the corpus albicans. In atretic follicles, intense staining was shown by the theca interna, whereas granulosa cells did not show any significant staining for EGF and EGFR.

Theca cells are known to produce EGF, which induces thecal cell proliferation (Skinner and Coffey, 1988). In contrast to this, EGF alone or in the presence of FSH does not induce granulosa cell proliferation. However, in the presence of TGFβ alone or IGF-I plus TGFβ, it induces cell proliferation (Bendell and Dorrington, 1990). It is likely that EGF of thecal origin controls granulosa cells' responsiveness to FSH in a paracrine manner.

Unlike IGF-I, EGF does not stimulate the expression of cytochrome P450 aromatase. Further, EGF increases IGFBP-1 secretion from granulosa cells in a dose-dependent manner (Angervo et al., 1992). This is also in contrast to the action elicited by IGF-I, which is known to suppress IGFBP secretion (Mason et al.,1992).

Further, EGF has been reported to have a luteinizing effect on human granulosa cells. There occurs a marked increase in the response to oestradiol when granulosa luteal cells are exposed to EGF (Richardson et al., 1989). EGF may induce luteinization directly or indirectly. The indirect action of EGF may be mediated through induction of IGFBP-1 to counteract the proliferation-inducing activity of IGFs. The ability of EGF to augment spontaneous maturation of immature oocytes was shown by significant increases in the percentages of metaphase II oocytes when unstimulated oocyte-cumulus complexes were incubated with EGF (Gomez et al., 1993).

Transforming Growth Factors (TGFs): Theca cells have been shown to express TGFα, a 50-amino-acid-long polypeptide which shares 30% sequence homology with EGF and interacts with the same receptors as EGF (Marquardt et al., 1984). TGFα produced by thecal cells has both paracrine and autocrine actions on cell proliferation within the growing follicle as TGFα stimulates the growth of both granulosa and theca cells (Skinner and Coffey, 1988).

TGFβ are multifunctional growth regulators which can either stimulate or inhibit cellular proliferation *in vitro*, depending on the cell type and the presence of other growth factors (Roberts et al., 1988). Transcripts for three TGFβs—TGFβ 1, 2 and 3—have been identified in ovarian cells (Flanders et al., 1991). TGFβ is synthesized by thecal/interstitial cells (Skinner et al., 1987). Human follicular fluid also contains TGFβ (Ruegsegger et al., 1988).

In vitro studies have demonstrated the effect of TGFβ on steroid synthesis in both granulosa and theca cells. TGFβ has been shown to inhibit androgen synthesis and stimulate progesterone accumulation (Magoffin et al., 1989). It may also augment FSH secretion from the anterior pituitary and potentiate FSH-mediated increase of LH receptor levels, aromatase activity and progesterone production in cultured granulosa cells (Ying et al., 1986a,b).

The sensitivity of the theca and interstitial cells to TGFβ is increased by IGF-I (Magoffin et al., 1989). *In vitro* studies have demonstrated that these factors act as potent stimulators of oocyte maturation. It is also speculated that TGFβ and other growth factors may participate in the selection of the dominant follicle and meiotic maturation during follicular development (Feng et al., 1988).

Fibroblast Growth Factor (FGF): FGFs are known to regulate the proliferation and differentiation of mesodermal and neurectodermal cells (Burgess et al., 1989). Basic FGF (βFGF) is abundant in ovaries, whereas acidic FGF (αFGF) is found mostly in neuronal tissues (Slack et al., 1989). Granulosa cell-derived βFGF may play an active intermediary role in regulating the growth and maturation of the developing follicle and the corpus luteum. βFGF may also have a role in the development of thecal vasculature in the preovulatory follicle and during luteal development because of its angiogenic properties (Gospodarowicz and Ferrera, 1989). FGF has been shown to inhibit FSH-induced aromatase activity, FSH-mediated induction of LH receptors and FSH-stimulated progesterone synthesis (Baird and Hsueh, 1986). It is likely that βFGFs exerts autocrine regulatory actions on granulosa cell growth and differentiation.

Inhibins and Activins: Inhibins are gonadal peptides which inhibit gonadotrophin secretion, especially of FSH, by the pituitary (Mason et al.,

1985). Inhibin exists as inhibin A and inhibin B in human follicular fluid (Mason et al., 1986). Both forms are composed of two subunits—similar α subunits and dissimilar β subunits. Expression of inhibin in granulosa cells is regulated by FSH (Woodruff et al., 1987).

Activins are structurally related dimers of the β subunits, representing activin A and activin B (Ling et al., 1985). In contrast to the suppressive action elicited by inhibins on FSH secretion, the activins stimulate FSH secretion. Binding sites for activin have been demonstrated on granulosa cells (Sugino et al., 1988).

Circulatory inhibin levels are maximal in the luteal phase (McLachlan et al., 1987), and the regulation of FSH secretion by inhibin occurs primarily in the luteal phase (Reddi et al., 1990). It has been suggested by Hillier and Miro (1993) that activin acting at the early stages of antral follicles may sensitize granulosa cells to the action of FSH, and thereby, may play a role in follicular recruitment.

Leucocytes and Cytokines

The presence of large populations of tissue-bound leucocytes and dramatic changes in the specific localization of leucocyte populations during different stages of the menstrual cycle have been observed in the ovary.

Macrophages: Since macrophages are known for their ability to secrete cytokines, eicosanoids, vasoactive amines and tissue-remodelling enzymes, they are supposed to be involved in the process of tissue remodelling at ovulation, luteinization and luteolysis. This was supported by the studies demonstrating a large number of macrophages in the follicle wall at ovulation and in the corpus luteum, with an increase towards the stage of luteolysis (Brannstorm et al., 1994; Wang et al., 1992a; Lei et al., 1991). Further, macrophage-derived products have been shown to stimulate progesterone production in human granulosa lutein cells (Halme et al., 1985). This may be one of the several events which lead to ovulation since progesterone is known to facilitate the process of ovulation.

Granulocytes: The presence of eosinophilic granulocytes in the human ovary has not been studied. However, neutrophilic granulocytes or neutrophils are reported to be present in high numbers in the human follicle wall at ovulation, and also in the human corpus luteum of the menstrual cycle (Brannstorm et al., 1994). Also, a preovulatory rise in neutrophil chemotactic activity was noticed in human follicular fluid (Herriot et al., 1986).

Lymphocytes: Lymphocytes of both the B and T types mediate a variety of immunological functions, like the production of antibodies, cytotoxicity reactions and modulation of the immune response. Human preovulatory follicular fluid and the preovulatory follicle wall were reported to contain T lymphocytes (Brannstorm et al., 1994). As compared to peripheral blood, an increased ratio of T suppressor (CD8+) to T helper (CD4+) cells was reported in ovarian follicular fluid (Hill et al., 1987). It is likely that a high proportion of CD8+ cells is required for the prevention of autoimmunity in the ovary (Lipscomb et al., 1979). Further, the presence of a high number of CD8+ cells is indicative of active immunoregulation occurring in the human ovary to maintain ovarian self-tolerance (Hill, 1991).

A low and constant number of T lymphocytes was found in the corpus luteum of the menstrual cycle (Wang et al., 1992a). B lymphocytes were undetectable and natural killer cells were present in very low numbers in the human corpus luteum tissue (Brannstrom et al., 1994).

Lymphocytes secrete various cytokines. These cytokines have the potential to influence the function of corpus luteum cells.

Interleukin (IL-1): IL-1 has been shown to be present in significant amounts in human follicular fluid. The circulating IL-1 levels are elevated during the post-ovulatory phase in regular menstrual cycling women (Cannon and Dinarello, 1985). In addition to IL-1, its receptor and antagonist have also been identified in the human ovary (Hurwitz et al., 1991).

Studies in rodent models suggest that intraovarian IL-1 plays a crucial role in ovulation. A significant increase in IL-1β mRNA is found at ovulation in the rat ovary (Hurwitz et al., 1992). At this ovulatory stage, only thecal cells express IL-1 and just before follicle rupture, granulosa cells also express IL-1 and its receptor (Simon et al., 1994a,b).

Tumor Necrosis Factor α (TNFα): In human ovary, TNFα is present in the healthy follicle at the time of antrum formation. In the corpus luteum, TNFα is localized in the large lutein-like cells and paraluteal cells, and also in the cytoplasm of the small paraluteal cells (Terranova et al., 1991). TNFα is also reported to be present in human follicular fluid (Wang et al., 1992b).

TNFα appears to negate the FSH effects as it inhibits FSH-induced aromatization and accumulation of progestagen derivatives (Adashi et al., 1990). TNFα also inhibits FSH-stimulated cholesterol side chain cleavage and 3β hydroxysteroid dehydrogenase synthesis (Adashi et al., 1992). TNFα is known to increase human chorionic gonadotrophin (hCG)-stimulated progesterone production and prostaglandin production in granulosa luteal cells (Terranova et al., 1991; Wang et al.,1992b).

Interferons (IFNs): IFNs are a heterogeneous group of peptides with antiviral, antiproliferative and immunoregulatory actions. It has been shown that IFN γ exerts an inhibitory effect on progesterone production by human luteal cells stimulated by hCG (Wang et al., 1992c). However, the cellular origin of IFNs in the ovary and their mechanisms of action are at present not understood.

Prostaglandins

There are several reports which suggest that prostaglandins play a critical role in the process of ovulation. Receptors for prostaglandins are known to be present on luteal cells (Powell et al., 1979). Both granulosa and theca cells produce prostaglandins in response to LH. Inhibitors of prostaglandin synthesis have been shown to inhibit follicular rupture.

Prostaglandin F2α is produced locally in the ovary (Patwardhan et al., 1985). Prostaglandin F2α has been shown to inhibit basal and hCG-stimulated progesterone synthesis in the corpus luteum (Bennegard et al., 1992). It has been suggested that prostaglandin F2α in association with oxytocin, also known to be secreted by the corpus luteum, leads to regression of the human corpus luteum. When oxytocin is injected locally into the corpus luteum of women with normal menstrual cycles, there occurs a rise in prostaglandin F2α metabolites, with a fall in serum progesterone levels. This effect was completely abolished by an inhibitor of prostaglandin synthesis, indicating that the luteolytic effect of oxytocin is prostaglandin-mediated (Bennegard et al., 1992).

The ovary, a multicompartmental organ with variable biological properties, responds to cyclic pituitary gonadotrophin secretions. The ovary produces not only oestrogen and progesterone, but also a multitude of regulatory peptides and growth factors. Some of these factors, like inhibin, have extra ovarian functions, while others, like cytokines and growth factors, regulate intraovarian function by modulating steroidogenesis, differentiation and remodelling of different ovarian cell types. The interaction between various follicular compartments of the ovary in a highly integrated manner leads to the production of a fertilizable ovum. Successful fertilization of the ovum in the oviduct is followed by embryo development, a major part of which occurs in the uterus.

3. UTERUS

The organ where the implantation of the fertilized egg takes place is the uterus. During each menstrual cycle, the uterus first prepares to receive and transport the spermatozoa from the cervix to the oviduct, and subsequently, it prepares to receive the conceptus from the oviduct and nourishes it. The uterus consists of three parts: (i) the perimetrium or serosa, a mesothelium of simple squamous cells plus a thin layer of aereolar tissue; (ii) the myometrium, a thick layer consisting of three layers of smooth muscle cells and associated connective tissue fibres and matrix; and (iii) the endometrium, a complex layer which is the innermost lining of the uterus and is nearest to the uterine lumen.

Like all other hormone-dependent female reproductive organs, the uterus, especially the endometrium, also undergoes periodic changes in response to rhythmic variations in the levels of circulating oestrogen and progesterone. In every cycle, the endometrium anticipates the arrival of a fertilized egg and gets ready for the implantation. If it does not encounter the egg, it sulks and regresses and leaves the body in the form of menstrual bleeding.

However, its remnants again start on an optimistic note and a new cycle of growth, proliferation and differentiation takes place.

Being an end organ in the hormonal cascade, the endometrium reflects the culmination of monthly physiological events. In fact, the endometrium has been used by clinicians to assess whether the female reproductive functions are optimal, in general. In the following section, we will look at the cellular architecture of endometrial tissue and the changes it undergoes during different phases of the natural menstrual cycle.

3.1. Endometrium

The endometrium is composed of simple tubular glands and cellular vascular stroma (Fig. 3.7). There are two components—a basal layer or basalis, which is normally refractory to hormonal stimulation; and the second layer, the functionalis, which responds to the hormonal changes during the normal ovulatory cycle. This component is regularly sloughed off and regenerated during the reproductive years. However, there are no sharp lines of demarcation between the functionalis and basalis, and also between the basalis and myometrium.

Basalis

The stroma in the basal endometrium is more densely cellular than in the functionalis. The glands are less evenly distributed in the basalis as compared to those in the functionalis. Nucleocytoplasmic ratios are high. Lymphocytes and lymphoid aggregates are common. Thick-walled arteries are also seen. There is a narrow zone where the basalis blends with the myometrium, and there is an intermingling of stromal cells and smooth muscle cells.

Functionalis

During a normal menstrual cycle, the functionalis follows a cyclic pattern of growth, differentiation and shedding. This cycle ends every 28 days if no pregnancy occurs.

It is customary to mark the first day of menstruation as the day of commencement of the menstrual cycle. In some countries, the day of ovulation is regarded as the first day of the cycle. The cyclical changes in the endometrium may be described either in terms of profound morphological changes, or alternatively, in terms of the ovarian hormonal secretion (Fig. 3.8).

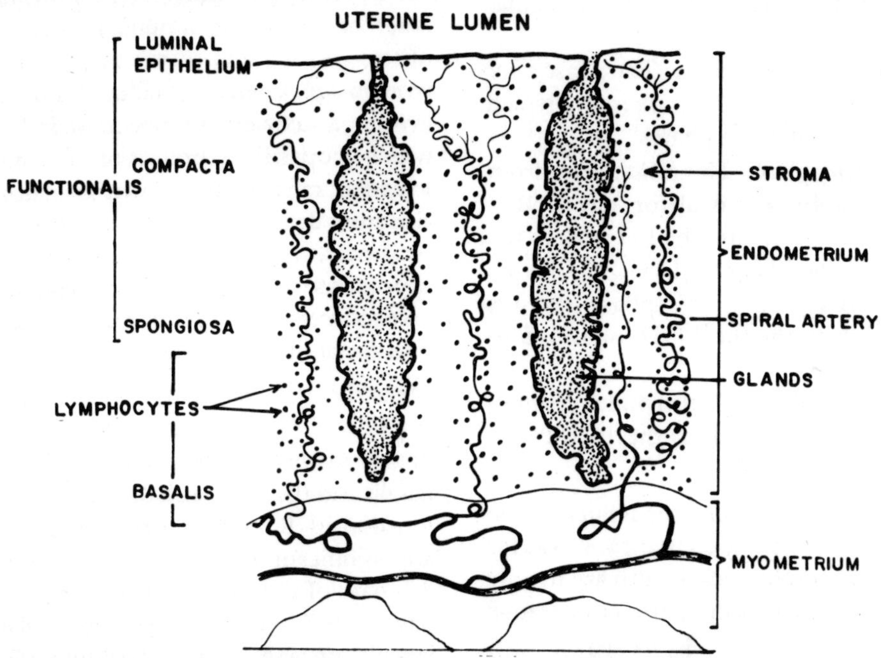

Fig. 3.7. Schematic representation to demonstrate organization of different uterine layers

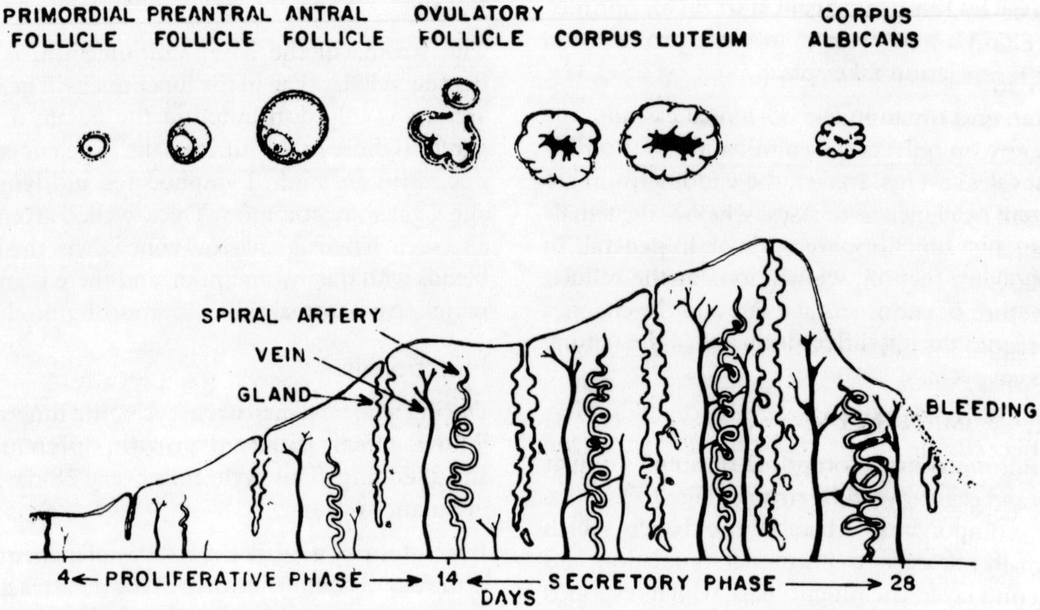

Fig. 3.8. Cyclical changes in the endometrial structure with respect to follicular development in the ovary

The normal menstrual cycle can be broadly classified into two phases.

(a) The proliferative or follicular phase: This corresponds to the phase of ovarian follicular growth prior to ovulation.

(b) The secretory or luteal phase: The phase after ovulation has occurred. This phase is divided into the three following phases:

(i) Early secretory phase: This phase spans from the 2nd to the 4th post-ovulatory day (POD), or from the 2nd day after the LH peak to the 4th day after the LH peak (LH+2 to LH+4).

(ii) Mid-secretory phase: This phase extends from the 5th to the 9th POD, or LH+5 to LH+9.

(iii) Late secretory phase: This includes changes occurring from the 10th to the 14th POD, or LH+10 to LH+14.

In the normal menstrual cycle, the length of the secretory phase is remarkably constant and lasts for 14 days. Variations in the cycle length are usually due to changes in the length of the proliferative phase, which may vary from 8 to 21 days.

Many women have regular menstrual cycles throughout their reproductive life, their monthly ovulation varying by a day or so. In others, the cycles are disturbed or vary in length. They may be extremely long or anovulatory in women with primary or secondary amenorrhoea. Proliferative phases shorten and secretory phases lengthen as women age. Ovulatory failure (anovulation) may involve a deficient sequence of folliculogenesis, which jeopardizes pregnancy or causes hectic, irregular, infrequent or absent ovulatory events. It also arises through inadequate inputs to the gonads or aberrant central nervous system responses. Inappropriate development of the endometrium can lead to infertility, repetitive miscarriages and dysfunctional uterine bleeding.

Menstruation, which lasts for approximately 5 days, is followed by the postmenstrual or proliferative phase. At this time, the uterus is lined only by a basalis and the residuum of the deeper part of the functionalis. Regrowth starts even in the absence of any significant levels of hormones on the 3rd and 4th days of the cycle. Between the 5th and 14th day, there is synchronous stromal, glandular and vascular growth. The endometrium also increases in thickness and this continues till ovulation.

3.2. Hormonal Changes During Menstrual Cycle

We saw in the previous section that during the proliferative phase, ovarian follicular growth occurs in response to oestrogen secreted by the granulosa and thecal cells of the developing follicle. The oestrogens act by binding to the oestrogen receptors which are present in abundance in the uterine tissue. Oestrogens also induce the synthesis of progesterone receptors.

At the beginning of the oestrogenic phase or proliferative phase of the cycle, progesterone receptors are at a low level and progesterone, therefore, has little effect on the uterus. Since the time taken for the ovarian follicles to develop and mature tends to vary between cycles and between women, and as the changes are less pronounced, the proliferative phase is not easy to date with any degree of precision.

In a typical 28-day cycle, ovulation occurs on the 14th day, designated LH+0. The day of ovulation can be precisely determined only by estimating daily plasma hormone levels or LH surge, as ovulation is immediately preceded by a midcycle LH surge.

Following ovulation and the subsequent development of the ovarian follicle into the mature corpus luteum, there occurs a rapid rise in progesterone secretion (Fig. 3.9), and this initiates the progestogenic or secretory phase of the menstrual cycle. Progesterone levels are highest 3 to 4 days after ovulation. However, the progesterone levels seen within 1.5 days of ovulation are sufficient to induce detectable endometrial changes. Progesterone stimulates the glandular secretory changes, stromal maturation or decidualization and differentiation of the spiral arteries. However, these changes occur only when progesterone receptors are present on the endometrium. This, in turn, is dependent on adequate oestrogen secretion in the proliferative phase.

Progesterone levels remain high until 2 or 3 days before the end of the cycle. The levels start declining in the absence of pregnancy and as the corpus luteum degenerates.

Now we will see how the individual components of endometrial tissue respond to hormonal variations in a normal menstrual cycle.

3.3. Changes In Endometrial Morphology During Menstrual Cycle

A. Epithelial Cells

(a) Glands: Endometrial glands are made of tall columnar cells, arranged as a simple epithelium. They have large round or oval nuclei, with their

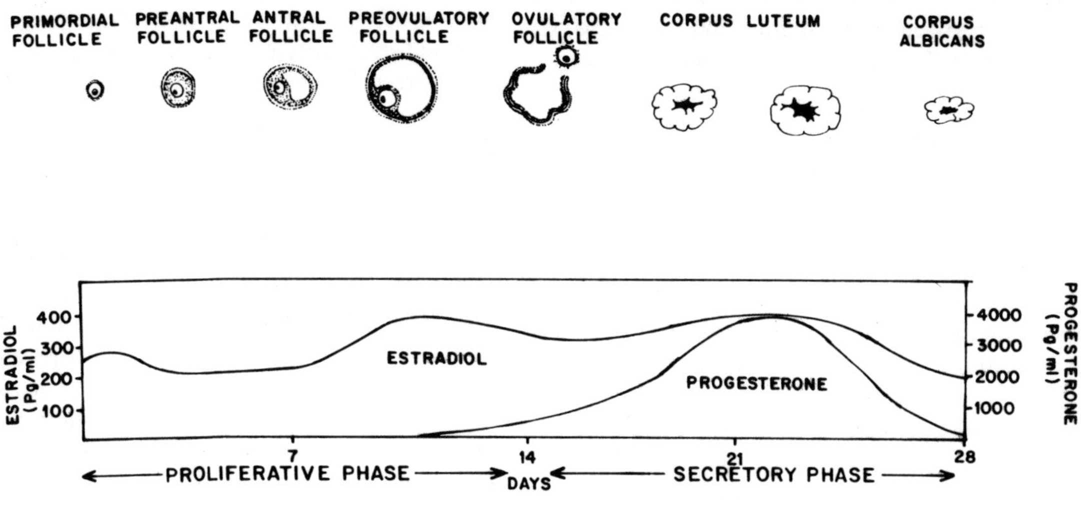

Fig. 3.9. Cyclical changes in the hormonal levels in a regular menstrual cycle

long axis oriented along that of the cell. Endometrial glands extend through the full depth of the endometrium, from the lumen of the uterus to the myometrium. The basal part of the glands, which lies in the basalis, is retained at menses (Ferneczy, 1976), while the remaining gland, located in the functionalis, is lost every month in a non-pregnant reproductive cycle. However, others are of the view that most of the endometrium is conserved and re-epithelialization occurs only in regions of the localized damage (Wilborn and Flowers, 1984).

Significant morphological changes seen in the endometrial glands can be correlated with the ovarian cycle. Gland formation begins soon after menstruation ends and mitoses are seen in the early proliferative phase. Gland cell mitoses are less common in the secretory phase. Glandular mitoses decrease from about 23 per 1,000 cells on day LH-3 (three days before the LH surge) to about 7 per 1,000 cells on day LH+3, after which they virtually cease (Johannisson et al., 1982). On the other hand, the diameter of the glandular lumen increases from about 50 μm on day LH+0 in the proliferative phase to 100 μm on day LH+8 in the secretory phase (Johannisson, 1985). However, the volume of endometrial glandular transudation and secretion is greater during the proliferative phase and reaches a peak around the time of ovulation. Hence, the term 'secretory' may be a misnomer (Johannisson, 1985).

The relatively straight, narrow tubular glands become more tortuous and distended in the late proliferative phase. The glands also lengthen. During the second half of the proliferative phase, both the surface and glandular epithelium are tall and columnar, with sharp luminal borders, probably because of sparse, short and blunt surface microvilli.

There occurs little variation in gland cell height and nuclear volume during the early secretory phase. The proportion of the cell made up of nucleus is reduced significantly due to the rapid accumulation of secretory material in subnuclear vacuoles after ovulation (Johannisson,1985; Dockery et al., 1988a). On about day LH+3, basal accumulation of secretory material causes the nucleus, usually located in a basal position, to be pushed upwards to the centre of the cell. This happens at slightly different times in adjacent cells, giving the nuclei a stratified appearance, a phenomenon termed pseudostratification by Noyes (1950).

Attempts to determine the day of ovulation by looking at endometrial morphology (especially progestagenic effect on the endometrial glands and the accumulation of glycogen and glycoproteins in epithelial cells) often lead to spurious findings as these events may not be true post-ovulatory events. However, it has been recommended that the appearance of uniform subnuclear vacuolation in the glands in the functionalis and smoothening of the pseudostratification of glands should be checked to ascertain whether ovulation has occurred. On day LH+6, the contents of the basal vacuole are transported to the cell apex, where they are released into the lumen. With this, the nucleus returns to its basal position.

B. Stroma

Stroma also undergoes changes, which are as dramatic and well coordinated as those seen in the epithelium. In the early proliferative phase, stromal cells are similar to undifferentiated fibroblasts (Verma, 1983). Stromal mitoses range from about 2 per 1,000 cells on day LH-10 to a peak of about 10 per 1,000 cells around ovulation (Johannisson, 1985). This declines to a significantly low level on day LH+6 and a second peak occurs just before menstruation (Noyes et al., 1950). Other cellular changes are infiltration by leucocytes from about day LH+10 through to the end of menstruation, increased stromal cell density from days LH+2 to LH+6, stromal oedema (maximal about day LH+8), and the formation of predecidual cells from about day LH+9 onwards (Noyes et al., 1950; Dockery et al., 1990).

In contrast to the remarkable morphological changes in the glands, little change is observed in the stromal cells during the first post-ovulation week, except that the stromal nuclei are slightly larger and vesicular. Stromal proliferation also increases under the influence of progesterone. The stromal cells become larger and plumper. Within the stromal tissues, the characteristic spiral arteries become fully developed.

In a non-conception cycle, when the endometrium does not get a chance to see a fertilized egg, the glands of the functionalis begin to involute about one week after ovulation. The luminal secretion tends to disappear gradually and the distended glands collapse to produce the crenated or saw-tooth outline characteristics of the late secretory phase. Degenerative changes in the epithelium and nucleus are observed on about the 8th or 9th POD. However, these regressive changes in the epithelium are accompanied by progressive changes in the stroma and vasculature. It has been speculated that these progressive changes in the stroma are caused by the mid-luteal rise in plasma oestrogen. At about the 9th or 10th POD, the spiral arteries and arterioles of the functionalis are more prominent due to true growth of the vessels, as well as enlargement and vesiculation of the nuclei and swelling of the cytoplasm in the predecidual stromal cells around the vessels. The degree of predecidualization increases significantly by the11th or 12th POD. Around this time, stromal oedema in the midzone of the endometrium becomes prominent, thus delineating the spongiosa, whereas progressive predecidualization of the upper layer of the endometrium demarcates the compacta, a solid zone of swollen stromal cells.

Blood vessels and immune cells are the other two components of the stroma.

Blood Vessels: Stromal blood vessels also show structural changes during different phases of the menstrual cycle. Blood vessels proliferate in response to the thickening endometrium and there is an increase in capillary luminal size towards the end of the secretory phase (Sheppard and Bonnar, 1980). Increased vascular permeability in the mid-secretory phase may be a cause of stromal oedema (Cornillie et al., 1985). The collapse or spasmic contraction of spiral arteries is a major factor regulating the events involved in the loss of part or all of the endometrium during menstruation.

Endometrial Leucocytes: The endometrium hosts a wide spectrum of immunocompetent cells, i.e., T lymphocytes, macrophages and endometrial granulated lymphocytes. These play a significant role during implantation by releasing immunosuppressive factors at the fetal-maternal interface, altering maternal endometrial lymphocyte populations and producing maternal blocking antibodies against, antigens of the semiallogeneic fetus (Houwert-De-Jong et al., 1990).

T lymphocytes: During both the proliferative and secretory phases, endometrial T lymphocytes (CD3+ cells) display three different patterns of distribution: intraepithelial, interstitial and lymphoid aggregates in the basalis. In all three areas, the majority of CD3+ cells are CD8+ (T suppressor/cytotoxic), and the ratio of CD8+ to CD4+ (T helper/inducer) cells is approximately 4:1 (Morris et al., 1985). The predominance of CD8+ leucocytic subset among CD3+ cells has also been reported by another group (Marshall and Jones, 1988). In a recent study, the endometrial leucocyte subpopulations were characterized in the biopsies obtained at different days following the LH surge. CD3+ cells increased significantly from day LH+4 to day LH+7 and this increase was contributed by a significant increase in the number of CD8+ cells. In the peri-implantation phase (LH+7), 22% of endometrial stromal leucocytes were found to be CD8+ cells and only 8% were CD4+ cells.

It is likely that the T lymphocytes in the endometrium and the decidua are involved in both immunosuppression and immunostimulation, and thereby, these cells contribute to successful implantation and placental development.

B lymphocytes: In contrast to T cells, only 2%–3% of the leucocytes (CD45+ cells) in the endometrium of normal fertile women are B lymphocytes (CD22+ cells). B lymphocytes have been observed either isolated in the stroma, or as a part of lymphoid aggregates. No significant change was observed in the number of B cells from day LH+4 to day LH+13 (Klentzeris et al., 1992). Occasional B cells are seen in lymphoid aggregates of the basalis and their number remains unaltered during the menstrual cycle. This suggests that the role of B lymphocytes in the reproductive performance of normal fertile women may be insignificant.

Endometrial granulated lymphocytes (eGLs): Granular endometrial stromal cells, also termed K cells, are reported to be present in both the pregnant and non-pregnant human endometrium. These cells contain a round reniform or oval, densely stained nucleus, often eccentric in position. Their cytoplasm contains a variable number of acidophilic and phloxinophilic granules. It has been observed that the eGLs have an unusual antigenic phenotype: CD45+, CD56+, CD3-, CD2+, CD38+, CD7+, CD4-, CD8, CD16-, CD57-, and these cells belong to a group of large granular lymphocytes. Further, it has been reported that at the time of implantation, the majority of endometrial leucocytes are CD56+, CD16-, CD2+, CD3-, HLADR- and morphologically similar to large granular lymphocytes. Now it is well established that the eGLs are migrating cells of bone marrow origin within the group of large granular lymphocytes. The number of eGLs is significantly higher in the late secretory phase and early pregnancy than in the proliferative endometrium (Bulmer et al., 1991). After the first trimester of pregnancy, the number of granulated decidual cells declines and they are virtually absent at term.

Stromal concentration of eGLs (CD56+, CD38+ cells) increases significantly from day LH+7 to day LH+10 and from day LH+10 to LH+13. At day LH+13, approximately 55% of stromal leucocytes are granulated lymphocytes. It is believed that eGLs differentiate ***in situ*** from bone marrow- derived precursors. ***In situ*** proliferation of eGLs explains the significant increase in their number from day LH+7 to day LH+13.

It has been speculated that eGLs in the human decidua may have an immunosuppressive role. They have been shown to have a natural killer activity and non-MHC-restricted cytotoxicity. It is possible that the lytic activity of eGLs may be directed towards the control of the trophoblast invasion during implantation and early pregnancy development.

Macrophages: Macrophages (CD14+,CD68+) constitute a significant proportion of endometrial leucocytes. Macrophages are located primarily around glands, dispersed in the stroma and occasionally between surface and glandular epithelial cells. It has been reported that macrophages can suppress the activation of lymphocytes and the subsequent generation of functional killer cells (Lala et al., 1986). These may also be involved in antigen presentation. Macrophages increase significantly in number from day LH+10 to day LH+13 in the secretory-phase endometrium (Kamat and Isaackson, 1987; Bulmer et al., 1991; Klentzeris et al., 1992). Macrophages synthesize and secrete a wide spectrum of cytokines, including tumour necrosis factor (TNF), granulocyte-colony stimulating factor (G-CSF), and macrophage-colony stimulating factor (M-CSF). Receptors for these molecules have been seen on the placenta. Nonspecific defence against infection and phagocytosis of tissue debris are two roles proposed for the endometrial macrophages.

Natural killer cells: Natural killer cells (CD56+, CD16+) constitute only 3.4% of stromal leucocytes in the proliferative phase (Bulmer et al., 1991). CD16+ cells comprise 2% of the bone marrow-derived cells in the secretory endometrium and show significant change from day LH+4 to day LH+13 (Klentzeris et al., 1992).

C. Luminal Epithelial Cells

The most relevant changes induced by oestrogens and progesterone are stromal reorganization in the endometrium, as indicated by the classical histological techniques. However, the uterine luminal surface epithelium, which is directly implicated in uterine secretion, spermatozoa transport and egg implantation, also undergoes changes during the menstrual cycle (Wynn, 1977). However, the cyclical changes expressed by luminal cells are less pronounced than those seen in glandular cells (Cornillie et al., 1985).

3.4. Endometrial Changes During Pregnancy

Successful implantation requires a well-coordinated interaction between an appropriately developed embryo and the hormone-primed endometrium. The embryo (morula stage) reaches the uterus 3 to 4 days after fertilization and develops into the blastocyst some hours later. The blastocyst loses its zona pellucida on coming in contact with the endometrium (Falck-Larsen,1978).

The first attachment event of the blastocyst is apposition to the luminal epithelium of the endometrium. Progressive adhesion of the blastocyst involves changes in the luminal epithelium surface and establishment of intercellular contact. The microvilli of the blastocyst cell membranes and the luminal epithelium flatten, and both surfaces become closely associated (Enders,1976).

Adherence is followed by invasion of and fusion with the endometrium by the trophoblastic cells of the blastocyst on day 11. There develops in the maternal endometrial tissue a corresponding specialized and vascularized region, which makes an intimate contact with the conceptus. This zone of intimate contact between mother and conceptus is called the placenta. This initial contact between the mother and conceptus causes profound changes in the stromal tissue underlying the epithelium. Moreover, this effect is seen over an extensive area of the endometrium. The stromal tissue underlying the conceptus shows an increased vascular permeability, oedema and compositional change in the intercellular matrix, a progressive sprouting and ingrowth of capillaries. The stromal reaction triggered by contact with the blastocyst is termed decidualization and it prepares the major endometrial component of the placenta, the decidua.

Soon after implantation, cytotrophoblastic cells of the blastocyst encircle the developing conceptus. Streamers of these cells infiltrate the decidua basalis. Capillaries and venules are breached by the conceptus around the 12th post-conception day. Invasion of the main spiral arteries is completely achieved by the 30th day by menstrual dating. The endovascular cytotrophoblast infiltrates into the wall of the artery, replaces the endothelium and causes much structural alteration to the vessel wall with the deposition of fibrinoid. The maternal blood vessels are eroded so deeply that the trophoblast cells bathe in maternal blood. The uterine glandular tissue and the decidual tissue in close proximity to the invading trophoblast are destroyed. Breakdown products (lipids, carbohydrates, nucleic acids and proteins) of these tissues are taken up by the conceptus and passed to the adjacent developed blood vascular system for utilization by the growing embryo.

It has been proposed by some researchers that the decidual tissue exerts a restraining influence over the conceptus to control its invasion into the maternal tissue. Blastocyst invasion is much more aggressive and penetrating whenever the decidual response is inadequate due to some uterine pathology or implantation at nonuterine ectopic sites.

At about the 16th week of gestation, clumps of cytotrophoblast may be seen in the lumens of the myometrial spiral arteries. In the second half of pregnancy, the affected vessels gradually become more distended and tortuous, emptying into the intervillous space of the fetal placenta and nonelastic fibrinoid and reparative fibrous tissue, replacing much of the musculo-elastic tissue of the affected vessels. Interestingly, the corresponding veins do not undergo the same morphological changes, even though syncytial giant cells may be found in their immediate vicinity.

The difference in the morphology of the endometria from the 7th to the 14th post-ovulatory day, between the cycle where conception has occurred and the one where it has not occurred, is not well documented. This may be attributed to non-access of histopathologists to gestational (especially at very early stage of pregnancy) endometrial samples. The data available on the gestational endometrium is based on samples obtained from spontaneous and induced abortions usually some weeks later.

3.5. Endometrial Changes During Menstruation

In the event of implantation failure, there occurs a decline in the corpus luteum function and menstruation ensues. Menstruation can be regarded as shedding of the functional layer of the endometrium which has failed to achieve its primary function (implantation), so that the tissue can prepare itself for implantation in the next cycle. There is still no consensus on the significance of menstruation. It might exert an antipathogenic or antimicrobial effect, provide a means of eliminating defective embryos or be a means of establishing a conducive environment for the embryo.

With the onset of luteolysis at approximately three days prior to menstruation, the progesterone level falls. As a result, lysosomes in the endometrium become unstable and release phospholipase which, in turn, acts on phospholipids to produce arachidonic acid and thereby leads to the synthesis of increasing amounts of prostaglandins. The prostaglandins so produced constrict the spiral arterioles supplying the functionalis of the endometrium, causing ischaemia and necrosis of that layer. The increased coiling and constriction of the spiral arterioles is considered to be important for the haemostasis of menstrual bleeding. On the other hand, straight arteries which supply the basalis are not affected by prostaglandins and the basal endometrium remains unaffected by menstruation.

Vascular changes of the spiral arterioles induce many changes in the endometrium prior to the onset of the menstruation. There occurs stromal haemorrhage and an increase in the number of stromal granulocytes. The functionalis undergoes shrinkage and its constituents—glands and stroma—fragment and crumble. Finally, menstruation starts with the shedding of the degenerated functionalis. The extent to which the endometrium is shed at menstruation is a subject of extensive debate. The most commonly held view is that in the normal cycle, the whole of the functionalis is sloughed off, whereas the basalis is saved so that it regenerates to give rise to the functionalis in the next cycle. However, others contend that only the compacta, with portions of the spongiosa, is sloughed off and the remaining spongiosa involutes to participate with the basalis in the regeneration process in the subsequent cycle.

3.6. Post-Menopausal Endometrium

As the reproductive phase of a women ends, a significantly high number of the ovarian follicles are used up, resulting in diminishing supply of oestrogen from the involuting ovaries. Further, there is increased urinary excretion of the pituitary gonadotrophins. Although there occurs oestrogenic production by the adrenal cortices and certain ovarian stromal cells, these amounts are not sufficient to prevent the endometrium from involution and atrophy after menopause.

3.7. Morphological Changes During The Induced Ovulatory Menstrual Cycle

In women with infertility and oligomenorrhoea, ovulation is induced with pharmacological agents to increase the chances of conception. The pharmocological agent of choice for the induction of ovulation in most women is clomiphene citrate, a synthetic weak oestrogen. Clomiphene citrate acts by competing with endogenous circulating oestrogens for oestrogen-binding sites in the hypothalamus. It has been shown to block the normal negative feedback of the endogenous oestrogens and produce a significantly increased pulse frequency of GnRH. The pulse frequencies of LH and FSH also increase, leading to oocyte maturation and an associated increase in oestradiol production. The rise in FSH is the key to follicular development and ovulation. Some data suggest that clomiphene may also act directly on the pituitary and ovary.

Eden et al. reported that endometrial thickness was reduced during the follicular phase in clomiphene-treated women (1989). This was supported by other studies demonstrating clomiphene-induced corpus luteum inadequacy. However, endometrial biopsies were found to be usually in phase during clomiphene therapy, even after multiple consecutive treatment cycles, and progesterone levels were higher during clomiphene-induced ovulations as compared with those achieved during spontaneous cycles.

3.8. Endometrial Structure And Dating

Typical endometrial structural changes during the menstrual cycle are utilized for histological dating. The proliferative and secretory phases are characterized by typical architectural patterns of cells and tissues in an endometrium. These may not always be homogeneous, since variations may exist in different parts of the uterus and between women.

The classical technique of Noyes et al. is used to examine the endometrial development in females with infertility. This technique related to a standardized menstrual cycle of 28 days, hence a standardized luteal phase of 14 days. However, the range of the normal luteal phase duration is actually 11.3 to 17.0 days (Lenton et al., 1984).

Dating has been virtually the only method of assessing the endometrium, and its limitations are well recognized. It is imprecise and invasive, provides no biochemical evidence of a receptive environment and does not predict implantation. Diagnostic variations arise between observers (65%), in duplicate diagnoses by the same observer (27%), and through regional differences (98%). This is especially true with biopsies taken in the late luteal phase or taken during different cycles from the same patient. Endometrial biopsies classified as normal by light microscopy may be abnormal ultrastructurally. Although some improvement in the precision of dating can be achieved by relating the characterization of the biopsy to the succeeding onset of menstruation rather than the last menstrual period, a more physiological approach is to use the LH surge as the reference point (Li et al., 1987). This method reduces the frequency of diagnosed chronological abnormalities. The chronological maturation of the endometrium with reference to the LH surge can be assessed by studying both glandular and stromal characteristics (Li et al., 1988). Morphometric features, such as the volume fraction of gland occupied by the gland cell, the amount of stromal predecidual reaction, the amount of secretion in the gland lumen, the amount of pseudostratification of the gland cell and the number of mitoses per 1,000 gland cells, can also be studied to establish a better correlation between the histologically and chronologically determined dates (Li et al., 1988).

The frequency of finding retarded endometrium in women with normal fertility (2.9%) was shown to be different from that of women with unexplained infertility (20%) (Li, 1988). It was also found that 50% of the cases with retarded endometrium were associated with a subnormal progesterone profile, whereas the other 50% were associated with a normal progesterone profile. It is possible that a receptor or post-receptor defect causes the failure of normal endometrial development in response to a normal progesterone stimulus in the latter group (Keller et al., 1979).

3.9. Biochemical Markers To Assess Endometrial Receptivity

The histological criteria for evaluating endometrial function in the luteal phase or histological dating was first established by Noyes et al. (1950). Theoretically, endometrial dating is an *in vivo* assay of oestrogen and progesterone for endometrial morphology and maturation. However, there seems to be no clinical benefit solely by histological dating of the endometrium, as demonstrated by random results obtained in an analysis of successive endometrial biopsies of infertile patients with three or more biopsy specimens from separate cycles (Balasch et al., 1992). Further, no clear correlation was found between serum progesterone concentrations and endometrial histological characteristics (Batista et al., 1993). A comparison of various morphological parameters of the endometrium in fertile and infertile subjects during the peri-implantation period revealed almost no differences between the two groups. This was further confirmed by a report demonstrating histologically normal endometria in infertile women with minimal and mild endometriosis and hydrosalpinges (Lessey et al., 1994). In addition, many hormone replacement regimes for donor oocyte embryos result in an out-of-phase and yet, receptive endometrium. These observations suggested that the classical histological dating relying on endometrial morphology is only a crude indicator of uterine receptivity, and there is a need to develop more objective and improved tests for assessing endometrial receptivity. This prompted researchers to investigate the expression of various biochemical markers, e.g., steroid hormone receptors, growth factors/cytokines, adhesion molecules and other secretory proteins, during the peri-implantation period and their potential as tools to assess the receptivity of the endometrium, especially for the management of infertility. Moreover, these markers were expected to reflect more specifically the uterine receptivity as compared to the morphology of the endometrium.

Steroid Hormone Receptors

There occur changes in oestradiol and progesterone receptors in the human endometrium throughout a normal menstrual cycle. The exponential rise in preovulatory oestrogen production stimulates cellular expression of cytoplasmic oestrogen receptor (OR) and progesterone receptor (PR), whereas the progesterone rise during the luteal phase down-regulates the expression of PR in the endometrial epithelium (Milogram et al., 1973; Brenner et al., 1974).

The loss of epithelial PR was shown to coincide with maximum endometrial receptivity. This was supported by a report demonstrating persistent and abnormally high epithelial PR levels in luteal phase deficiency patients (Lessey et al., 1995). However, it has been shown that women with endometriosis had normal downregulation of PR but still failed to conceive (Lessey et al., 1994). Recent studies by Classen Linke et al. (1995) have also suggested that the timing of steroid expression may not prove a useful marker system for assessing endometrial receptivity.

Cytokines/Growth Factors

Growth factors/ cytokines also seem to play a role in endometrial differentiation (Tabibzadeh, 1991; Findlay and Salamonsen, 1991). These factors can act as intermediaries in the endometrial response to steroids, as well as in paracrine interactions with the placenta. This may explain why direct steroid hormone receptor-mediated activation of transcription cannot apply to all gene products (Beato, 1989). Some progesterone-activated products (e.g., secretory mucin) increase within 1–2 days of exposure to the hormone, whereas others (e.g., α2-PEG) may take as long as one week and do not correlate with the expression of steroid receptors.

Several studies have been carried out to analyse the expression of different cytokines and growth factors, e.g., Leukaemia inhibitory factor (LIF) (Bhatt et al., 1991; Kojima et al., 1994; Arici et al., 1996) Interleukin-1 (De et al., 1993; Simon et al., 1997), and Interleukin-6 (Tabibzadeh et al., 1995), in the endometrium. These factors were found to have increased expression in the luteal phase of a normal menstrual cycle in humans.

Heparin-binding epidermal growth factor (HB-EGF), a member of the epidermal growth factor family, was found to be expressed maximally during the secretory phase of the menstrual cycle, and its levels were low in the pregnant endometrium and high in placental tissues. This report was suggestive of the fact that HB-EGF may have an important function in the implantation of the human blastocyst (Yoo et al., 1997). Further, several growth factors, including epidermal growth factor, were shown to increase the expression of integrins, considered to be the most promising markers of uterine receptivity (Somkuti et al., 1997). However, expression of HB-EGF appeared unaffected in the Hoxa10⁻, homeobox gene mutant mice demonstrating the failure of implantation (Benson et al., 1996).

Transforming growth factor β (TGF-β), a polypeptide involved in a variety of physiological and pathophysiological processes such as implantation of the embryo, has been speculated to have some role in the predecidualization of human endometrial stromal cells during the late secretory phase of the non-fertile, ovulatory cycle, and in the completion of decidualization during fertile cycles after blastocyst implantation. TGFβ has been shown to influence proliferation and differentiation of the embryo, regulate embryonic proteolytic activity and modulate the maternal embryonic immune response (Polli et al., 1996).

In baboons, progesterone has been shown to stimulate the endometrial production of IGF-binding protein-1 (IGFBP1), which is the major secretory product of the primate decidualized endometrium (Fazleabas et al., 1994). This binding protein may modulate the functions of the somatomedins IGF-1 and IGF-2 in the decidua. In human endometrial cell culture IGF-I, its receptor and the IGF-binding proteins 1–4 are all localized to the epithelial cells and show the highest expression at the early/mid-secretory phase of the cycles (Tang et al., 1991). However, at present, these data are purely correlative.

Among these growth factors/cytokines, only LIF has shown some promise as a receptivity marker. Expression of LIF was shown to increase approximately six times in the secretory phase (Charnock-Jones et al., 1994). Further, treatment with an anti-implantation agent, e.g., mifepristone, was shown to reduce endometrial glandular LIF expression in fertile females (Danielsson et al., 1997). It has been shown that the endometrium of most of the infertile women whose eggs did not implant despite their oocytes having undergone a successful IVF, or explants from women suffering from an unexplained infertility, secreted much less LIF as compared to explants from the endometrium of fertile women, suggesting a causal relationship between LIF deficiency and the failure of implantation (Delage et al., 1995). Further, the amount of LIF in uterine flushings from women with unexplained infertility was found to be significantly lower than in those from normal fertile women (Laird et al., 1997). However, it has been shown in Cyclooxygenase (Cox$^-$) knock out mice that though LIF production remains normal, implantation still fails to take place. This suggested that LIF may not be the only receptivity marker.

Further, the role of other cytokines like IL-1 and TNFα in implantation is still controversial. Most of the studies on the role of cytokines/growth factors have been carried out in rodent models. We may not infer from animal studies, however, that in humans, too, the same set of endometrial genes is implicated in endometrial receptivity and implantation. For example, despite the data that amphiregulin may be important in implantation in the mouse (Das et al., 1995), no immunoreactivity for amphiregulin could be detected in the gestational endometria throughout the entire pregnancy in humans (Lysiak et al., 1995). Therefore, a great amount of work still needs to be carried out in primates to identify potential receptivity markers to delineate the period in the luteal phase when the endometrium is most receptive to an incoming embryo, i.e. implantation window.

Cell Adhesion Molecules

As the first step in implantation involves the attachment of the trophoblast to the surface epithelium of the endometrium (Aplin, 1991a; Tabibzadeh and Babaknia, 1995), some groups focused their attention on the role of cell adhesion molecules in implantation. Trophinin and Tastin, a novel cell adhesion complex, was shown to be expressed in the human endometrial surface epithelium on day 16/17 of the menstrual cycle, i.e., during the early secretory phase of the human endometrium (Fukuda et al., 1995). Further, extracellular matrix (ECM) proteins, known to be involved in cell adhesion, e.g., collagen type IV, fibrenectin and laminin, were found to be absent in endometria from females with unexplained infertility, suggesting defects in the distribution of certain ECM glycoproteins (Bilalis et al., 1996).

Among the cell adhesion molecules, MUC-1, a glycoprotein, seemed attractive as a resistance marker of uterine receptivity since it was found to have some role in selecting only healthy embryos and thereby imposing a barrier to the implanting embryo (Lightenberg et al., 1990). This was supported by the report demonstrating a reduction in the abundance of MUC-1 in an endometrium with recurrent spontaneous miscarriage (Serle et al., 1994). However, exploiting MUC-1 as a marker of uterine receptivity was limited by its heterogeneous expression, leading to mosaicism within the normal epithelial cell population (Campbell et al., 1988).

Expression of the integrins, another class of adhesion molecules in the endometrium, is characterized by temporal and spatial changes during the menstrual cycle. The integrins $\alpha_v\beta_3$ (the vitronectin receptor), $\alpha_1\beta_1$ (a collagen laminin receptor) and $\alpha_4\beta_1$ (a fibronectin receptor) exhibit increased expression during the luteal phase of the human menstrual cycle. The $\alpha_v\beta_3$ is perhaps a good receptivity marker as it was found to be expressed aberrantly in the endometrium of women with reproductive failure. Lack of expression of β_3 integrin was also observed in females who had recurrent implantation failure, even after at least four attempts at stimulated cycles of IVF. Further, $\alpha_v\beta_3$ was found to be absent in infertile women with minimal endometriosis, even in the presence of normal luteal phase progesterone levels (Lessey et al., 1994).

Till date, only integrins have been extensively studied as a potential receptivity marker, but it is not yet resolved as to how these integrins, especially $\alpha_v\beta_3$, which appear on the uterine luminal epithelium on day 24 of the cycle, i.e. the day when the 'implantation window' closes, facilitate endometrial-embryonic interaction. Further, the aberrant expression of integrins in the endometrium, especially from infertile cases with a normal hormonal profile, is intriguing.

Besides cytokines/growth factors and cell adhesion molecules, some other molecules also have been investigated for their potential role in implantation.

Heat Shock Proteins

Alpha crystallin β chain, a member of the heat shock family, was found to be absent in the proliferative phase in the human endometrium. It appears first in the secretory phase, followed by a progressive increase and peak in the late secretory endometrium (Gruidl et al., 1997). However, its function in the endometrium is not yet known.

Vasoactive Substances

It has been suggested that the uterine response at nidation is inflammatory in nature (Finn, 1986). This led to the speculation that prostaglandins (PG) may be involved in implantation. Inhibition of implantation confirmed this when PG synthesis was blocked in animal models (Kennedy, 1990; Smith, 1991). The activity of PG synthetase, an enzyme required for PG synthesis, was found to be essentially higher in luminal and glandular epithelial cells than in stromal cells of endometrial tissues in humans and monkeys during the peri-implantation period (Rees et al., 1982; Ghosh et al., 1996). Though a large body of data is available on the endometrial PGs in primates, the role of PGs in the process of blastocyst implantation in humans is still not clear.

Secretory Proteins

Uterine fluid contains a mixture of plasma-derived components and endometrial secretions. Many of the endometrial secretions are derived from the apical secretory activity of the glandular and luminal epithelial cells. The epithelial secretions are carbohydrate-rich (Aplin, 1991b). Glycan biosynthesis and epithelial secretory activity are present in the proliferative phase. This gives rise to a greatly increased secretory output, including glycogen, which originates in the cytoplasm and appears to escape from cells by an apocrine route. Secretory glycoconjugates are presumably transferred from Golgi to secretory vesicles and thence to the lumen by exocytosis.

Mucins constitute a quantitatively significant proportion of the secretory products. The polymorphic epithelial mucin (MUC-1) is present in epithelial cells and to a restricted extent, in gland secretions in the proliferative phase. There occurs an increase in MUC-1 expression during the secretory phase.

Another major secretory product of the late secretory phase endometrial epithelial cells is α2-PEG—pregnancy-associated endometrial α-2 globulin, also termed placental protein 14 (PP-14) or progestogen-associated endometrial protein. The production of PP-14 begins in the mid-secretory phase (6 days after the LH peak) and increases in the late secretory phase. Very high concentrations of PP-14 are found in the uterine fluid during the late secretory phase (Waites et al., 1988; Julkunen et al., 1990). In the first trimester, PP-14 synthesis continues to increase and its levels are maximum in the maternal serum during 8–10 weeks (Bell, 1986). It has been suggested that PP-14 may act as a binding protein for ligand transport to the fetus in early pregnancy.

The 27 kDa human heat shock protein (hsp 27) appears in the glandular epithelium of the endometrium during the late proliferative phase and in the luminal epithelium during the mid-secretory phase (Ciocca et al., 1983). Decidual stromal cells also express hsp 27, which shows strong homologies to the low-molecular-weight heat shock proteins of Drosophila and the mammalian α-crystallins (Fuqua et al., 1989).

Histones H2A, H2B and H3, as detected by uterine secretion electrophoresis, were found to appear as characteristic markers of the receptive stage of the luteal phase (Beier-Hellwig et al., 1994). Placental protein PP-12 (insulin-like growth factor binding protein 1) is the other secretory protein which was initially characterized as an endometrial protein (Than et al., 1993; Seppala and Titinen, 1995). Concepts have been proposed to develop blood tests to detect these endometrial proteins as markers of the functional stage of the endometrium. So far, however, no such reliable blood test is available since the peripheral blood plasma levels do not accurately reflect a substantial synthesis and lumenal release of endometrial proteins (Todorow et al., 1995).

Most of the endometrial markers identified to date seem to be regulated by a progesterone rise in the luteal phase. The more direct evidence for this suggestion comes from the studies conducted on artificially created adequate and inadequate secretory endometria in rhesus monkeys (Okulicz et al., 1996).

It would be interesting to analyse whether an infertile endometrium, with and without luteal insufficiency, in humans presents a similar under-

or over-representation of progesterone-dependent genes. These studies are expected to give some clues to the role of local factors in the regulation of progesterone-dependent genes in infertile females, especially in those with unexplained infertility.

COMMENTS

The functional network between the ovary and the uterus, and its regulation via endocrine and paracrine factors determine the fate of a male gamete, i.e. sperm, in the female reproductive tract. The success of various reproductive events, e.g., the interaction between an egg and a sperm resulting in fertilization, implantation of the fertilized egg or development of the implanted embryo, is primarily governed by the functional synchronization between the hypothalamus-pituitary, the ovary and the uterus. Any disharmony between the ovarian and endometrial cycles, caused either by organic anomalies or functional defects, may lead to reproductive failure in women.

This chapter provides basic information on the structural and functional roles of the ovary and uterus in a natural menstrual cycle. The authors have attempted to review information on the structure of different cellular components, the structural and functional changes, and finally, the expression of various paracrine factors, i.e., cytokines and growth factors, in response to the changing endocrine milieu in these two organs.

ACKNOWLEDGEMENTS

The authors wish to thank Mrs Shobha Waradkar and Mr Prasanna Chavan for typing the manuscript. The authors also thank Ms Vishakha Patil for the skilful art work.

REFERENCES

Ackermann, R.C. and W.J. Murdoch (1993). 'Prostaglandin-induced apoptosis of ovarian surface epithelial cells', *Prostaglandins*, **45**: 475–85.

Adashi, et al. (1990). 'Cytokine-mediated regulation of ovarian function: Tumor necrosis factor alpha inhibits gonadotropin-supported progesterone accumulation by differentiating and luteinized murine granulosa cells', *Am. J. Obstet. Gynecol.*, **164**: 889–99.

Adashi, E.Y. et al. (1992). 'Local tissue modification of follicle stimulating hormone action', in A.R. Genazzami, F. Petraglia (eds.) *Hormones in Gynoecological Endocrinology*, Parthenon Publishing, Carnfors, UK, pp. 255–60.

Angervo, M. et al. (1991). 'Insulin-like growth factor binding protein-1 inhibits the DNA amplification induced by insulin-like growth factor 1 in human granulosa-luteal cells', *Hum. Reprod.*, **6**: 770–73.

______(1992). 'Epidermal growth factor stimulates production of insulin-like growth factor binding protein-1 in human granulosa-luteal cells', *J. Endocrinol.*, **134**: 127–31.

Aono, T. et al. (1976). 'Progesterone advancement of oestrogen-induced luteinizing hormone release during the mid-follicular phase in normal cyclic women', *J. Endocrinol.*, **71**: 451–2.

Aplin, J.D. (1991a). 'Implantation, trophoblast differentiation and haemochorial placentation: Mechanistic evidence *in vivo* and *in vitro*', *J. Cell. Sci.*, **99**: 681–92.

______. (1991b). 'Glycans as biochemical markers of human endometrial secretory differentiation', *J. Reprod. Fertil.*, **91**: 525–41.

Arici, A. et al. (1996). 'Modulation of the levels of transforming growth factor beta messenger ribonucleic acids in human endometrial stromal cells', *Biol. Reprod.*, **54**: (2): 463–9.

Baird, A. and A.J.W. Hsueh (1986). 'Fibroblast growth factor as an intraovarian hormone: Differential regulation of steroidogenesis by an angiogenic factor', *Regul. Pept.*, **16**: 243–50.

Baird, D.T. (1987). 'A model for follicular selection and ovulation: Lessons from superovulation', *J. Steroid. Biochem.*, **27**: 15–23.

Baker, T.G. (1982). 'Oogenesis and ovulation', in C.R. Austin, R.V. Short (eds.) *Reproduction in mammals*, 2nd ed., Cambridge University Press, Cambridge, pp. 17–45.

Balasch, J. and J.A. Van Rell (1987). 'Corpus luteum insufficiency and infertility, a matter of controversy', *Hum. Reprod.*, **2**: 557–67.

Balasch, J. et al. (1992). 'The usefulness of endometrial biopsy for luteal phase evaluation in infertility', *Hum. Reprod.*, 7: 973–7.

Batista, M.C. et al. (1992a). 'Delayed endometrial maturation induced by daily administration of the antiprogestin RU 486: A potential new contraceptive therapy', *Am. J. Obstet. Gynecol.*, **167**: 60–65.

______(1992b). 'Evidence for a critical role of progesterone in the regulation of the midcycle gonadotropin surge and ovulation', *J. Clin. Endocrinol. Metab.*, **74**: 565–7.

______(1993). 'Midluteal phase endometrial biopsy does not accurately predict luteal function', *Fertil. Steril.*, **59**: 294–300.

Beato, M. (1989). 'Gene regulation by steroid hormones', *Cell*, **56**: 335–44.

Beier, H.M. (1974). 'Oviductal and uterine fluids', *J. Reprod. Fertil.*, **37**: 221–37.

Beier-Hellwig, K. et al. (1994). 'Hormone regulation and hormone antagonist effects on protein patterns of human endometrial secretion during receptivity', *Ann NY Acad. Sci.*, **734**: 143–150.

Bell, S.C. (1986). 'Secretory endometrial and decidual proteins: Studies and clinical significance of a maternally derived group of pregnancy associated serum proteins', *Hum. Reprod.*, **1**: 129–43.

Bell, S.C. and J.W. Keyte (1988). 'N-terminal amino acid sequence of human pregnancy-associated endometrial alpha-1 globulin, an endometrial insulin-like growth factor (IGF) binding protein—evidence for two small molecular weight IGF binding proteins', *Endocrinol.*, **12**: 1202–4.

Bendell, J.J. and J.H. Dorrington (1990). 'Epidermal growth factor influences growth and differentiation of rat granulosa cells', *Endocrinol.*, **127**: 533–40.

Bennegard, B. et al. (1992). 'Oxytocin and prostaglandin F2a in human luteolysis', in H.J.T. Coelingh Bennink, et al. (eds.) *Local regulation of ovarian function,* An Eric K Fernstrom Symposium, Parthenon Publishing, pp. 323–6.

Benson, G.V. et al. (1996). 'Mechanisms of reduced fertility in Hoxa-10 mutant mice: Uterine homeosis and loss of maternal Hoxa-10 expression', *Dev.*, **122** (9): 2687–96.

Bhatt, H. et al. (1991). 'Uterine expression of leukaemia inhibitory factor coincides with the onset of blastocyst implantation', *Proc. Natl. Acad. Sci.*, **88**: 11408–12.

Bilalis, D.A. et al. (1996). 'Immunohistochemical localization of extracellular matrix proteins in luteal phase endometrium of fertile and infertile patients', *Hum. Reprod.*, **11** (12): 2713–18.

Brannstrom, M. et al. (1994). 'Localization of leukocyte subsets in the human follicle wall and in the corpus luteum throughout the menstrual cycle', *Fertil. Steril.*, **61**: 488–95.

Brenner, R.M. et al. (1974). 'Cyclic changes in oviductal morphology and residual cytoplasmic estradiol binding capacity induced by sequential estradiol progesterone treatment of spayed rhesus monkeys', *Endocrinol.*, **95**: 1094.

Bulmer, J.N. et al. (1991). 'Granulated lymphocytes in human endometrium, histochemical and immunohistochemical studies', *Hum. Reprod.*, **6**: 791–8.

Burgess, W.H. and T. Maciag (1989). 'The heparin-binding (fibroblast) growth factor family of proteins', *Annu. Rev. Biochem.*, **58**: 575–606.

Cambell, S. et al. (1988). 'Expression of a secretory product by microvillous and cilliated cells of the human endomertial epithelium *in vivo* and *in vitro*', *Hum. Reprod.*, **3**: 927–34.

Cannon, J.G. and C.A. Dinarello (1985).'Increased plasma interleukin-1 activity in women after ovulation', *Science*, **227**: 1247–9.

Charnock-Jones, D.S. et al. (1994). 'Leukaemia inhibitory factor mRNA concentration peaks in human endometrium at the time of implantation and the blastocyst contains mRNA for receptor at this time', *J. Reprod. Fertil.*, **101**: 421–6.

Clocca, D.R. et al. (1983). 'Evidence for modulations of 27 K protein in human endometrium during the menstrual cycle', *J. Clin. Endocrinol. Metabol.*, **57**: 496–9.

Classen-Linke, I. et al. (1995). 'Expression of progesterone and estrogen receptors in human endometrial cells in culture', *Exp. Clin. Endocrinol.*, **103**: 113.

Cornillie, F.J. et al. (1985). 'Normal human endometrium', *Gynecol. Obstet. Invest.*, **20**: 113–29.

Danielsson, K.G. et al. (1999). 'The effect of various doses of mifepristone on endometrial leukaemia inhibitory factor expression in the midluteal phase—an immunohistochemical study', *Hum. Reprod.*, **12**: (6) 1293–7.

Das, S.K. et al. (1995). 'Amphiregulin is an implantation specific progesterone-regulated gene in the mouse uterus', *Mol. Endocrinol.*, **9**: 691–705.

De, M. et al. (1993). 'Expression of interleukin-1, interleukin-6 and tumor necrosis factor α in mouse uterus during the peri-implantation period of pregnancy', *J. Reprod. Fertil.*, **97**: 83–9.

Delage, G. et al. (1995). '*In vitro* endometrial secretion of human interleukin for DA cells/leukaemia inhibitory factor by explant cultures from fertile and infertile women', *Hum. Reprod.*, **10**: (9). 2483–8.

Deutinger, J. et al. (1988). 'Elevated tissue type plasminogen activator in human granulosa cells correlate with fertilizing capacity', *Hum. Reprod.*, **3**: 597–9.

di Zerega, G.S. and G.D. Hodgen (1981). 'Folliculogenesis in the primate ovarian cycle', *Endocr. Rev.*, **2**: 27–49.

Dockery, P. et al. (1988). 'An examination of the variation in timed endometrial biopsies', *Hum. Reprod.*, **3**: 715–20.

Dockery, P. et al. (1990). 'A morphometric study of the human endometrial stroma during the peri-implantation period', *Hum-Reprod.*, **5**: 112–6.

Eden, J.A. et al. (1989). 'The effect of clomiphene citrate on follicular phase: Increase in endometrial thickness and uterine volume', *Obstet. Gynecol.*, **73**: 187–90.

EI-Roeiy, A. et al. (1992). 'Localization and expression of insulin-like growth factor binding proteins (IGFBPs) 1–6 in normal and polycystic (PCO) human ovaries', Proceedings of the 48th Annual Meeting of the American Fertility Society, November 2–5, 0–020.

EI-Roeiy, A. et al. (1993). 'Localization and expression of insulin like growth factor I (IGF-I) and IGF-II and the IGF-I, IGF-II and insulin receptor genes and localization of gene products in the human ovary', *J. Clin. Endocrinal. Metab.*, 77: 1411–18.

Enders, A.C. (1976). 'Anatomical aspects of implantation', *J. Reprod. Fertil.*, **25**: 1.

Erickson, G.F. et al. (1985). 'The ovarian androgen producing cells: A review of structure/function relationships', *Endocr. Rev.*, **6**: 371–99.

Erickson, G.F. et al. (1989). 'Insulin like growth factor I regulates aromatase activity in human granulosa and granulosa luteal cells', *J. Clin, endocrinol. Metab.*, **69**: 716–24.

Falck-Larsen, J. (1978). 'Aspects ultrastructuraux de l' ovoimplantation humaine', in F. du Mesnil, et al. (eds.), *I implantation de l' oeuf* Masson, Paris.

Fazleabas, A.T. and H.G. Verhage (1994). 'Expression and regulation of insulin like growth factor binding protein I and retinol binding protein in the baboon (*Papio anubis*) uterus', in S.R. Glasser, et al. (eds.), *Endocrinology of embryo endometrium interaction*, Plenum, New York, pp. 57–75.

Feng, P. et al. (1987). 'Hormonal control of epidermal growth factor receptors by gonadotrophins during granulosa cell differentiation', *Endocrinol.*, **120**: 1121–6.

Feng, P. et al. (1988). 'Transforming growth factor-beta stimulates meiotic maturation of the rat occyte', *Endocrinol.*, **122**: 181–6.

Ferenczy, A. and C. Bergerson (1991). *Ann NY Acad. Sci.*, **622**: 6–27.

Ferneczy, A. (1976). 'Surface ultrastructural response of the human uterine lining to hormonal environment: A scanning microscopic study', *J. Clin. Endocrinol. Metabol.*, **21**: 566–72.

Findlay, J.K. and L.A. Salamonsen (1991). 'Paracrine regulation of implantation and uterine function', Bailliere's *Clin. Obstet. Gynaecol.*, **5**: 117–31.

Fink, G. (1979). 'Feedback actions of target hormones on hypothalamus and pituitary with special reference to gonadal steroids', *Am. Rev. Physiol.*, **41**: 571–85.

Finn, C.A. (1986). 'Implantation, menstruation and inflammation', *Biol. Reprod.*, **61**: 313–28.

Flanders, K.C. (1991). 'Transforming growth factor b: A multifunctional regulatory peptide with actions in the reproductive system', in D.W. Schomberg (ed.), *Growth Factors in Reproduction,* New York, Springer-Verlag, New York, pp. 23–37.

Franchimont, P. et al. (1979). 'Inhibin: From concept to reality' *Vitamins and Hormones,* **37**: 243–302.

Fukuda, M.N. et al. (1995). 'Trophinin and tastin, a novel cell adhesion molecule complex with potential involvement in embryo implantation', *Journal*, **9** (10): 1199–1210.

Fuqua, S.A. et al. (1989). 'Induction of the progesterone regulated 24K protein by heat shock', *Cancer Research.*, **49**: 4126–9.

Geisthorel, F. et al. (1989). 'Expression of insulin like growth factor II (IGF-II) messenger ribonucleic acid (mRNA) but not IGF-I mRNA in human preovulatory granulosa cells', *Hum. Reprod.*, **4**: 899–902.

Ghosh, D. et al. (1996). 'The involvement of prostaglandins (PGF2a and PGE2) during receptivity, implantation and decidualization in the rhesus monkey.'

Gomez E, et al. (1993). 'Oocyte maturation in humans: The role of gonado-tropins and growth factors', *Fertil. Steril.*, **60**: 40–6.

Gospodarowicz, R.E. and N. Ferrara (1989). 'Fibroblast growth factor and the control of pituitary and gonad development and function', *J. Steroid Biochem.*, **32**: 183–91.

Greep, R.O. (1963). 'Histology, histochemistry and ultrastructure of the adult ovary', in H.G. Grady, D.E. Smith (eds.), *The Ovary*, Williams and Wilkins Baltimore.

Gregg, D.W. (1990). 'Estradiol-induced increase in number of goandotropin releasing hormone receptors in cultured ovine pituitary cells', *Biol. Reprod.*, **43**: 1032–6.

Gruidl, M. et al. (1997). 'The progressive rise in the expression of alpha crystallin b chain in human endometrium is initiated during the implantation window: Modulation of gene expression by steroid hormones', *Mol. Hum. Reprod.*, **3** (4): 333–42.

Guidice, L.C. et al. (1991). 'Human granulosa contain messenger ribonucleic acids encoding insulin-like growth factor-binding proteins (IGFBPs) and secrete IGFBPs in culture', *Fertil. Steril.*, **56**: 475–80.

Halme J. et al. (1985). 'Peritoneal macrophages modulate human granulosa-luteal cell progesterone production', *J. Clin. Endocrinol. Metab.*, **61**: 912–16.

Herriot, D.M. et al. (1986). 'Pregnancy related chemotactic activity of human follicular fluid', *Fertil. Steril.*, **45**: 196–201.

Hey, N.A. et al. (1995). 'MUC-1 in secretory phase endometrium: Expression in precisely dated biopsies and flushings from normal and recurrent miscarriage patients', *Hum. Reprod.*, **10**: 2655–62.

Hill, J.A. et al. (1987). 'Detection of T8 (suppressor/cytotoxic) lymphocytes in human ovarian follicular fluid', *Fertil. Steril.*, **47**: 460–67.

Hill, J.A. (1991). 'Cellular immune mechanisms of early reproductive failure', *Semin. Perinatol.*, **15**: 225–9.

Hillier, S.G. et al. (1977). 'Androgenic stimulation of progesterone production by granulosa cells from preantral ovarian follicles: Further *in vivo* studies using replicate cell cultures', *Endocrinol.*, **100**: 1539–49.

Hillier, S.G. and F. Miro (1993). 'Inhibin, activin and follistatin: Potential roles in ovarian physiology', Ann *N. Acad. Sci.*, **687**: 29–38.

Holly, J.M. et al. (1990). 'Insulin-like growth factor binding proteins in follicular fluid from normal dominant and cohort follicles polycystic and multicystic ovaries', *Clin. Endocrinol.*, **33**: 53–64.

Houwert-Dejong, M.H. et al. (1990). 'The immunology of normal pregnancy and recurrent abortion', in H.J. Huisjes, T. Lind (eds.), *Early Pregnancy Failure*, Churcill Livingstone, Edinburgh, pp. 27–38.

Hurwitz, A. et al. (1991). 'Endocrine and autocrine mediated regulation of rat ovarian (theca-interstitial) interleukin-1β (Beta) gene expression: gonadotropin dependent preovulatory acquisition', *Endocrinology*, **129**: 3427–9. .

Hurwitz, A. et al. (1992). 'Human intraovarian interleukin-1 (IL-1) system: Highly compartmentalized and hormonally dependent regulation of the genes encoding IL-1, its receptor, and its receptor antagonist', *J. Clin. Invest.*, **88**: 1746–54.

Illingworth, P.J. et al. (1991). 'The source of inhibin secretion during the human mensturel cycle', *J. Clin. Endocrinol. Metab.*, **72**: 667–73.

——— (1985) *In vitro* formulation in the human corpus luteum. *Prostaglandins* ,1985; **30**: 91–6.

Jalkanen, J. et al. (1989). 'Regulation of insulin-like growth factor-binding protein-1 production in human granulosa-luteal cells', *J. Clin. endocrinol. Metab.*, **69**: 1174–9.

Jesionowska, H. et al. (1990). 'Determination of insulin and insulin-like growth factors in the ovarian circulation', *Fertil. Steril.*, **53**: 88–91.

Johannisson, E. (1985). 'Cyclical changes in endometrial morphology', in R.P. Shearman (ed.), *Clinical Reproductive Endocrinology*, Churchill Livingstone, Edinburgh, pp. 128–64.

Johannisson, E. et al. (1982). 'Morphometric analysis of the human endometrium in relation to peripheral hormone levels', *Fertil, Steril.*, **38**: 564–71.

——— (1985) '*In vitro* formulation in the human corpus luteum', *Prostaglandins*, **30**: 91–6.

Julkunen, M. et al. (1988). 'Primary structure of human insulin-like growth factor-binding protein/placental protein 12 and tissue-specific expression of its mRNA', *FEBS Lett.*, **236**: 295–302.

Julkunen, M. et al. (1990). 'Identification by hybridization histochemistry of human endometrial cells expressing mRNAs encoding a uterine b lactoglobulin homologue and insulin-like growth factor-binding protein-1', *Mol. Endocri.*, **4**: 700–07.

Kamat, B.R. and P.G. Isaackson (1987). 'The immunocytochemical distribution of leukocytic sub-population in human endometrium', *Am. J. Path.*, **127**: 66–73.

Keller, D.W., W.G. Wiest, F.B. Askin et al. (1979). 'Pseudocorpus luteum insufficiency, a local defect of progesterone action on endometrium stroma', *Clinical Andocrine and meta*, **48**: 127–32.

Kennedy, T.G. (1990). 'Eicosanoids and blastocyst implantation', in M.D. Mitchell (ed.), *Eicosanoids in Reproduction*, CRC Press, Boca Raton, Florida, pp. 123–38.

Klentzeris, L.D. et al. (1992). 'Endometrial lymphoid tissue in the timed endometrial biopsy: Morphometric and immunohisto-chemical aspects', *Am J. Obstet. Gynec.*, **167** (3): 667–74.

Knobil, E. (1980). 'The neuroendocrine control of the menstrual cycle', *Rec. Prog. Horm. Res.*, **36**: 53–88.

Koistinen, R. et al. (1987). 'Purification of placental protein PP-12 from human amniotic fluid and its comparison with PP-12 from placenta by immunological, physicochemcial and somatomedin-binding properties', *Clin. Chim. Acta.*, **164**: 293–303.

______(1990). 'Human granulosa cells contain insulin-like growth factor binding protein (IGFBP-1) mRNA', *Clin. Endocrinol.*, **32**: 635–40.

Kojima, K. et al. (1994). 'Expression of leukaemia inhibitory factor in human endometrium and placenta', *Biol. Reprod.*, **50**: 882–7.

Laird, S.M. et al. (1997). 'The production of leukaemia inhibitory factor by human endometrium: Presence in uterine flushings and production by cells in culture', *Hum. Reprod.*, **12** (3): 569–74.

Lala, P.K. et al. (1986). 'Immunological role of the cellular constitutes of the decidua in the maintenance of semiallogenic pregnancy', *Ann NY Acad. Sci.*, **476**: 183–205.

Ledger, W.L. et al. (1992). 'Inhibition of ovulation by low dose mifepristone (RU 486)', *Hum. Reprod.*, **7**: 495–504.

Lee, Y-L. et al. (1988). 'Insulin-like growth factor (IGF) binding protein complementary deoxyribonucleic acid from human HPG2 hepatoma cells: Predicted protein sequence suggests an IGF binding domain different from those of the IGF and IGF II receptors', *Mol. endocrinol.*, **2**: 404–11.

Lei, R.M. et al. (1991). 'Quantitative cell composition of human and ovine corpora lutea from various reproductive states', *Biol. Reprod.*, **44**: 1148–56.

Lenton, E.A. (1990). 'Gonadotrophins of the menstrual cycle and ovulation', in R.G. Edwards (ed.) *Establishing a Successful Human Pregnancy*, Raven Press, New York, p. 33.

Lenton, E.A. et al. (1984). 'Normal variations in the length of the luteal phase: Identification of the short luteal phase', *Br. J. Obstet Gynaecol.*, **91**: 685–9.

Lessey, B.A. et al. (1974). 'Further characterization of endometrial integrins during the menstrual cycle and in pregnancy', *Fertil. Steril.*, **62**: 497–506.

Lessey, B.A. et al. (1995). 'Integrins as markers of uterine receptivity in women with primary unexplained infertility', *Fertil Steril.*, **63**: 535–42.

Li T.C. (1988). 'A morphometric study of endometrial development in the luteal phase and its regulation by progesterone in fertile and infertile women', Ph.D. thesis, University of Sheffield.

Li, T.C. et al. (1988). 'How precise is histologic dating of endometrium using the standard dating criteria?', *Fertil. Steril.*, **51**: 759–63.

Li, T.C. et al. (1987). 'A comparison between two methods of chronological dating of human endometria biopsies during the luteal phases and their correlation with histologic dating', *Fertil. Steril.*, **48**: 928–32.

Lightenberg, M.J.L. et al. (1990). 'Episialin a carcinoma associated mucin is generated by a polymorphic gene encoding splice variants with alternative amino termini', *J. Biol. Chem.*, **265**: 5575–8.

Ling, N. et al. (1985). 'Isolation and partial characterization of a Mr 32000 protein with inhibin activity from porcine follicular fluid', *Proc. Natl. Acad. Sci.*, USA, **82**: 7217–21.

Lipscomb, H.L. et al. (1979). 'The effect of neonatal thymectomy on the induction of autommune orchitis in rats', *J. Reprod. Immunol.*, **1**: 209–17.

Liu, J.H. and S.S.C. Yen (1983). 'Induction of midcycle gonadotropin surge by ovarian steroids in women: an initial evaluation', *J. Clin. Endocrinol. Metab.*, **57**: 797–802.

Loutradis, D. et al. (1991). 'Preovulatory effects of the progesterone antagonist mifepristone (RU486) in mice', *Hum-Reprod.*, **6**: 1238–40.

Louvet, J.P. et al. (1975). 'Evidence for a role of androgens in follicular maturation', *Endocrinol.*, **97**: 366–72.

Lysiak, J.J. et al. (1995). 'Localization of amphiregulin in the human placenta and decidua throughout gestation: Role in trophoblast growth', *Placenta*, **16**: 359–66.

Macnaughton, J. et al. (1992). 'Age-related changes in follicle stimulating hormone, luteinizing hormone, estradiol and immunoreactive inhibin in women of reproductive age', *Clin. Endocrinol.*, **36**: 339–45.

Magoffin, D.A. et al. (1989). 'Transforming growth factor β (Beta) promotes differentiation of ovarian thecal-interstitial cells but inhibits androgen production', *Endocrinol.*, **125**: 1951–8.

Marquardt, H. et al. (1984). 'Rat transforming growth factor type 1: Structure and relation to epidermal growth factor', *Science*, **223**: 1079–82.

Marshall, R.J. and D.B. Jones (1988). 'An immunohistochemical study of lymphoid tissue in human endometrium', *J. Gynec. Path.*, **7**: 225–35.

Maruo, T. et al. (1993). 'Expression of epidermal growth factor and its receptor in the human ovary during follicular growth and regression', *Endocrinol.*, **132**: 924–31.

Mason, H.D. et al. (1993). 'Insulin-like growth factor-I inibits production of IGF binding protein-I while stimulating estradiol secretion in granulosa cells from normal and polycystic ovaries', *J. Clin. Endocrinol. Metab.*, **76**: 1275–9.

Mason, H.D. et al. (1992). 'Inhibitory effects of insulin-like growth factor-binding proteins on steroidogenesis by human granulosa cells in culture', *Mol. Cell. Endocrinol.*, **89**: R1–R4.

Mason, A.J. et al. (1985). 'Complementary DNA sequences of ovarian follicular fluid inhibin show precursor structure and homology with transforming growth factor-b', *Nature*, **318**: 659–63.

Mason, A.J. et al. (1986). 'Structure of two human ovarian inhibins', *Biochem. Biophys. Res. Commun.*, **135**: 957–64.

McLachlan, D. et al. (1987). 'Circulating immunoreactive inhibin levels during the normal human menstrual cycle', *J. Clin-Endocrinol. Metab.*, **65**: 954–61.

Menon, M. et al. (1985). 'Estradiol potentiationof gonadotropin-releasing hormone responsiveness is mediated by an increase in goandotropin releasing hormone receptors', *Am. J. Obstet. Gynecol.*, **151**: 534–40.

Milogram, E. et al. (1973). 'Mechanisms regulating the concentration and the conformation of progesterone receptor (s) in the uterus', *J. Biol. Chem*,. **248**: 6366.

Monroe, S.T. et al. (1972). 'Regulation of human gonadotropins XII: Increase in serum gonadotropins in response to estradiol', *J. Clin. Endocrinol. Metab.*, **34**: 298–305.

Mori, T. et al. (1977). 'Inhibition of ovulation in immature rats by anti progesterone antiserum', *J. Endocri.*, **73**: 185–6.

Morris, H. et al. (1985). 'Endometrial lymphoid tissue: An immunological study', *J. Clin. Pathol.*, **38**: 644–52.

Naftolin, F. et al. (1972). 'Plasma and pituitary lutenizing hormone and peripheral plasma estradiol concentrations in the normal esterous cycle of the rat and after experimental manipulation of the cycle', *J. endocrinol.*, **53**: 17–30.

Nilsson, L. et al. (1982). 'Recruitment of an ovulatory follicle in the human following follicle-ectomy and lute-ectomy', *Fertil. Steril.*, **37**: 30–34.

Noyes, R.W. et al. (1950). 'Dating the endometrial biopsy', *Fertil. Steril.*, **1**: 3–25.

Okulicz, W.C. et al. (1996). 'Analysis of differential genes regulation in adequate versus inadequate secretory-phase endometrial complementary de-oxyribonucleic acid populations from the rhesus monkey', *Endocrinol.*, **137**: 4844–50.

Patwardhan, V.V. and A. Lantheir (1985). 'Luteal phase variations in endogenous concentrations of prostaglandins PGE and PGF and in the capacity for their *in vitro* formulation in the human corpus luteum', *Prostaglandins*, **30**: 91–6.

Pavelka, V.R. et al. (1972). 'Die ultrastrucktur der menschlichen Eizelle des Graafshen Follikels', *Wien Klin Wshr.*, **84**: 305.

Pearlstone, A.C. et al. (1992). 'Ovulation induction in women age 40 and over: The importance of basal follicle stimulating hormone level and chronological age', *Fertil. Steril.*, **58**: 674–9.

Permezel, J.M. et al. (1989). 'Acute effects of progesterone secretion in the follicular phase of the menstrual cycle', *J. Clin, Endocrinol. Metab.*, **68**: 960–56.

Polli, V. et al. (1996). 'Transforming growth factor beta 1 in the human endometrium', *Gynecol-Endocrinol.*, **10**: 297–302.

Powell, W.S. et al. (1979). 'Prostaglandin F2α receptor in human corpora lutea', *Lancet*, **6**: 1120–22.

Ramasharma, K. et al. (1986). 'Identification of insulin

like growth factor II in human semina and follicular fluids', *Biochem. Biophys. Res. Commun.*, **140**: 536–42.

Reddi, K. et al. (1990). 'Circulating bioactive follicle stimulating hormone and immunoreactive imhibin during the normal human menstrual cycle', *Clin. Endocrinol.*, **33**: 547–57.

Rees, M.C.P. et al. (1982). 'Immunohistochemical localisation of cyclooxygenase in human uterus', *Protaglandism*, **23**: 207–14.

Richards, J.S. et al. (1987). 'Ovarian follicular development: From physiology to molecular biology', *Recent Prog-Horm. Res.*, **43**: 231–73.

Richardson, M.C. et al. (1989). 'Augmentation by epidermal growth factor of basal and stimulated progesterone production by human luteinized granulosa cells', *J. Endocrinol.*, **121**: 397–402.

Roberts, A.B. et al. (1988). 'Transforming growth factor b: Biochemistry and roles in embryogenesis, tissue repair and remodeling and carcinogenesis', *Recent Prog. Horm. Res.*, **44**: 157–93.

Romern, A. et al. (1986). 'Results of *in vitro* fertilization attempts in women 40 years and over, the Norfolk experience', *Fertil. Steril.*, **47**: 130–36.

Ruegsegger Veit, C. and R.K. Asoian (1988). 'Identification of transforming growth factor-b in human ovarian follicular fluid', [Abstract] *Endocrinol.*, **122**: 1227.

Sallam, H.N. et al. (1983). 'The incidence of mature follicles in spontaneous and induced ovarian cycles', *Lancet*, **i**: 357.

San Roman, G.A. and D.A. Magoffin (1993). 'Insulin-like growth factor-binding proteins in healthy and atretic follicles during natural menstrual cycles', *J. Clin. Endocrinol. Metab.*, **76**: 625–32.

Seppala, M. and A. Titinen (1995). 'Endometrial responses to corpus luteum products in cycles with induced ovulation: Theoretical and practical considerations', *Hum. Reprod.*, (Suppl 2): 67–76.

Seppala, M. et al. (1984). 'Human preovulatory follicular fluid, luteinized cells of hyperstimulated preovulatory follicles and corpus luteum contain placental protein 12 (PP-12)', *J. Clin. Endocrinol. Metab.*, **58**: 505–10.

Serle, E. et al. (1994). 'A morphological and immunohistochemical study of endometrial development in the peri-implantation phase of women with recurrent miscarriage', *Fertil. Steril.*, **62**: 989–96.

Sheppard, B.L. and J. Bonnar (1980). 'The development of vessels of the endometrium during the menstrual cycle', in E. Diczfalusy, et al. (eds.), *Endometrial Bleeding and Steroidal Contraception,* Pitman Press, Bath, England, pp. 65–77.

Shivers, B. et al. (1983). 'Absence of oestradiol concentration in cell nuclei of LHRH-immunoreactive neurons', *Nature*, **304**: 345–7.

Simon, C. et al, (1994a). 'Immunohistochemical localization of the interleukin-1 system in the mouse ovary during follicular development, ovulation and luteinization', *Biol. Reprod.*, **50**: 449–57.

Simon, C. et al. (1994). 'Embryonic implantation in mice is blocked by interleukin-1 receptor antagonist', *Endocrinol.*, **134**: 521–8.

Simon, C. et al. (1997). 'The interleukin-1 system and human implantation', *Am J. Reprod. Immunol.*, **37** (1): 64–72.

Skinner, M.K. et al. (1987). 'Ovarian thecal cells produce transforming growth factor-b which can regulate granulosa cells growth', *Endocrinol.*, **121**: 786–92.

Skinner, M.K. and R.J. Coffey Jr. (1988). 'Regulation of ovarian cell growth through the local production of transforming growth factor-alpha by thecal cells', *Endocrinol.*, **123**: 2632–8.

Slack, J.M.W. (1989). 'Peptide regulatory factors in embryonic development', *Lancet*, **1**: 1312–15.

Smith, S.K. (1991). 'The role of prostaglandins in implantation', *Bailliere's Clin. Obstet. Gyanecol.*, **5**: 73–93.

Snyder, B.W. et al. (1984). 'Inhibition of ovulation in rats with epostane, an inhibitor of 3 b hydroxysteroid dehydrogenase', *Proc. Soc. Exp. Biol. Med.*, **176**: 238–42.

Somkuti, S.G. et al. (1997). 'Epidermal growth factor and sex steroids dynamically regulate a marker of endometrial receptivity in Ishikawa cells', *J. Clin. Endocrinol. Metab.*, **82** (7): 2192–7.

Steinkampf, M.P. et al. (1988). 'Effects of epidermal growth factor and insulin-like growth factor I on the levels of mRNA encoding aromatase cytochrome P–450 of human ovarian granulosa cells', *Mol. Cell. Endocrinol.*, **59**: 93–9.

Stewart, C.L. et al. (1992). 'Blastocyst implantation

depends on maternal expression of leukaemia inhibitory factor', *Nature*, **359**: 76–9.

Sugino, H. et al. (1988). 'Identification of a specific receptor for erythroid differentiation factor on follicular granulosa cell', *J. Biol. Chem.*, **263**: 15249–52.

Tabibzadeh, S. (1991). 'Human endometrium: An active site of cytokine production and action', *Endocrine Review*, **12**: 272–90.

Tabibzadeh, S. and A. Babaknia (1995). 'Signals and molecular pathways involved in implantation, a symbiotic interaction between blastocyst and endometrium involving adhesion and tissue invasion', *Mol. Hum. Reprod.*, **18**: 1579–1602.

Tabibzadeh, S. et al. (1995). 'Progressive rise in the expression of interleukin-6 in human endometrium during menstrual cycle is initiated during the implantation window', *Hum. Reprod.*, **10** (10): 2793–9.

Tang, X.M. et al. (1991). 'Insulin-like growth factor I-(IGF-I), IGF-I receptors and IGF binding proteins 1–4, in human uterine tissue: Tissue localization and IGF-I action in endometrial stromal and myometrial smooth muscle cells *in vitro*', *Biol. Reprod.*, **50**: 1113–25.

Terranova, P.F. et al. (1991). 'Tumor necrosis factor a: Localization and actions within the preovulatory follicle', in D.W. Schomberg (ed.), *Growth Factors in Reproduction*, Springer-Verlag, New York, pp. 63–78.

Terzakis, J.A. (1965). 'The nucleolar channel system of human endometrium', *J. Cell. Biol.*, **27**: 293–304.

Than, G.N. et al. (1993). 'Advances in pregnancy-related protein research: Functional and clinical applications', CRC, Boca Raton.

Tilly, J.L. et al. (1992). 'Apoptosis in atretic ovarian follicles is associated with selective decreases in messenger ribonucleic acid transcripts for gonadotropin receptors and cytochrome P-450 aromatase', *Endocrinol.*, **131**: 1670–76.

Todaro, G.J. et al. (1980). 'Transforming growth factors produced by certain human tumor cells: Polypeptides that interact with epidermal growth factor receptors', *Proc. Natl. Acad. Sci.* USA, 77: 5158–62.

Todorow, S. et al. (1995). 'PP-14 concentration fluctuations in human uterine fluid used for monitoring endometrial function of infertility patients', *Hum. Reprod.*, **10**: 33.

Tsang, B.K. et al. (1979). 'Androgen biosynthesis in human ovarian follicles: Cellular source, gonadotrophic control and adenosine 3'5' mono-phosphate mediation', *J. Clin, Endocrinol. Metabol.*, **48**: 153–8.

Turner, I.M. et al. (1989). 'Regulation of inhibin subunit gene expression by FSH and estradiol in cultured rat granulosa cells', *Endocrinol.*, **125**: 2790–92.

Van Look, P.F.A. et al. (1977). 'Hypothalamic-pituitary-ovarian function in perimenopausal women', *Clin. Endocrinol.*, **7**: 13–31.

Verma, V. (1983). 'Ultrastructural changes in human endometrium at different phases of the menstrual cycle and their functional significance', *Gynecol. Obstet Invest.*, **15**: 193–212.

Voutilainen, R. and W.L. Miller (1987). 'Coordinate tropic hormone regulation of mRNAs for insulin like growth factor II and the cholesterol side chain cleavage enzyme P450scc in human steroidogenic tissues', *Proc. Natl. Acad.Sci.* USA, **84**: 1590.

Waites, G.T. et al. (1988). 'Immunohistological localization of the human endometria secretory protein pregnancy associated endometrial a1-globulin, an insulin-like growth factor binding protein, during the menstrual cycle', *J. Clin. Endocrinol. Metab.*, **67**: 1100–104.

Wang, L.J. et al. (1992a). 'Distribution of leukocyte subpopulations in the human corpus luteum', *Hum. Reprod.*, **7**: 197–206.

Wang, L.J. et al. (1992b). 'Tumor necrosis factor a in the human ovary: Presence in follicular fluid and effects on cell proliferation and prostaglandin production', *Fertil Steril*, **58**: 934–40.

Wang, H.Z. et al. (1992c). 'Inhibitory effect of interferon and tumor necrosis factor in human luteal function *in vitro*', *Fertil. Steril.*, **58**: 934–40.

Wilborn, W.H. and C.E. Flowers (1984).'Cellular mechanisms for endometrial conservating during menstrual bleeding', *Sem. Reprod. Endocrinol.*, **2**: 307–42.

Wynn, R. (1977). 'Histology and Ultrastructure of the human endometrium', in R. Wynn (ed.), *Biology of the uterus,* R. Plenum Press, New York.

Woodruff, T.K. (1987). 'Rat inhibin: Molecular cloning of a and b subunit complementary deoxyribonucleic acids and expression in the ovary', *Mol. Endocrinol.*, **1**: 561–9.

Yoo, H.J. et al. 1997. 'Temporal and spatial regulation

of expression of heparin binding epidermal growth factor like growth factor in the human endometrium: A possible role in blastocyst implantation', *Dev. Genet.*, **21** (1): 102–108.

Ying, S-Y (1988). 'Inhibins, activins and follistatins: Gonadal proteins modualting the secretion of follicle stimulating hormone', *Endocr. Revs.*, **9**: 267–93.

Ying, S-Y, et al. (1986a). 'Type beta transforming growth factor (TGF-b) is a potent stimulator of the basal secretion of follicle stimulating hormone (FSH) in a pituitary monolayer system', *Biochem. Biophys. Res. Commun.*, **135**: 950–56.

Ying, S-Y, et al. (1986b). 'Inhibin and beta type transforming growth factor (TGF-b) have opposite modulating effects on the follicle stimulating hormone (FSH)-induced aromatase activity of cultured rat granulosa cells', *Biochem. Biophys, Res. Commun.*, **136**: 969–75.

4

Folliculogenesis and Ovarian Stimulation in Assisted Reproduction

Marc Dhont

INTRODUCTION

It is well established that the success of IVF is dependent on the number and the quality of eggs that can be obtained per cycle. The use of GnRH agonists proved to be one of the major advances in the development of reliable schemes for follicular stimulation. Recombinant gonadotrophins and GnRH antagonists have recently been introduced. It is still too early, however, to decide whether these agents will fundamentally change our strategy of ovarian stimulation. Nevertheless, both for the induction of mono-ovulation and for the multifollicular stimulation, an understanding of the basic mechanisms of follicular growth and the intimate relationship between follicular maturation and hormonal signals is mandatory. This chapter will address both the fundamental aspects of follicular maturation and the practical procedures that are being used to obtain multifollicular development.

Notwithstanding the remarkable progress, many problems remain unsolved. While the number of oocytes that are obtained with a stimulation protocol can easily be quantified, the quality of oocytes can be assessed only by indirect means. So, much less is known about the quality of oocytes obtained by using different stimulation protocols. Why is it that notwithstanding a high fertilization figure, only one out of every five embryos is able to implant? Can this figure be enhanced by better stimulation schemes? What is the reason for the tremendous individual variation in ovarian response? Will we ever be able to get more oocytes out of poor responders?

FOLLICULOGENESIS

The Ovarian Clock

Every species has its own quotum of eggs that are developed for optimal reproductive purposes. Germ cells are enveloped within a somatic structure, a follicle that forms the interphase between the egg and the body. The intricate coexistence of the follicle and the egg forms the basis of the mechanisms that allow for the species specific number of oocytes to be developed per reproductive cycle. The follicle communicates with the oocyte and the body to regulate the needs for reproduction. The cyclic process of egg maturation is regulated by an external clock which resides in the hypothalamus, and an internal clock which is dictated by the inherent cyclic nature of follicular ripening. The external clock consists of a monotonous pulsatile secretion of a releasing hormone that keeps the pituitary secretion of gonadotrophins tuned to feedback by the follicle. The growth of the follicle is associated with the production of oestrogens, which have a triple function: feedback with the pituitary to tell about the progress of oocyte ripening; intra-ovarian regulation of oocyte ripening; and preparation of the target organs, mainly the lower genital tract and the endometrium, for meeting of the gametes, fertilization and implantation to occur.

Monofollicular development is an obvious characteristic of primates. This quotum is regulated by intrinsic mechanisms determining the number of follicles which will be allowed to go through the final stages of maturation. Through a balance of feedback mechanisms, the development of only one mature egg is the goal of the female cycle.

At the time of puberty, about 400,000 eggs are present in the ovary. By an intrinsic and as yet unknown mechanism, some of these oocytes, enclosed in their primordial follicle, undergo a process of growth. It is estimated that follicular growth takes about 300 days between the stage of primordial follicle till the moment of ovulation (Gougeon, 1986). For most of this period, the growth of these follicles is independent of the hormonal milieu; they keep growing independently of the hormonal state, whether a woman is pregnant or taking hormonal contraceptives. At a given stage of growth—the antral stage—the follicles become sensitive to FSH for further development. This coincides with the beginning of a menstrual cycle. The number of follicles that can be selected for further growth varies among individuals and in general, diminishes with age. Recruitment of a number of follicles occurs at the beginning of the cycle. After a few days, one follicle takes precedence and accelerates its production of oestrogen and inhibin which, in their turn, depress the pituitary secretion of FSH, halting the further development of the recruited follicles. In most circumstances, the most advanced follicle becomes dominant and by its hormonal production, impedes the other follicles from further development. These will undergo the process of atresia. Timed and optimal stimulation enables the recruitment of all follicles that have become gonadotrophin-dependent, but it cannot supersede the individual quotum of follicles that are ready for stimulation.

The Role Of FSH And LH

The availability of pure FSH and LH preparations, and the possibility of suppressing the pituitary secretion of gonadotrophins have allowed for the investigation of the separate roles of FSH and LH in follicular maturation. According to the two-cell, two-gonadotrophin model, during follicular maturation, LH serves mainly to promote the production by the theca cells of androgens, which are the substrate for transformation to oestrogens by the granulosa cells in response to FSH (Ryan and Petro, 1966). Besides its effect on thecal steroidogenesis, LH has a major role in the process of oocyte maturation, ovulation and the formation and functioning of the corpus luteum.

Actuated by the removal of the negative feedback at the end of the cycle, the early rise of FSH increases the FSH receptors on the granulosa cells, which start producing oestrogens. Oestrogens are essential for preparing the genital tract for fertilization and implantation, and for communicating with the feedback regulation of gonadotrophin secretion. It was previously thought that they also played a major role in the intrafollicular events of growth and maturation. However, ovulation induction in patients with congenital defects in oestrogen biosynthesis and experimental data using aromatase inhibitors have indicated that oestrogens are not essential for follicular and oocyte maturation (Rabinovici et al., 1989). This can be explained by the fact that the intrafollicular activity of oestrogens is mediated by a number of peptide growth factors which are all modulated by FSH (Erickson, 1997). These findings question the role of LH, at least in stimulated cycles, in the process of follicular maturation. Excessive LH levels, both in spontaneous and stimulated cycles, have been shown to have a deleterious effect on oocyte and embryo quality (Shoham et al., 1993).

Oogenesis

Primordial germ cells originate in the gut endoderm and migrate through the dorsal mesentery into the genital ridges, and then start mitotic proliferation, after which they enter meiosis up to the diplotene stage (4n DNA). They remain in a meiotic resting state until the onset of ovulation at puberty. Meanwhile, however, several primordial follicles start growing and undergo significant changes in size and structure. Granulosa cells, initially forming a single layer of spindle-shaped cells, start dividing and form a multilayered cuboidal cell sheet. In addition, the oocyte enlarges from 0.02 mm to 0.10 mm and secretes a mucoid substance containing glycoproteins, which form the zona pellucida. Granulosa cells surrounding the zona pellucida form gap junctions with the oocyte (corona radiata), allowing for cell-to-cell communication and synchronization of oocyte maturation. The zona pellucida has a role in the binding of sperm cells and provides the mechanism for preventing polyspermy. Further development of the follicle includes the formation of an antrum and a layer of cells endowed with the enzymatic machinery for steroidogenesis (the theca cell layer). At this time, antral follicles are ready to start their further growth and maturation when an adequate gonadotrophin stimulus is at hand. Oocytes from antral follicles are competent to resume meiosis after isolation from their follicles, which indicates that oocyte maturation is inhibited by a substance, called the oocyte maturation inhibitor. A distinction should be made between the nuclear and cytoplasmic maturation of the oocyte, which normally are synchronized but there are examples of dissociation of the two events. Nuclear maturation is a two-step process which is set in motion by the rise of LH. The first step consists of the breakdown of the germinal vesicle and completion of the first meiotic division, followed by extrusion of the first polar body. The second step is the entering of the second meiotic division, which is arrested at metaphase II until fertilization occurs. Cytoplasmic maturation refers to the processes that prepare the egg for sperm penetration, activation, formation of pronuclei and preimplantation development. The formation and release of cortical granules, which is necessary to prevent polyspermy, is one of the manifestations of cytoplasmic maturation. Elucidation of the factors responsible for cytoplasmic maturation has gained vital importance for progress in *in vitro* maturation of oocytes (Eppig, 1996).

These are the essential ingredients of the process of follicular and oocyte maturation that will be of interest for understanding the different stimulation protocols.

THE SPONTANEOUS CYCLE

Although the first IVF baby was conceived after oocyte retrieval in a spontaneous cycle, it soon became apparent that follicular stimulation and the availability of more than one oocyte provided a number of advantages, and improved the success rate of IVF. This has been proved over the years and most, if not all, centres are now using one method or another to recover an optimal number of oocytes. Besides the fact that in a spontaneous cycle, only one oocyte can be retrieved, there are also a number of other inconveniences associated with IVF in a spontaneous cycle. Oocytes are fertilizable and hence, should be recovered when mature, i.e. at the time of ovulation when they are at metaphase II. Unless the ovulatory LH surge is monitored at regular intervals, the exact timing for oocyte retrieval is uncertain. But monitoring of the LH surge is an exhausting task both for the patient and the physician because it should be performed every four hours day and night. No wonder that most, if not all, IVF centres have abandoned the idea of retrieving eggs in a spontaneous cycle.

FOLLICULAR STIMULATION IN IVF

The principles of ovulation induction in anovulatory patients and those of follicular stimulation for IVF are totally different, although the same stimulatory drugs can be given. In the former case, anovulation is due to a decreased or inappropriate gonadotrophin secretion and the aim of the treatment is to restore the imbalance very precisely to induce the growth and maturation of a single follicle. IVF patients mostly have an ovulatory cycle and the purpose of the stimulation is to get a reasonable number of follicles and eggs by giving an extra stimulation.

In the early eighties, clomiphene citrate and gonadotrophins, alone or in combination, were used for this purpose. Although the average number of mature oocytes that could be obtained varied between 4 and 8, the problem of the timely detection of a spontaneous LH surge persisted. This inconvenience could be circumvented by stimulation of the ovaries with gonadotrophins, while at the same time, suppressing the pituitary with GnRH agonists. Several advantages of the combination of pituitary suppression and ovarian stimulation are apparent. There was no longer any need to monitor the LH surge, nor signs of premature luteinization. The number of oocytes was, on an average, larger than with previous schemes and the timing of oocyte retrieval appeared to be not so critical, allowing for practical arrangements for monitoring and oocyte retrieval. Hormonal monitoring, a basic requirement in non-desensitized patients, could even be passed by. In fact, it was proven that stimulation could be monitored by ultrasonography alone.

NUMBER OF OOCYTES AND SUCCESS RATE

The success of IVF and ICSI is correlated with the number of oocytes that can be retrieved (Fig. 4.1). There are several factors that can explain this relationship. There is the fact that the number of oocytes decreases with age, which in itself is negatively correlated with the success rate of IVF (Fig. 4.2). Given the fact that fertilization rates vary between 60 and 80%, the probability of ending up with two to three good-quality embryos increases with the number of oocytes. On the other hand, there is evidence that the quality of the oocyte is not necessarily related to the quantity of oocytes. The overall pregnancy rate does not increase any further when the number of oocytes retrieved is in excess of 20. There is also the paradoxical fact

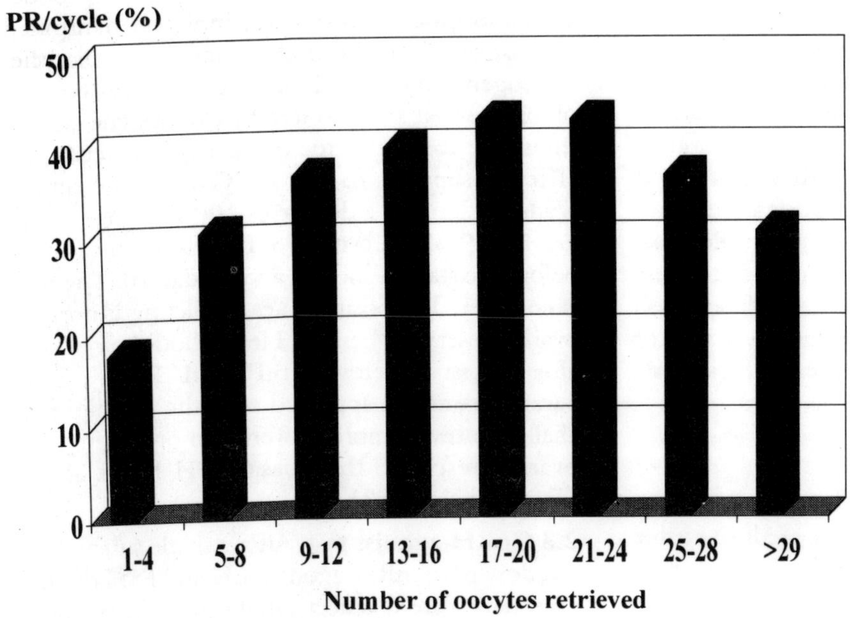

Fig. 4.1. Relation between number of oocytes retrieved and pregnancy rates (PR) per cycle. (Data were derived from 4,500 IVF cycles performed over the last 7 years at our infertility centre, using mainly the short protocol reported in the text.)

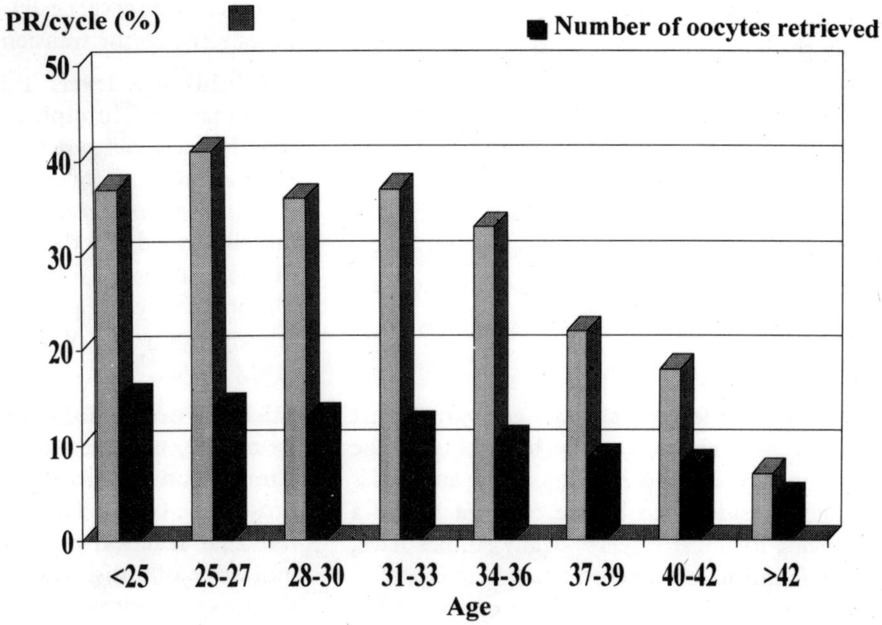

Fig. 4.2. Relation between age of the patient, number of oocytes retrieved and pregnancy rates (PR) per cycle. (Data were derived from 4,500 IVF cycles performed over the last 7 years at our infertility centre, using mainly the short protocol reported in the text.)

that the reproductive success of a fertile couple in the spontaneous cycle, where a single egg is ovulated, is, on an average, higher than the success rate of IVF after replacing one embryo.

Determinants And Prediction Of Ovarian Response

Several parameters which might predict the outcome of ovarian stimulation have been investigated. There are three types of predictors: history of the patient (age, previous pelvic surgery, endometriosis, previous response to stimulation), hormonal estimators of the ovarian reserve and the presence of antral follicles and the ovarian volume measured by ultrasound. Although most of these parameters are able to distinguish between poor and normal responders, they are unfortunately not able to assist in choosing the most appropriate stimulation protocol, which, to a large extent, still depends on trial and error. In fact, the most reliable predictor of the ovarian response is the previous response, provided optimal stimulation was given.

1. Patient's Characteristics

Although on average, age is an excellent predictor of the ovarian response, its positive predictive value is rather poor because chronological age may be different from biological age.

Nevertheless, although age alone cannot adequately predict the outcome of ovarian stimulation, it is a distinct predictor for the outcome of IVF. Pregnancies after IVF beyond the age of 42, even in women who are still able to produce a fair number of oocytes, are extremely rare.

It is well known that patients with previous pelvic surgery are at risk of a poor ovarian response. Adhesions and compromised vascularization are the two main culprits (Molly et al., 1987).

2. Hormonal Predictors

2.1 Basal FSH levels: It is well established that FSH is slightly elevated at the beginning of the cycle in women beyond 35 years of age and this is generally considered to be the consequence of a diminished follicular reserve. Many studies have, indeed, found an inverse correlation between FSH levels between day 2 and 5 of the cycle and the subsequent response to ovarian stimulation. There are two problems with the determination of FSH as a predictor of the ovarian response. Every centre has to establish its own reference values because depending on the kit one is using, figures can be different. Moreover, a poor response as a sign of impending ovarian failure has been reported to occur without any elevation of FSH (Fahri et al., 1997).

2.2 Clomiphene citrate challenge test: The principle of the clomiphene challenge test is that the oestrogen and inhibin B production of the cohort of follicles that are recruited by clomiphene citrate should be able, by virtue of the negative feedback effect, to suppress FSH levels. Clomiphene citrate is administered at a dosage of 100 mg a day, from day 5 to 9 of the cycle. FSH levels are measured before the start of the test and on day 10. The test is considered as positive, i.e. predicting a normal ovarian reserve, when FSH levels both before and after the test are below 10 mIU/mL. From a comparative study, it appeared that the clomiphene challenge test is more powerful in predicting the ovarian response than basal FSH levels alone (Tanbo et al., 1992).

2.3 GnRH-agonist test: After a single subcutaneous dose of a GnRH-agonist, LH and FSH rise for a few days (flare-up effect). In the presence of a normal ovarian reserve, oestradiol levels should double in response to the transient rise of LH and FSH.

2.4 Inhibin B levels: Inhibin B is produced by follicular and luteinized granulosa cells, and together wih oestradiol, suppresses the pituitary FSH secretion. Because decreased levels of inhibin B signal an impending ovarian failure, it was initially hoped that their level would be a measure of the number of follicles that can be recruited. Unfortunately, the predictive value of inhibin B is not superior to that of the other parameters (Sharara et al., 1998).

2.5 Basal oestradiol levels: High oestradiol levels (> 50 pg/mL) at the beginning of follicular stimulation are considered to be an adverse prognostic factor. They result from a precipitous follicular reaction to raised FSH levels and are indicative of a disturbed feedback, or at least of the onset of monofollicular development. It is, therefore, recommended to cancel the current cycle when high oestradiol levels are found at the start of stimulation.

3. Ultrasound

The number of antral follicles that can be visualized decreases with age and has been correlated with the number of oocytes that can be obtained following stimulation. A correlation has also been reported between the ovarian volume and the ovarian response. The greatest value of visualization of the ovary before starting stimulation, however, lies in the detection of polyfollicular ovaries and other abnormalities.

STIMULATION PROTOCOLS

1. Clomiphene Citrate and hMG

Three types of stimulation protocols without pituitary suppression are available. They consist of the administration of either clomiphene citrate or hMG alone, or a sequential combination of both. The low cost of clomiphene citrate and the limited number of ampoules of hMG needed are the advantages of these protocols. No difference in oocyte yield or pregnancy rates was observed when clomiphene was used at a dosage of 50 mg or 100 mg a day for 5 days. When used in combination with clomiphene citrate, hMG is started at the end of the treatment with clomiphene citrate and is given at a dosage of 2 ampoules a day for five days on an average. When used alone, hMG is given at a dosage of 2 ampoules a day, starting on day three of the cycle. The duration of treatment varies between 8 and 12 days, and the average number of mature oocytes that can be retrieved varies between 4 and 8.

These protocols were used mainly in the eighties. They have been replaced in most centres by protocols using GnRH-agonists because of a number of drawbacks, mainly the occurrence of an unpredictable LH surge, premature luteinization and the limited number of oocytes recruited. In a prospective randomized study, it was shown that both the number of oocytes and pregnancy rates were significantly higher in patients treated with GnRH-agonist/hMG compared to clomiphene citrate and hMG, and that the difference in pregnancy rates was totally accounted for by the excess number of oocytes in the former group (Dhont et al., 1995).

It remains to be seen whether clomiphene and/ or hMG alone will regain their importance in follicular stimulation for IVF with the advent of GnRH-antagonists.

2. GnRH-agonists and HMG

GnRH-agonists for follicular stimulation in IVF were introduced in the mid-eighties and they are now being used in more than 90% of all IVF cycles. Their main purpose is control of the pituitary secretion of LH to avoid premature LH surges, premature luteinization and raised LH levels, which are thought to have a deleterious effect on oocyte quality. Unfortunately, along with the suppression of LH levels, FSH levels also are shut down, necessitating a higher dose of exogenous hMG. The supplementary cost of extra ampoules of hMG should be added to the expense of the GnRH-agonist itself, making the modern type of follicular stimulation rather expensive.

GnRH-agonists exert a biphasic action on gonadotrophin secretion: during the first days of treatment, they stimulate the pituitary and can, by virtue of this effect, initiate follicular growth. The different stimulation protocols are conceived either to avoid the initial stimulating effect (long protocols), or to take advantage of the so-called flare-up effect of GnRH-agonists on gonadotrophin secretion (short protocols). Different protocols for GnRH-agonist/hMG stimulation have been reported, depending mainly on the timing of GnRH-agonist administration and the duration of agonist treatment. In the so-called long protocol, GnRH-agonists are given several weeks before starting stimulation to ensure a maximal shut-down of the pituitary secretion of gonadotrophins. Both long- and short-acting GnRH-agonists can be used for this purpose. In short protocols, follicular stimulation by hMG is started simultaneously with short-acting GnRH-agonists.

2.1 Long protocol: In a long protocol, GnRH-agonists are given several weeks in advance of follicular stimulation in order to completely suppress the pituitary and to avoid any remaining follicular activity which might have resulted from the initial flare-up effect. Theoretically, the timing of the start of GnRH-agonist treatment would not matter, provided it is given long enough to suppress completely all follicular activity. For practical purposes, however, the length of the pretreatment period is limited to two or three weeks, which renders it mandatory to start the GnRH-agonist either at the beginning of the cycle or during the middle of the luteal phase.

Timing of administration: Administration of a GnRH-agonist at the beginning of the cycle may initiate follicular ripening and, therefore, can give rise to the formation of a functional cyst, which can persist until the time stimulation should start. Provided oestradiol levels are basal at this time, the persistence of such a cyst has no effect on subsequent stimulation (Herman et al., 1990).

Timing during the luteal phase has the advantage that the pituitary is more suppressed by the combined action of luteal progesterone and oestradiol levels, making the flare-up reaction to GnRH-agonist administration less pronounced. A further advantage is that a normal menstruation intervenes before a new wave of endometrial proliferation starts. A worrying complication of timing during the luteal phase is, however, that occasionally a spontaneous pregnancy can occur. Although no deleterious effects of GnRH-agonists during early pregnancy have been reported, this complication should be avoided.

The advantages of luteal phase administration without the risk of pregnancy can be obtained by treating the patient with an oral contraceptive, starting at the beginning of the cycle. The GnRH-agonist is administered after the woman has been on the oral contraceptive for one or two weeks, or even longer. Stimulation with hMG is started one week after cessation of the oral contraceptive. We have shown that, using this method, the flare-up effect is even less than when administered in the luteal phase and functional cysts arise very exceptionally. A further advantage of this procedure is that all IVF procedures can be scheduled a long time in advance (Dhont et al., 1995).

2.2 Short protocols: A great diversity of short protocols has been reported, depending on the dosage and the duration of the GnRH-agonist treatment (Balasch and Howles, 1999). The main rationale behind the short protocol, however, is to take advantage of the flare-up effect in order to boost the initial recruitment of follicles by a combined stimulation of both exogenous and endogenous gonadotrophins.

The classical scheme consists of a short-acting GnRH-agonist, given from day three of the cycle, along with exogenous gonadotrophins till the time of oocyte retrieval. A number of variations on the classic short protocol have been reported, such as the ultra-short protocol in which the duration of GnRH-agonist treatment is limited to the first three days of stimulation. We ourselves have been using an intermediate type of short protocol where the treatment (triptorelin, 0.100 mg a day, SC) is given only for seven days. In practice, most patients are put on an oral contraceptive for a variable duration of time, like in the long protocol, and the GnRH-agonist is started five days after cessation of the oral contraceptive. Stimulation with gonadotrophins is started two days later.

2.3 Dose of gonadotrophins: The dose of gonadotrophins should be adapted to the characteristics of the patient (previous response, age, number of antral follicles in basal condition) and the protocol that is used.

As a rule and for evident reasons, the dose of gonadotrophins in the long protocol is about 50% higher than in the short protocol. From our own extensive experience both with the long and the short protocol, the following rules can be recommended.

Normal responders: Treatment is started with three (long protocol) or two ampoules of hMG (short protocol), and continued at the same dose unless follicular growth (monitored by ultrasound and determination of oestradiol concentrations after seven and ten days of stimulation) appears to come to a standstill prematurely. In that case, the dose should be doubled.

Hyper-responders: Treatment is started with two ampoules both in the short and long protocol, and adapted according to the results of the monitoring.

Poor responders: Given the need for higher doses of hMG in poor responders, we invariably apply the short protocol and start with 4 to 6 ampoules a day. There is no proof that higher doses are effective in poor responders.

3. GnRH-Antagonists

It has taken a long time to develop GnRH-antagonists with an acceptable incidence and severity of side-effects. Some preparations have now become available for clinical use and a few more are on the way. Altough the ultimate effect is the same, the mechanism of action of GnRH-antagonists is different from that of agonists. The latter occupy the GnRH receptors of the gonadotrophic cells and, after an initial stimulatory effect on gonadotrophin secretion, eventually downregulate them, leading to the inability of the gonadotrophic cells to respond to subsequent GnRH stimulation. Antagonists compete with the endogenous GnRH for the receptor and, when given in a sufficient dose, temporarily and immediately shut down the secretory activity of the gonadotrophic cells. Their activity lasts only for a few days. In contrast with GnRH-agonists, the antagonists are given after several days of stimulation with hMG, either as a single large dose when the follicles reach a diameter of 14 mm, or as multiple smaller doses which are continued till the time of oocyte retrieval (Felberbaum and Diedrich, 1999).

It is still too early to decide whether the antagonists, combined with clomiphene citrate and/or hMG, will have any advantage over the use of GnRH-agonists, or whether there will be specific indications for their use.

4. Recombinant FSH

Although they have served well without any serious adverse effects over the last thirty years, urinary gonadotrophins are a very impure mixture of proteins, with varying degrees of FSH and LH ratios. The advent of recombinant gonadotrophins should certainly be hailed as a big step in the development of reliable protein hormone preparations and this innovation will certainly pave the way for the development of other purified hormones. These purified preparations have been of great help in elucidating the respective roles of LH and FSH in follicular maturation. Although a certain amount of LH is necessary for optimal follicular growth, the primordial role of FSH has been clarified. Prospective studies comparing purified urinary FSH with recombinant FSH have shown a marginal benefit in terms of the number of oocytes and overall pregnancy rates (Howles and Wikland, 1999). The cost of the new gonadotrophins, however, raises the question whether in the current state of affairs, they can stand the test of a cost-benefit assessment for the patient.

Luteal Phase Support

After pituitary downregulation with GnRH-agonists, the endogenous secretion of LH might be insufficient to support the corpus luteum till the time of implantation. Randomized studies have, indeed, shown that luteal support increases pregnancy rates in downregulated IVF cycles. The aim of the luteal support is to maintain a critical level of progesterone. This may be achieved either by intermittent intramuscular injections of hCG (1.500 units every three days, starting on the fifth day of the oocyte retrieval), or by giving progesterone, either intramuscularly (50 mg daily) or vaginally (200 to 600 mg daily). There seems to be no advantage in terms of pregnancy rates between the indirect support with hCG or the direct supplementation with progesterone. The route of administration of the latter, vaginally or intramuscularly, does appear to be equivalent. When a woman is considered to be at risk of developing ovarian hyperstimulation syndrome, progesterone should be the treatment of choice. Although some authors extend the luteal support throughout the first trimester of pregnancy, there is no scientific evidence that this precaution is necessary (Akande et al., 1996).

CONCLUSION

It is sometimes argued that IVF can restore fertility to the level we see in young fertile couples. This is partially correct, considering the fact that the average pregnancy rates per cycle of 30% following IVF are comparable to those seen in young fertile couples. It remains frustrating, however, that contrary to what happens in nature, we have to depend on maximal ovarian stimulation and the replacement of at least two embryos to obtain this result. These requisites continue to make IVF a costly and, for many people, inaccessible treatment for infertility. Moreover, the ensuing pregnancies are unfortunately compounded by a high perinatal risk, mainly due to the high incidence of multiple pregnancies. Although optimal stimulation schemes are, for the time being, a necessary complement to efficient IVF treatment, the ultimate improvement should come from attention and research into quality rather than quantity.

REFERENCES

Akande, A.V. et al. (1996). 'The choice of luteal support following pituitary down regulation, controlled ovarian hyperstimualtion and *in vitro* fertilisation', *Br. J. Obstet. Gynaecol.*, **103**: 963–6.

Balasch, J. and C.M. Howles (1999). 'GnRH-agonists: Which one to use?' in Z. Shoham, et al. (eds.), *Female Infertility Therapy, Current Practice,* Martin Dunitz, London, pp. 189–202.

Dhont, M. et al. (1995). 'Prospective randomised study of clomiphene citrate and gonadotrophins versus goserelin and gonadotrophins for follicular stimulation in assisted reproduction', *Hum. Reprod.*, **10**: 791–7.

Eppig, J.J. (1996). 'The ovary: oogenesis', in S.G. Hillier, et al. (eds.), *Scientific Essentials of Reproductive Medicine,* W.B. Saunders Company, London, pp. 147–159.

Erickson, G.F. (1997). 'Control of follicular development', in R.A. Lobo et al. (eds.), *Infertility, Contraception, and Reproductive Endocrinology,* 4th ed. Blackwell Science., Malden, Massachusetts, pp.159–173.

Fahri, J. et al. (1997). 'Non-response to ovarian stimulation in normogonadotrophic, normogonadal women: A clinical sign of impending onset of ovarian failure pre-empting the rise in basal follicle stimulating hormone levels', *Hum. Reprod.*, **12**: 241–3.

Felberbaum, R. and C. Diedrich (1999). 'The use of GnRH antagonists in IVF', in Z. Shoham et al. (eds.), *Female Infertility Therapy, Current Practice,* Martin Dunitz, London, pp. 203–12.

Gougeon, A. (1986). 'Dynamics of follicular growth in the human: A model from preliminary results', *Hum. Reprod.*, **2**: 81–7.

Herman, A. et al. (1990). 'Follicle cysts after menstrual versus midluteal administration of gonadotropin-releasing hormone analog in *in vitro* fertilization', *Fertil. Steril.*, **53**: 854–8.

Howles, M.C. and M. Wikland (1999). 'The use of recombinant human FSH in *in vitro* fertilization', in Z. Shoham et al. (eds.), *Female Infertility Therapy, Current Practice,* Martin Dunitz, London pp. 103–114.

Molly, D. et al. (1987). 'Performance of patients with a "frozen pelvis" in an *in vitro* fertilization program', *Fertil. Steril.*, **47**: 450–55.

Rabinovici, J. et al. (1989). '*In vitro* fertilization and primary embryonic cleavage are possible in 17 alpha-hydroxylase deficiency despite extremely low intrafollicular 17 beta-estradiol', *J. Clin. Endocrinol. Metab.*, **68**: 693–7.

Ryan, K.J. and Petro Z. (1966). 'Steroid biosynthesis by human ovarian granulosa and theca cells', *J. Clin. Endocrinol. Metab.*, **26**: 46–52.

Sharara, F.I. et al. (1998). 'The detection of diminished ovarian reserve in infertile women', *Am. J. Obstet. Gynecol.*, **179**: 804–12.

Shoham, Z. et al. (1993). 'Luteinizing hormone: Its role, mechanism of action, and detrimental effects when hypersecreted during the follicular phase', *Fetil. Steril.*, **59**: 1153–61.

Tanbo, T. et al. (1992). 'Prediction of response to controlled ovarian hyperstimulation: A comparison of basal and clomiphene citrate-stimulated follicle-stimulating hormone levels', *Fertil. Steril.*, **57**: 819–24.

5

Oocyte Maturation: In Vivo and In Vitro

Pravin Goud, Anuradha Goud and Marc Dhont

INTRODUCTION

In the current programmes of assisted reproduction, ovarian stimulation is an essential component, the purpose of which is to retrieve a large number of mature oocytes of an optimum quality. Ovarian hyperstimulation is also compounded by high cost, patient inconvenience, need for repeated ultrasonographic monitoring and the risk of ovarian hyperstimulation. Recently, concerns have also been raised about the long-term effects of ovulation induction.

Retrieval of immature oocytes from the unstimulated ovary and their subsequent maturation in culture is an attractive alternative to ovarian stimulation. Recent successes in achieving live births in experimental and farm animals, as well as in humans, are encouraging in this regard. Apart from offering just an alternative to ovarian stimulation, this also gives an opportunity to study the process of oocyte maturation and the oocyte factors that determine successful embryogenesis. Knowledge of these factors could improve the process of assessment of oocyte and embryo quality, and also help design new strategies in assisted reproduction. Besides, this technique could be a practical and possibly also more acceptable alternative for the oocyte donors who currently need to undergo ovarian stimulation.

Another issue of recent clinical interest is that of young patients undergoing ablative procedures for the treatment of malignancies. Application of cryopreservation techniques to preserve the ovarian tissue could offer such patients a chance to preserve their fertility by subsequent thawing and autotransplantation or *in vitro* maturation (IVM) at a later date.

In spite of all these advantages, IVM is still far from being a routine application in clinical practice. The main contention is the low success rate of pregnancy with the *in vitro* matured oocytes, in comparison to their *in vivo* matured counterparts from stimulated cycles (Fig. 5.1). This is mainly related to the suboptimal quality of cytoplasmic maturation. Therefore, future research should be concentrated on understanding the physiology and pathophysiology of oocyte maturation, and on devising strategies to improve the quality of oocyte maturation.

This chapter is devoted to discussing the physiological mechanisms involved in oocyte maturation *in vivo*, and to the review of the current techniques of *in vitro* maturation and their scope for clinical application.

HUMAN OOCYTE: PECULIAR CHARACTERISTICS

The human oocyte exhibits a remarkable phenomenon of reductional divisions (meiosis), necessary to create the haploid gamete during meiotic maturation. The diploid condition is then restored when a spermatozoon unites with the mature oocyte during fertilization. The process of meiosis in the oocyte is also distinctly marked by the peculiar arrest periods that are not seen in the male germ cells. Furthermore, the zygote inherits almost the whole of its cytoplasm from the oocyte and

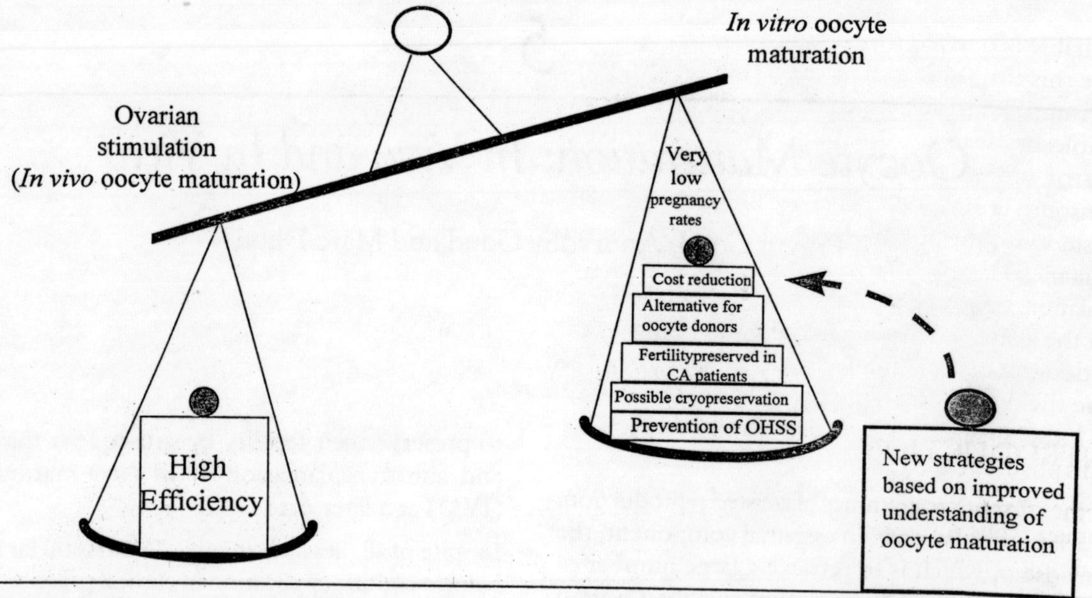

Fig. 5.1. Practical aspects of *in vivo* and *in vitro* oocyte maturation in humans. The very low pregnancy rate after the transfer of the embryos derived from *in vitro* matured oocytes is a major setback for its clinical applicability

the early preimplantation embryo is thence dependent on the maternally transcribed RNA until the activation of its own genome.

These characteristics make the oocyte perhaps the most important cell in the body. The recent successes obtained in cloning certain mammals have further highlighted the enormous potential of the oocyte to remodel, transform and even reprogramne a somatic cell nucleus virtually from any phase of the cell cycle (Wilmut et al., 1997; Wakayama et al., 1998). Although the technology of cloning to develop embryos is still far from being used for application in humans and also in the stage of infancy in other mammals, this issue nevertheless underscores the important role played by the oocyte in controlling the reproduction. It is, therefore, very essential to have some insight into the origin, growth and development of the oocyte.

ORIGIN, GROWTH AND DEVELOPMENT OF THE FEMALE GAMETE

Generally, the term 'oocyte maturation' is applied to the period between the resumption of meiosis in an oocyte, which was arrested in the dictyate stage of meiotic prophase I, and the stage of second metaphase (M II), when the oocyte undergoes a re-arrest, awaiting penetration by a spermatozoon. However, in order to understand these penultimate events of development, it is necessary to know something about the origin and development of the oocyte.

The major milestones in the development of the female germ cells are: (a) differentiation of the germ cells from the rest of the cellular population; (b) migration from the site of origin to lodge in the developing gonad; (c) further development characterized by initial mitosis, which gradually ceases with the initiation and arrest of meiosis; (d) decline in the gamete number, starting from mid-gestation; and (e) re-initiation of meiosis following the preovulatory gonadotrophin surge, and its transient re-arrest preceding ovulation and fertilization. The phenomena (a) and (b) occur during the embryonic period, (c) occurs mainly during the fetal period, whereas (d) and (e) encompass almost the entire reproductive span of a woman.

FORMATION AND MIGRATION OF THE GERM CELLS

The stage of embryology during which the germ cells and the somatic cells differentiate is not precisely known in humans. Most of the information available is derived from studies in mice, in whose case this timing is considered to occur during the peri-implantation period. Germ cells first become visible by histo-cytochemical staining on the 8th day of mouse development (Chiquoine, 1954; Ginsburg et al., 1990). They are found immediately posterior to the primitive streak in the extra-embryonic mesoderm of the yolk sac. Later, during gastrulation, these primordial germ cells (PGC) migrate via the allantois to lodge in the mesoderm and the endoderm of the primitive streak. Finally, they pass into the developing hind gut and dorsal mesentery to lodge in the developing nephro-gonadal ridge. This phenomenon occurs on day 26 in humans. The PGC can be distinguished from the surrounding somatic cells with the help of alkaline phosphatase staining. However, the male and the female cells cannot be distinguished by morphological or any other known cytochemical marker.

The PGC undergo some mitotic divisions by the time they colonize in the developing gonad. This sojourn of the germ cells is regulated mainly by the following: (a) a mass movement mainly related to growth of the surrounding tissues in the developing embryo; (b) independent movement assisted by self-propulsion and tissue invasion, a behaviour similar to that of the metastatic cells from a malignant tumour; and (c) a transmembrane receptor and its ligand, the stem cell factor or steel factor (SCF). The PGC express the *c-kit* receptor in a developmentally regulated manner, while the SCF is expressed by the surrounding embryonic cells. The binding of SCF to c-kit and also that of one other factor—the leukaemia inhibitory factor (LIF)—to its receptors on the PGC promote their survival (Pesce et al., 1993). Recently, another factor, basic fibroblast growth factor (bFGF), was shown to play a role in regulating the development of the PGC (Resnick et al., 1998). Additionally, there may be several other factors that play a role in the maintenance of the PGC that are yet to be revealed. Further movement of the PGC and their orientation in the final destination may be modulated by the chemotactic substances released from the gonadal ridge (Donovan, 1994). One candidate to play this role is the transforming growth factor-ß (TGF-ß).

Dynamics of the Germ Cell Population

The female germ cells at this stage are called the oogonia. In humans, oogonia undergo several rounds of mitotic divisions almost throughout the fetal period, before starting meiosis. This step is very crucial as oogonia are the stem cell precursors of oocytes and their number, therefore, determines the number of oocytes in the postnatal ovary. The oogonia disappear after birth and that also marks the cessation of mitosis in the germ cells. In fact, the germ cells undergo a dramatic decline from 6–7 million during mid-gestation to around 1 million at birth (Baker, 1963). The number further dwindles to only about 200–300 thousand by the time puberty is attained. This is attributed to the cell death that occurs during mainly the fetal period, exceeding the rate of division. The cell division totally ceases postnatally, while the phenomenon of cell-death continues (Gosden, 1995; Coucouvanis et al., 1993; De Pol et al., 1997). A further drop in the germ cell number occurs throughout the reproductive age of women because only about 600 are destined to ovulate.

Further Growth and Development of the Oocyte and the Follicle

The process of meiosis starts during prenatal development. After a few rounds of mitosis, some oogonia enter meiosis. In fact, during mid-gestation, the fetal ovary shows the presence of both mitosis as well as meiosis in the germ cells. The primary oocyte found in the fetal ovary undergoes DNA synthesis and enters the prophase of meiosis I. This process encompasses various phases, including the pairing of homologous chromosomes and the formation of chiasmata. Growth gets arrested in diplotene as primordial follicles form. These are units of meiosis-arrested, resting-stage oocytes, surrounded by a single layer of cuboidal cells. They start appearing from around 22 weeks of gestation.

During the prophase of the first meiotic division, homologous chromosomes are still paired together. This stage is called the dictyate stage or dictyotene, which is characterized by the presence of a germinal vesicle (GV) that persists until just before ovulation.

At birth, the ovary is densely packed with oocytes within the primordial follicles. However, a number of growing follicles may also be found in the neonatal ovaries.

GROWTH AND RECRUITMENT OF FOLLICLES

Overall, an ovary contains two broad categories of oocytes, namely, growing oocytes and fully grown oocytes. The former are unable to respond to the maturation signals, while the latter respond to the gonadotrophic signal and can progress to metaphase II (M II). The transition from category (a) to category (b) entails a complex process involving structural and biochemical changes (Fulka et al., 1998). This transition confers on the oocytes the ability to undergo GV breakdown and resume and complete meiosis. Therefore, this process is called acquisition of meiotic competence. The immature GV-stage oocytes acquire the competence at some stage during their development. The most notable features of this gradual transition from growing to fully grown oocytes are as follows: (a) enlargement of the GV, prominence of the nucleoli, with change in their configuration from diffuse fibrillogranular to dense; (b) ribosomal RNA synthesis; (c) multiplication of mitochondria; (d) formation of cortical granules; and (e) formation of the zona pellucida from pools of fibrillar material between the oocyte and its surrounding cells. Cytoplasmic extensions connecting the oocyte with the follicular cells, however, persist, traversing the newly formed zona pellucida (Motta et al., 1994). Finally, the end of this transition is marked by the end of nucleolar transcription and the synthesis of proteins needed for oocyte maturation. The oocytes then become sensitive to the gonadotrophin stimulus.

The mRNA acquired during this period is selectively sequestered in the form of ribonucleoproteins, and is translated during the final steps of oocyte maturation and during the early embryonic period. Also, the mitochondria formed during the oocyte growth phase persist to function throughout the embryonic period and no new mitochondria are formed until the hatched blastocyst stage. Defective storage, recruitment, storage and poly-A tail processing of the maternal mRNA, as well as intrinsic or extrinsic factor-related damage to the mitochondria can, therefore, result in failure of oocyte maturation and arrested embryogenesis. Hence, the step of acquiring meiotic competence has enormous implications for the success of oocyte maturation and embryo development. Although the mechanisms that control this process are yet to be understood, the c-kit ligand plays a major role during this phase (Ismail et al., 1996; Tanikawa et al., 1998). Also, there may be a number of other local paracrine factors or putative intra-ovarian regulators involved in the process of acquisition of meiotic maturation.

THE PENULTIMATE EVENTS OF MEIOTIC MATURATION

The term 'meiotic maturation' generally refers to the resumption of meiosis in an oocyte that was arrested in the dictyate stage of meiotic prophase I. Morphologically, these events are represented by the breakdown of the germinal vesicle (GVB) and asymmetric cytoplasmic division of the oocyte, resulting in the extrusion of the first polar body (Fig. 5.2). Here, the oocyte remains arrested in the metaphase of the second meiosis until sperm penetration, fertilization and the following events that mark the initiation of embryonic development. The events related to the nuclear changes are peculiar in that the chromosome and the DNA content of the oocyte are halved (Fig. 5.2). Also, the transition between meiosis I and II is peculiar because the progression of the cell cycle occurs without DNA replication between these two stages. Finally, a truly haploid ootid does not exist in mammals because the final reduction in the chromosome number does not occur until fertilization. These nuclear events are encompassed in the term: 'nuclear maturation'. Nonetheless, these events are also paralleled by certain changes occurring in the cytoplasm. These changes prepare the oocyte to undergo the events related to fertilization and activation of embryonic development.

Currently, the following are considered to be the components of cytoplasmic maturation.

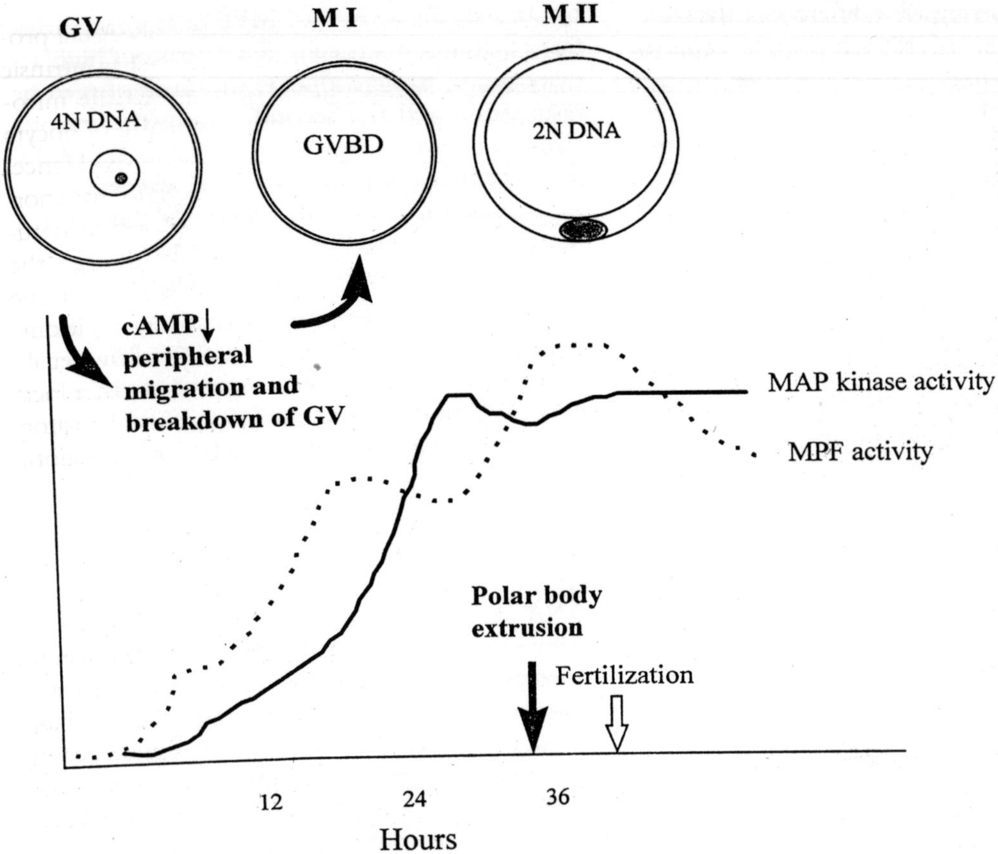

Fig. 5.2. Major events related to oocyte maturation. Resumption and rearrest of meiosis are controlled by the cell cycle factors. High activity of the M-phase promoting factor (MPF) ensures the occurrence of the reductional chromosome division between M I and M II without DNA replication

a) Events that ensure the occurrence of normal fertilization: (i) acquisition and redistribution of the calcium stores; (ii) increase in the number as well as redistribution of the receptor-operated calcium channels (Shiraishi et al., 1995; Mehlmann et al., 1996); (iii) peripheral migration of the cortical granules, in close proximity to the oolemma; and (iv) acquisition of the putative sperm nucleus decondensing factor that remodels the chromatin of the fertilizing spermatozoa (Ohsumi and Katagiri, 1991).

b) Cell cycle factor activation related to the meiotic maturation. The activity of these factors is closely associated with cytoskeletal dynamics, which, in turn, influences the normal progression of nuclear maturation.

c) Other events related to the synthesis/activation of certain molecules that are related to embryo development.

The events of nuclear and cytoplasmic maturation are at least partly independent, and the parallel occurrence of cytoplasmic and nuclear maturation is of paramount importance to ensure the occurrence of normal fertilization and embryogenesis. Sometimes, however, the two events may be dissociated, resulting either in the failure of fertilization of a mature M II-stage oocyte, or fertilization and triploid embryo development of an M I-arrested oocyte. Thus, the simultaneous occurrence of nuclear and cytoplasmic maturation is extremely important for ensuring the normalcy of embryonic development. Certain defects in embryonic development occurring after IVM could also be explained by the incomplete cytoplasmic maturation in an oocyte that has otherwise completed the nuclear events of maturation.

Cell Cycle Factors Related to Oocyte Maturation

The understanding of the molecular mechanisms of oocyte maturation has significantly improved in recent years. Barring a few differences, the basic molecular machinery of cell cycle control seems to be similar in a number of diverse species. Therefore, the paucity of data on human oocytes could be conveniently overcome with the data on the other species studied so far. The molecular mechanisms controlling meiosis and the regulation of the cell cycle, in general, began to be understood after the discovery of the meiosis-promoting or the M-phase-promoting factor (MPF) as an activity present in mature frog oocytes (Masui and Markert, 1971). The MPF was later found to be a heterodimeric protein complex (see Fig. 5.3) composed of a 34-kD P34cdc2 serine/threonine kinase and a 45-kD cyclin-B subunit (Dunphy et al., 1988; Gautier et al., 1988; 1990).

Cyclins were first characterized in marine invertebrate embryos. Their concentrations were shown to fluctuate according to the phase of the cell cycle (Evans et al., 1983). In accordance with the cell cycle phase-dependent fluctuations in the activity of the cyclins, MPF activity also undergoes similar changes during the cell cycle. Newly-assembled MPF is needed for each cell division and a degradation of MPF occurs at the end of each mitosis. These alterations in MPF activity occurring parallel with those in the cyclin-B build-up and degradation indicate that MPF activity is, in fact, controlled by cyclin-B activity. The human oocytes are known to contain cyclin-B1 mRNA (Heikinheimo et al., 1995).

In oocytes, the activity of MPF differs somewhat from that in somatic cells. Two peaks of high activity occur, namely, one at the time of meiotic resumption and the second during the meiotic arrest in the M II stage (see Fig. 5.2). High MPF activity between the M I and M II stages also ensures condensation of chromosomes and prevention of DNA replication, thereby permitting the reductional divisions of meiotic maturation.

The MPF is thought to be involved in the disassembly of the nucleus, condensation of the chromosomes, cytoskeletal rearrangements and arrest of transcriptional activity (see Fig. 5.3). The latter may be due to the inhibition of RNA polymerase II by MPF.

Histone H1 is a classical substrate for MPF. Hence, MPF is also referred to as histone H1 kinase. Histone H1 has an important role in packaging DNA into nucleosomes which constitute the primary structural units of the chromatin fibres. Phosphorylation of histone H1 probably plays a role in chromosome condensation during cell division. Nuclear lamins are also phosphorylated by the p34cdc2 kinase. Phosphorylation of pp60c-src kinase may be responsible for the cytoskeletal rearrangements during cell division.

Regulation of MPF Activity

Following the assembly of the cyclin B-p34cdc2 kinase complex, the MPF is maintained in an inactive stage via phosphorylation of specific amino

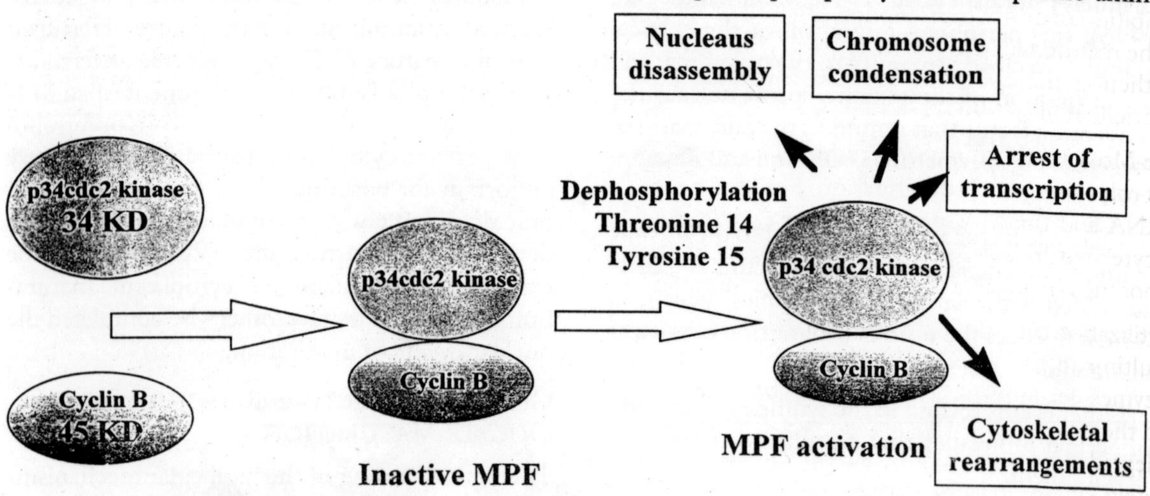

Fig. 5.3. Formation, activation and functions of the M-phase promoting factor (MPF)

acid residues of the p34 cdc2 kinase by the action of specific protein kinases (see Fig. 5.3).

Cdc25-phosphatase controls the coordinated dephosphorylation and activation of MPF. Besides acting on MPF, cdc25-phosphatase itself is also a target for the action of MPF, which enhances its activity via phosphorylation. This catalytic loop may be responsible for the rapid activation of MPF during oocyte maturation.

A protein kinase is believed to maintain the activity of MPF during the M II stage arrest until fertilization. This is the cellular counterpart of the viral oncogene mos (c-mos). This peculiar protein is selectively expressed in developing oocytes and pachytene spermatocytes, and in oocytes, it disappears after fertilization. Thus, the possible role of c-mos in maintaining the activity of MPF is based on the timing of its activity. Due to this role, c-mos protein is also called the cytostatic factor (CSF). The inhibition of c-mos expression in the somatic cells is probably due to a negative regulatory sequence in the promoter region of the c-mos gene, and also to a putative repressor protein expressed only in the somatic but not in the germ cells.

The proposed mechanisms connecting the activity of c-mos and MPF are: indirect activation of MPF via the mitogen-activated protein (MAP) kinase or cyclin-dependent kinase 2 (cdk2), and inhibition of proteolytic degradation of cyclin-B, leading to its accumulation between the M I and M II stages. Inhibition of c-mos transcription can lead to failure of the maintenance of the M II arrest, resulting in parthenogenetic activation (O'Keefe et al., 1991; Gabrielli et al., 1993).

The Mos protein thus seems to play a very important role during oocyte maturation. Both the c-mos mRNA and the Mos protein appear early during oocyte maturation, and polyadenylation of the c-mos mRNA is a central step in oocyte maturation.

Fertilization triggers Ca^{2+} oscillations in the oocyte, resulting in the activation of certain proteolytic enzymes, leading to the degradation of the c-mos and the cyclin-B. In *Xenopus* oocytes, the cyclin-B is degraded via the calcium/calmodulin-dependent protein kinase II (CaM kinase), and the Mos via a ubiquitin pathway (Lorca et al., 1993; Ishida et al., 1993). A similar mechanism may be active in mammalian oocytes.

Mitogen-activated protein kinases (MAPK), also called extracellular signal-regulated kinases (ERK), are intermediates in signal transduction pathways that are initiated by a variety of mitogens, such as growth factors, tumour promoters and proto-oncogene products. They are activated by phosphorylation of both tyrosine and serine/threonine residues by an upstream kinase-MAP kinase. MAP kinase is stimulated during meiotic maturation in a variety of species (Inoue et al., 1995). The process of MAP kinase activation has been studied in *Xenopus*, and it is indicated that the activation of this kinase occurs downstream of MPF and the proto-oncogene products—Ras and Mos. In mammals, MAP kinase was shown to get activated after GVBD, and the activity of MAPK persists during the transition from the M I to the M II stage (Verlhac et al., 1993). Two MAP kinases, of 42 kD and 44 kD each, are reported (Inoue et al., 1995). Currently, the mechanisms of action of MAPK in activating MPF are under investigation.

Spontaneous and Ligand-Induced Oocyte Maturation

Exactly which signals initiate oocyte maturation is not precisely known. The classical experiments performed by Pincus and Enzman (1935) and those by Edwards et al. (1965a, b) led to the presumption that the oocyte resides under an inhibitory signal from the surrounding somatic cell compartment of the follicle, and that removal of the oocyte from this inhibitory environment would lead to maturation. This mechanism is referred to as spontaneous oocyte maturation. However, this mechanism may be artifactual because the maturation occurring *in vivo* occurs secondary to a positive signal that follows the preovulatory LH surge. This putative signal is passed from the follicular somatic cell compartment to the oocyte, and overrides the meiotic arrest. Table 5.1 summarizes the salient features of spontaneous and ligand-induced oocyte maturation.

Cyclic AMP and Meiotic Arrest

Spontaneous maturation of oocytes can be prevented by supplementing the culture medium

Table 5.1. Certain Differences Between Spontaneous and Ligand-Induced Oocyte Maturation Mechanisms

Spontaneous oocyte maturation	Ligand-induced maturation
1. Passive resumption of meiosis secondary to removal of the oocyte from the putative inhibitory influence with the follicle.	1. Occurs secondary to a positive signal within intact follicle following the preovulatory LH surge.
2. A process occurring *in vitro*.	2. Occurs *in vivo* as well as *in vitro*.
3. May be considered to be artifactual.	3. Considered to be physiological.
4. Occurs secondary to the fall of cAMP within the oocyte because treatment with cAMP analogues, phosphodiesterase inhibitors or activators of cAMP can prevent spontaneous maturation.	4. Although fall in cAMP may also occur, the positive signal can override the cAMP-mediated meiotic arrest.
5. Independent of the intracellular phosphoinositide metabolism or Ca^{2+} rises.	5. Rise in the intracellular Ca^{2+}, possibly secondary to the activation of the phosphoinositide metabolism, may be involved in this mode of oocyte maturation.
6. Possible risk of discordance between nuclear and cytoplasmic maturation.	6. Synchronized activation of certain intracellular pathways result in the parallel occurrence of nuclear and cytoplasmic maturation.

with either an analogue of cAMP like dibutyryl cAMP, inhibitors of phosphodiesterase enzyme (PDE) like 3-isobutyl-1-methylxanthine (IBMX), or treating with activators of adenyl cyclase, like forskolin (Eppig and Downs, 1984; Schultz et al., 1983; Tornell et al., 1993). The meiotic arresting effect of cAMP on the oocytes may be mediated via the cAMP-dependent protein kinase (PKA) and the subsequent phosphorylation of specific proteins (Schultz et al., 1983).

The arrest of meiosis *in vivo* is maintained by certain putative factors in the follicular fluid and by the theca cell layer (Kotsuji et al., 1994). A heat-stable and a heat-labile low-molecular-weight peptide have been identified from porcine and bovine follicular fluids that have meiotic inhibitory action (Tsafariri et al., 1976; Gwatkin and Anderson, 1976). Other specific molecules that affect the meiotic arrest include steroids, fatty acid- linoleic acid and purines-hypoxanthine and adenosine (Racowsky, 1993; Homa and Brown, 1992; Downs et al., 1985; 1998; Eppig et al., 1985). Follicular fluid has the latter in concentrations high enough to prevent meiotic resumption. However, there may be several other factors present in the follicular fluid that could contribute to a similar inhibitory action.

Based on these findings, meiotic resumption may arise either due to a loss of the inhibitory input or due to positive stimulation. The action of the gonadotrophins is believed to be via binding to the cell surface receptors and the activation of adenyl cyclase, thereby increasing the cAMP. Indeed, a rise in the cAMP levels in the follicular cells occurs following gonadotrophin stimulation. However, it is accompanied by the decrease in the cAMP levels within the oocyte in the study specimen mouse and rat, but not in the hamster, sheep, rabbit and pig (Schultz et al., 1983; Aberdam et al., 1987; Racowsky, 1985; Moor and Heslop, 1981; Yoshimura et al., 1992; Mattioli et al., 1994). Furthermore, exposure of mouse cumulus-enclosed oocytes or follicles to moderate pulsing concentrations of cAMP results in GV breakdown (Dekel et al., 1988). Thus, the action of cAMP seems to be paradoxical. This could possibly be attributed to the relative levels of cAMP to which the follicular cells and oocytes are exposed. Also, the inhibitory action of cAMP is potentiated in cumulus-enclosed as opposed to denuded oocytes.

The loss of the inhibitory input during the preovulatory period may occur through one or several mechanisms, like dissociation between the follicular cells and the oocyte, increase in the activity of PDE leading to the accelerated metabolism of cAMP, and possibly decreased synthesis of cAMP. One possible theory is related to a putative inhibitory signal which is modified or inactivated following the gonadotrophin surge, leading to meiotic resumption (Dekel *et al.*, 1981). But the oocyte-follicle cell coupling does not seem to decrease before the onset of gonadotrophin-induced meiotic maturation (Moor et al., 1981; Motilik et al., 1986). However, a decreased metabolic and dye coupling have been noted to occur with GV breakdown in hamster and rat oocyte-cumulus complexes (Rackowsky and Satterlie, 1985; Dekel et al., 1988). Also, a reduction in the cumulus cell gap junction fractional area may occur in association with the GVB (Larsen et al., 1986). Nevertheless, these studies indicate that the uncoupling between the follicle cells and the oocyte follow, and not precede, the preovulatory gonadotrophin surge. On the other hand, the cumulus-cumulus cell and the cumulus-membrana cell gap junctions may be downregulated before those between the cumulus cell and the oocyte (Larsen et al., 1987; Racowsky and Baldwin, 1989; Wert and Larsen, 1990). Thus, the integrity of the gap junctions may be altered following the preovulatory gonadotrophin surge, leading to a decrease in the transfer of the putative inhibitory factor/s.

Another proposed mechanism behind meiotic resumption is the generation of a positive signal that overrides the existing inhibitory influence. This signal may be generated in the follicle cells and transferred to the oocyte (Downs et al., 1988). This positive signal has been identified in the frog and starfish as progesterone and l-methyladenine, respectively. A variety of ligands have been identified to have a similar action on mammalian oocytes *in vitro*. These agents include gonadotrophins, growth factors, phorbol ester, etc. These agents can act via a number of signal transduction pathways, with a possibility that these signals may converge finally to one common triggering pathway. The final event is the activation of MPF by specific protein phosphorylation and dephosphorylation.

Role of Ca^{2+} in Resumption of Meiotic Maturation

In many species, the control points of the meiotic and mitotic cycles are triggered by an increase in the intracellular Ca^{2+}. In mammalian oocytes, the role of Ca^{2+} is equally important. A series of Ca^{2+} transients that occur at fertilization lead to oocyte release from the meiotic arrest (meiotic exit). But the role of Ca^{2+} in triggering meiosis resumption and progression in the mammalian oocyte are not clearly defined. In the cells, Ca^{2+} is released from the intracellular stores in response to the second messenger, inositol 1, 4, 5-trisphosphate (IP3), which is a product of the hydrolysis of phosphotidyl inositol 4, 5 bisphosphate (PIP2). This is brought about by phospholipase C, either in response to a G-protein-mediated or a tyrosine kinase-mediated stimulus (Berridge, 1993). Similar mechanisms may be operative in the oocytes as well. Spontaneous Ca^{2+} oscillations are known to occur in fully grown immature mouse oocytes and their occurrence is correlated to the acquisition of meiotic competence (Carroll et al., 1992; Lefèvre et al., 1995; Deng et al., 1998). These oscillations have been noted to occur in the cytoplasm as well as the nucleus and are inhibited in the presence of dbcAMP (Lefèvre et al., 1995). One of the most likely modes of Ca^{2+} release during oocyte maturation is that occurring via the inositol 1, 4, 5-trisphosphate receptors (InsP3R). In GV-stage oocytes, these receptors are in the perinuclear region (Shiraishi et al., 1995; Mehlmann et al., 1996; Goud et al., 1999). Recently, these receptors were shown to be within the nucleus as well as cytoplasm of the GV-stage mouse oocytes, and the release of Ca^{2+} at these sites was shown to occur via the InsP3R (Pesty et al., 1998).

It is proposed that elevation of Ca^{2+} within the oocyte at meiosis resumption may occur secondary to the LH surge (Homa 1995). Apart from the activation of adenyl cyclase to increase the cAMP level, the preovulatory LH surge is also associated with a rapid turnover of phosphoinositide metabolism and the release of a secondary messenger, IP3, which, in turn, may release Ca^{2+} in the follicular cells (Davis et al., 1986). This mechanism explains the release of Ca^{2+} within the follicular cells secondary to LH, and also the release of Ca^{2+} within the oocyte that occurs after a 100–300-s delay (Mattioli et al., 1998). This signal is conducted to the oocytes via the cumulus cell-oocyte gap junctions and IP3 is the most likely mediator of this signal transduction. A similar mechanism may occur even after exposure of the oocyte-cumulus complexes to FSH or epidermal growth factor (EGF). Although the signal transduction for both these agents may be different (adenyl cyclase- and tyrosine kinase-mediated), both result in the mobilization of Ca^{2+} from the intracellular stores.

These findings, however, are specific for the positive signal-induced meiotic maturation and are quite different from the spontaneous oocyte maturation. Studies have been performed with Ca^{2+}-deficient media, Ca^{2+} chelators, Ca^{2+} channel blockers as well as Ca^{2+} ionophores. But the evidence of the role of Ca^{2+} in spontaneous maturation remains contradictory (Homa 1995). A recent study confirms this theory (Coticchio and Fleming, 1998).

CYTOSKELETAL REARRANGEMENTS DURING OOCYTE MATURATION

The cytoskeleton of the human oocyte consists mainly of microtubules and microfilaments. These cytoskeletal components undergo considerable changes during oocyte maturation. These changes are specific and related to the cell cycle phase. In the GV stage, the microtubules are restricted mainly to the periphery and to a small perinuclear region. This distribution changes after GVBD as the chromatin gets condensed and is surrounded by the microtubules. In an M I oocyte, the microtubules are restricted mainly to the spindle. However, treatment with a microtubul-enhancing agent, taxol, leads to the induction of foci of microtubule organizing centres (MTOC) in the cytoplasm. The number of these foci was found to increase during meiotic maturation (Battaglia et al., 1996; Kim et al., 1998). In the M II-stage oocyte, the microtubules are restricted to a barrel-shaped spindle oriented perpendicular to the oolemma, while the condensed chromosomes are arranged on the equatorial metaphase plate. Treatment with taxol induces MTOC in the cortical cytoplasm (Battaglia et al., 1996). However, these findings are somewhat different from the earlier reports (Pickering et al., 1988). Nevertheless, these differences could be partly explained by the extremely dynamic nature of MTOC, making them very sensitive to physical conditions during fixation.

Microtubules are involved in the process of chromosome separation during meiosis. During fertilization, they play an important role in bringing about the centripetal movement and approximation of the pronuclei. Any defects in microtubule activity could, therefore, lead to chromosomal abnormalities in the embryo (Nicolaidis and Petersen, 1998).

Microfilaments are made of actin. They are observed mainly around the nucleus and the cortex in the GV-stage oocyte. After GVBD, they are concentrated close to the chromatin and form thick and thin domains in the cortex. The chromosomes are in the thick microfilament domain (Kim et al., 1998). Microfilaments are involved in the migration and peripheral maintenance of meiotic chromosomes, spindle orientation and polar body extrusion. They also possibly play a role in the peripheral migration of the cellular organelles, like smooth endoplasmic reticulum (SER) and cortical granules (Mehlmann et al., 1995; Connors et al., 1998).

IN VITRO MATURATION OF OOCYTES FOR CLINICAL APPLICATION

Although the successful demonstration of the spontaneous maturation of mammalian and human oocytes dates back 60 years, success in obtaining live births from oocytes was achieved only around 15 years ago (Minato and Toyoda, 1983; Schroeder and Eppig, 1984; Eppig et al., 1996). Since then, the *in vitro* maturation technique has been successfully applied to a number of mammalian species (Bovine: Goto et al., 1988; Sirard et al., 1988; Fukuda et al., 1990; Pigs: Mattioli et al., 1989; Yoshida et al., 1993; Rat: Vanderhyden and

Armstrong, 1989). Since the last eight years, the technique has also been applied successfully in the human oocyte donation programme, for polycystic ovarian syndrome (PCOS) and for unstimulated cycle retrieval (Cha et al., 1991; Trounson et al., 1994; Barnes et al., 1995; 1996; Russell et al., 1997). Recent successes have also been obtained in achieving growth and maturation of oocytes from preantral follicles (Eppig et al., 1989; 1996; Spears et al., 1994; Roy and Treacy, 1993; Abir et al., 1997). There are certain occasions during stimulated cycles when there is a high risk of ovarian hyperstimulation syndrome (OHSS). The current strategies to tackle such a situation would include cycle cancellation, coasting or aspiration of all oocytes, fertilizing and cryopreservation of the embryos for transfer in a subsequent cycle. However, since hCG is a key precipitating factor in OHSS, withholding it could be one possible option. Retrieval of immature oocytes with subsequent maturation, fertilization and embryo transfer have resulted in successful pregnancies (Liu et al., 1997; Jaroudi et al., 1997).

Another promising area is that of ovarian tissue cryopreservation and autologous transplantation in patients undergoing ablative procedures for the treatment of malignancies. Recently, there has been some success in orthotopic insertion of cryopreserved and thawed ovarian tissue in non-human species. Similarly, an examination of human ovarian tissue after the freeze-thaw shows a substantial number of morphologically normal primordial follicles. The details of this, however, are beyond the scope of the current chapter and have been reviewed elsewhere (Newton, 1998).

IN VITRO MATURATION OF OOCYTES FROM UNSTIMULATED OVARIES

Early attempts at the application of IVM in humans to obtain mature, fertilizable oocytes date back several years (Edwards 1965a, b; Edwards et al., 1969). However, the first successful birth from IVM resulted only recently (Cha et al., 1991). Oocytes in the latter case were obtained from the ovaries of patients undergoing gynaecological surgery for benign conditions and the technique used consisted of aspiration of all follicles of 2–5 mm. Later, the technique of immature oocyte retrieval under ultrasound guidance was perfected by others, initially in patients with PCOS and later also in those without PCOS (Trounson et al., 1994; Barnes et al., 1995; 1996).

OOCYTE RETRIEVAL FROM AN UNSTIMULATED OVARY

Retrieval of oocytes in the initial successful attempts was easy because the source of material was from excised ovaries or from ovarian biopsies. This allowed for open examination and aspiration of follicles of 2–5 mm under vision. The technique used was simple, utilizing just a 21-guage needle attached to a syringe. However, the later attempts involved the use of a laparoscope and transvaginal ultrasound (Trounson et al., 1994). Recently, immature oocyte retrieval has been almost perfected with the use of transvaginal ultrasound (Russell et al., 1997; 1998).

The initial application of this technique involved patients with PCOS because visualization of the follicles was rather easy and a higher yield of immature oocytes was obtained in PCOS patients as well (Trounson et al., 1994). However, later, a similar oocyte retrieval could be successfully performed in non-PCOS patients as well (Russell et al., 1997). The technique of obtaining immature oocytes from an unstimulated ovary is somewhat different from the technique of ovum pick-up from stimulated ovaries that is used routinely today. Unstimulated ovaries are smaller, firmer, and are difficult to pierce due to their tendency of moving away from the needle. Therefore, the success of the technique depends more on anticipation and practice. Also, the follicles are smaller and the compact oocyte-cumulus may tend to remain adherent to the follicle wall. These problems are countered by using a specially designed oocyte pick-up needle, which is shorter in length, more rigid in structure and has a shorter bevel (Trounson et al., 1994). It is important also to lower the aspiration pressure to half of that used for stimulated ovaries, and to introduce the needle with the bevel facing downwards. This ensures complete emptying of the follicle and maximizes the chances of obtaining the oocyte. As the aspiration needle tends to get blocked, frequent flushing may be required.

The number of oocytes obtained using this technique is, however, also dependent on the age of the patient. The stage of the menstrual cycle, however, may not be relevant to the number of oocytes retrieved. However, it is suggested that the quality of the oocytes obtained may be suboptimal if the oocyte retrieval is performed after the emergence of a dominant follicle (Russell et al., 1998).

OOCYTE CULTURE: CHOICE OF MEDIA AND SUPPLEMENTS

An ideal culture medium should mimic the microenvironment of a preovulatory follicle. However, the complex interplay between the follicle cells and oocyte involves a number of known and unknown factors, which cannot be simulated *in vitro*. This process is further complicated by the dynamism of cellular coupling that occurs between the oocyte and follicular cells, and among the follicular cells. Unfortunately, the current knowledge of these dynamics has confined us to settle for a simple and static system for the culture of oocyte-cumulus complexes. Therefore, positive results of maturation indicate a remarkable flexibility of the oocyte to adjust to the *in vitro* conditions rather than to mimicry of the *in vivo* conditions. There is also a possibility of redundancy of oocyte maturation mechanisms that may have led to the success in achieving optimum oocyte maturation *in vitro*. Another confounding factor is the occurrence of spontaneous maturation and the difficulty in differentiating it from physiological maturation.

The contemporary system of *in vitro* culture involves creating an optimum environment for the maturing oocyte. Therefore, formulating a medium that satisfies all the needs of the oocyte is the main goal of this system. Most current maturation media contain a buffered isotonic solution that contains glucose, pyruvate, amino acids and supplements. Albumin or serum is the commonly used protein supplement. The initial successful protocols, however, had utilized follicular fluid as a supplement. The results of the latter were superior to those of fetal calf serum (FCS) as a supplement (Cha et al., 1991). However, using serum or follicular fluid carries a certain risk. Furthermore, systematic dissection of the media components is not possible due to the resultant undefined conditions (Bavister, 1995). It may, therefore, be preferable to use defined media supplemented with albumin or synthetic serum substitute rather than serum for predictable results (Russell et al., 1997; Goud et al., 1998).

Culture Media Supplements

A number of culture media supplements are suggested to mimic the *in vivo* events of oocyte maturation. These consist mainly of extra-nutritive supplements, gonadotrophins, steroids and growth factors. A number of the media available may be deficient in pyruvate and may instead contain only glucose. Oocytes require pyruvate as an energy source and depend on the presence of granulosa cells for the conversion of glucose into pyruvate (Biggers et al., 1967; Leese and Barton, 1985). Supplementation of the culture medium with gluamine, L-cysteine and cysteamine may improve the cytoplasmic maturation of oocytes (Kito and Bavister, 1997).

The addition of gonadotrophins improves the fertilization competence of IVM oocytes (Shalgi et al., 1979; Prins et al., 1987; Younis et al., 1989; Funahashi and Day, 1993; Zhang et al., 1993; Schramm and Bavister, 1995). In a recent report on the IVM of human oocytes, no difference was noted between gonadotrophin-supplemented versus unsupplemented media in terms of maturation, fertilization and cleavage (Trounson et al., 1998). However, these results could be partly explained by the presence of beneficial factors in the control medium (Chang's medium) because the addition of gonadotrophins to Chang's medium resulted in an improvement in the rates of maturation (Trounson et al., 1996). The possibility of the occurrence of spontaneous maturation is another factor that may have led to these results. Thus, gonadotrophins continue to constitute one of the most important components of the contemporary culture media. Similarly, 17 b-oestradiol was shown to exert a direct effect on maturing human oocytes by increasing the intracellular free Ca^{2+} and improving the fertilization and cleavage rates (Tesarik et al., 1995). Thus, supplementation of the culture medium with 17 b-oestradiol may be beneficial.

The addition of growth factors, especially Insulin-like growth factor-I (IGF-I) and epidermal growth factor (EGF), improves the nuclear as well as cytoplasmic maturation *in vitro* in a number of species, including human (Das et al., 1991; Gomez et al., 1993; Goud et al., 1998). The effect can be seen both in the presence as well as absence of the attached cumulus corona cells. Recently, supplementation of another intra-ovarian regulating peptide, Activin-A, was shown to have a similar positive role in accelerating human oocyte maturation *in vitro* (Alak et al., 1998).

GRANULOSA CELL AND OTHER CO-CULTURES

Co-culture systems are often used in IVF to improve the clinical pregnancy rates (Bongso et al., 1990). This technique involves culture of the embryo with the somatic cell monolayer. In the case of oocytes, the immature oocytes have been cultured along with the cumulus cells or with Vero cells (Dandekar et al., 1991; Janssenswillen et al., 1995). The mechanisms by which co-cultures possibly improve maturation could be either the secretion of certain factors, or by diluting the effect of growth inhibiting substances in the oocyte's microenvironment.

Maintenance of the cumulus corona cells that are attached to the oocytes throughout the culture period is of vital importance. These cells are attached to the oocytes, making intimate contact with these through gap junctions and desmosomal complexes (Motta et al., 1994). These gap junctions help in a selective transfer of macromolecules and beneficial factors to the oocytes, and help improve the rate of nuclear and cytoplasmic maturation of the oocytes (Brower and Schultz, 1982; Goud et al., 1998).

DYNAMICS OF OOCYTE MATURATION, FERTILIZATION AND EMBRYO DEVELOPMENT *IN VITRO*

Under physiological conditions, the maturation of human oocytes is completed within about 36 hours of the onset of the LH surge (Edwards 1965a). However, the reported dynamics of IVM in human GV-stage oocytes from unstimulated and stimulated ovaries are different (Fig. 5.4). Germinal vesicle breakdown, polar body extrusion and cumulus expansion occur after culture of the immature oocytes from both unstimulated and stimulated cycles (Fig. 5.5). But in the case of the latter, maturation occurs faster than in the former (Janssenswillen et al., 1995; Goud et al., 1998; Trounson et al., 1996). The faster rate of maturation in GV oocytes from stimulated ovaries may be explained by the possibility of exposure to the gonadotrophins *in vivo*; whereas the slower rate of maturation (compared to that of *in vivo* maturation) in oocytes from unstimulated ovaries may be related to the *in vitro* conditions. Furthermore, the occurrence of spontaneous maturation in these oocytes could be another factor related to these differences in the maturation dynamics.

Fertilization of IVM oocytes may be compromised due to the occurrence of zona hardening. This phenomenon may occur secondary to premature cortical granule loss. However, this could be countered with the help of certain agents, like serum or fetuin, in the culture media (Downs et al., 1986; Eppig et al., 1996). Thus, fertilization could be achieved either with standard insemination or intracytoplasmic sperm injection (ICSI). A significant improvement in the fertilization rates with ICSI was noted only in oocytes obtained from PCOS patients. Moreover, the rate of cleavage was lower among the fertilized oocytes from the PCOS group compared to the non-PCOS group, indicating that ICSI may have led to fertilization of developmentally incompetent oocytes (Trounson et al., 1996; 1998). Thus, the role of ICSI in the fertilization of IVM oocytes in non-male factor cases is doubtful.

The development of embryos derived from IVM oocytes is retarded in comparison to those derived from *in vivo*-matured oocytes. This is due to the more frequent cleavage arrests at the pronuclear stage and beyond the 8-cell stage (Trounson et al., 1996; 1998). The cause of these developmental arrests may be related to the defects in the process of cytoplasmic maturation. Recently, a difference in the Ca^{2+} responses was noted in oocytes matured *in vitro* and *in vivo* (Herbert et al., 1997). This could be one possible specific defect in the *in vitro*-matured oocytes compared to their *in vivo*-matured counterparts. Further investigations of the protein profile of *in vitro*-matured oocytes could reveal more specific information. Correction of these effects by optimizing the culture

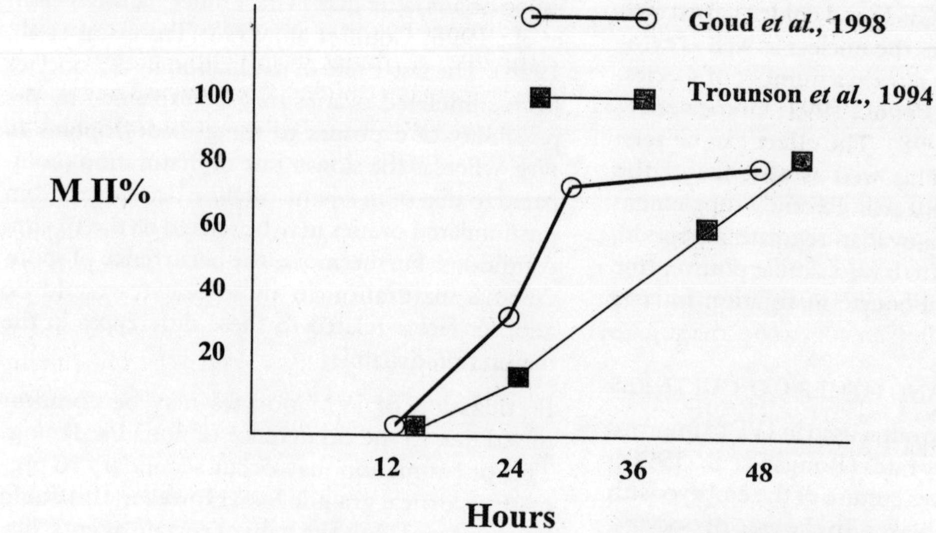

Fig. 5.4. Time course of *in vitro* maturation of oocytes obtained from unstimulated and gonadotrophin-stimulated ovaries (data derived from Trounson *et al.*, 1994 and Goud et al., 1998)

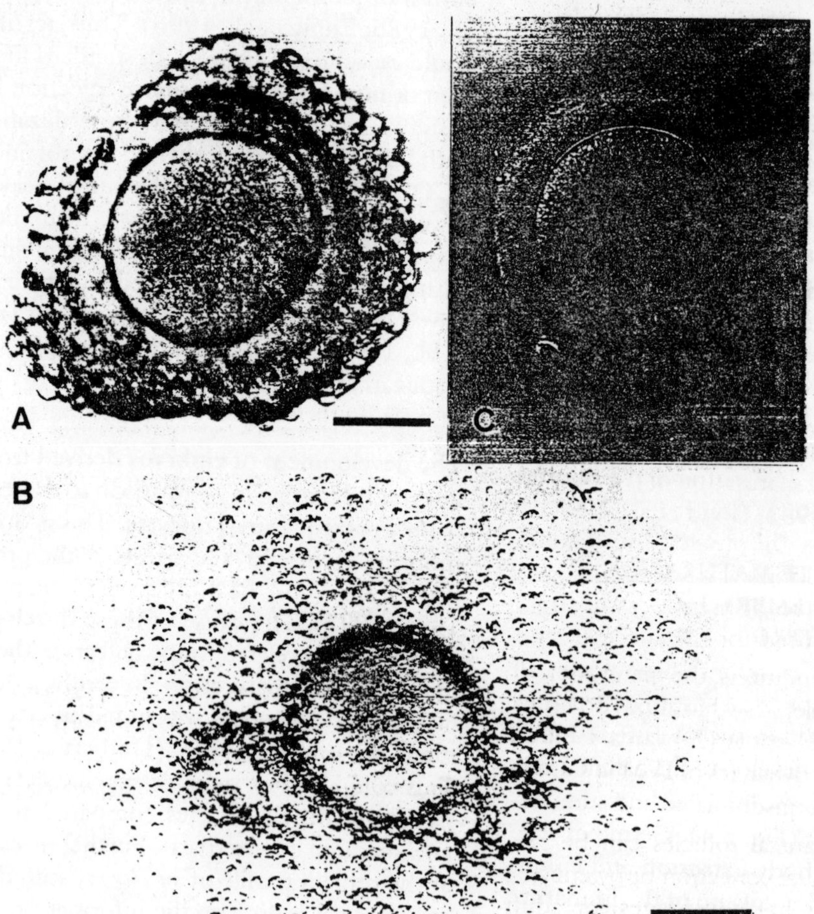

Fig. 5.5. Photomicrographs of a human oocyte through *in vitro* maturation. (A) A germinal vesicle (GV)-stage oocyte surrounded by a few compact layers of cumulus-corona cells. A slightly peripheral GV is indicated by an arrow. (B) The same oocyte after 30 h-culture in a maturation medium. Note the markedly expanded cumulus. (C) An *in vitro*-matured M II-stage oocyte. Original magnification = 320x. Solid bar corresponds to 50 μ

conditions would possibly improve the results of IVM in the future.

Application of the recently introduced improved culture media for human embryo development could be another approach to improving the outcome of IVM. Optimizing the culture medium could possibly salvage at least some oocytes that would have failed to develop in the conventional media (Gardner and Lane, 1998; Trounson et al., 1998). However, this remains to be investigated.

ISOLATION AND CULTURE OF OOCYTES FROM PREANTRAL FOLLICLES

The isolation and long-term culture of preantral follicles can develop preovulatory oocytes that mature, fertilize and cleave *in vitro*. This strategy has already been successful in obtaining live births in mice and has developed to various extents in different species, including humans (Eppig and Schroeder, 1989; Roy and Treacy, 1993; Hirao et al., 1994; Abir et al., 1997). However, precise reproduction of the dynamic *in vivo* conditions is extremely difficult *in vitro*. But even *in vivo*, the conditions within the follicles are more or less hypoxic and these follicles may perhaps be more tolerant to *in vitro* conditions than expected. Thus, preantral follicle isolation and long-term culture may have tremendous implications for clinical application. Currently, there are few reports on successful *in vitro* growth and maturation of human preantral follicles in culture (Abir et al., 1997). The limitations are related to the physical constraints in developing large antral follicular sizes comparable to the preovulatory sizes. Recently, a substrate-adherent system was used for the successful development of oocytes *in vitro* (Cortvrindt et al., 1996). Although the spherical shape of the follicle could not be maintained in such a system, mouse oocytes were shown to develop to the hatched blastocyst stage.

The isolation of preantral follicles can be performed either by manual dissection or by enzyme treatment. The latter has advantages for adult ovaries, which are firm, and the chances of having an intact basement membrane may be higher. But the overall recovery of small follicles, especially in the case of ovaries from young subjects or fetal ovaries, may be higher after enzyme treatment. It may be worthwhile to consider a combination of the two methods.

The methods used for culture may involve an organ culture or culture of multiple tissue fragments (Eppig et al., 1996). Nonetheless, this method has problems associated with the degeneration of the neighbouring follicles due to hypoxia and the complexity of the culture system. Besides, multiple follicles could be placed in groups, with or without direct contact, or cultured individually.

THE USE OF FETAL OVARIAN TISSUE

Fetal ovaries have a large number of oocytes and, therefore, could be considered as a potential source for obtaining oocytes. A number of studies have been performed in animals, mainly in mice. But the application of this technique in humans raises a number of ethical issues, which must be taken into account. These issues are mainly related to the source of the material and the proposed application of this tissue. Furthermore, other factors, like the gestational age of the fetus and the type of abortion (spontaneous or terminated), need to be considered. Generally, oocytes from terminations survive better in culture. Also, during the first trimester, most cells are oogonia and meiosis has not begun. However, it could be an important model to study the onset of meiosis. Furthermore, among the commonest terminations, congenital abnormalities form a large group in which oocyte development may be inherently abnormal.

Although the overall survival of the tissue may be better in comparison to adult tissues, development *in vitro* is compromised due to the current unavailability of optimal conditions for their long-term culture. Nevertheless, some progress has been made in non-human models, but further progress in research on fetal ovaries is marred by the paucity of appropriate tissues.

CONCLUDING REMARKS

In vitro maturation technology has taken a new turn in the last few years. There is a scope now to study and apply the technique of immature oocyte retrieval from unstimulated ovaries to clinical maturation. However, it is necessary to further investigate the factors involved during *in vivo* maturation and apply them to the *in vitro* system. This could significantly improve the quality of cytoplasmic maturation, which is lacking in the current systems.

The techniques of follicle culture and ovarian tissue cryopreservation have great potential for clinical application, and considerable progress has been made in the non-human species. Exploring the needs of the follicle in culture to support the growth of developmental competence of the emerging *in vitro*-matured oocyte will be a challenge in the future.

REFERENCES

Aberdam, E. et al. (1987). 'Maintenance of meiotic arrest in isolated rat oocytes by the invasive adenyl cyclase of Bordetella Pertussis', *Biol. Reprod.*, **36:** 530–35.

Abir, R. et al. (1997). 'Mechanical isolation and *in vitro* growth of preantral and small antral human follicles', *Fertil. Steril.*, **68:** 682–8.

Alak, B.M. et al. (1998). 'Activin A stimulates meiotic maturation of human oocytes and modulates granulosa cell steroidogenesis *in vitro*', *Fertil. Steril.*, **70:** 1126–30.

Baker, T.G. (1963). 'A quantitative and cytological study of germ cells in human ovaries', *Proc. Roy. Soc. B.*, **158:** 417–33.

Barnes, F.L. et al. (1995). 'Blastocyst development and birth after *in-vitro* maturation of human primary oocytes, intracytoplasmic sperm injection and assisted hatching', *Hum. Reprod.*, **10:** 3243–7.

Barnes, F.L. et al. (1996). 'Production of embryos from *in vitro* matured primary human oocytes', *Fertil. Steril.*, **65:** 1151–6.

Battaglia, D.E. et al. (1996). 'Changes in centrosomal domains during meiotic maturation in the human oocyte', *Mol. Hum. Reprod.*, **2:** 845–51.

Bavister, B.D. (1995). 'Culture of preimplantation embryos: Facts and artifacts', *Hum. Reprod. Update*, **1:** 91–148.

Berridge, M.J. (1993). 'Inositol trisphosphate and calcium signalling', *Nature*, **361:** 315–25.

Biggers, J.D. et al. (1967). 'The pattern of energy metabolism in the mouse oocyte and zygote', *Proc. Natl. Acad. Sci.* USA, **57:** 560–67.

Bongso, A. et al. (1990). 'Co-cultures: Their relevance to assisted reproduction', *Hum. Reprod.*, **5:** 893–900.

Brower, P.T. and R.M. Schultz (1982). 'Intercellular communication between granulosa cells and mouse oocytes: Existence and possible nutritional role during oocyte growth', *Dev. Biol.*, **90:** 144–53.

Carroll, J. and K. Swann (1992). 'Spontaneous cytosolic calcium oscillations driven by inositol trisphosphate occur during *in vitro* maturation of mouse oocytes', *J. Biol. Chem.*, **267:** 11196–201.

Cha, K.Y. et al. (1991). 'Pregnancy after *in vitro* fertilization of human follicular oocytes collected from nonstimulated cycles, their culture *in vitro* and their transfer in a donor oocyte program', *Fertil. Steril.*, **55:** 109–13

Chiquoine, A.D. (1954). 'The identification, origin, and migration of primordial germ cells in the mouse embryo', *Anat. Rec.*, **118:** 135–46.

Connors, S.A. et al. (1998). 'Involvement of the cysoskeleton in the movement of cortical granules during oocyte maturation and cortical granule anchoring in mouse eggs', *Dev. Biol.*, **200:** 103–15.

Cortvrindt, R. (1996). '*In vitro* maturation, fertilization and embryo development of immature oocytes from early preantral follicles from prepubertal mice in a simplified culture system', *Hum. Reprod.*, **11:** 2656–66.

Coticchio, G. and S. Fleming (1998). 'Inhibition of phosphoinositide metabolism or chelation of intracellular calcium blocks FSH-induced but not spontaneous meiotic resumption in mouse oocytes', *Dev. Biol.*, **203:** 201–9.

Coucouvanis, E.C. et al. (1993). 'Evidence that the mechanism of prenatal germ cell death in mouse is apoptosis.' *Exp. Cell Res.*, **209:** 238–43.

Dandekar, P. et al. (1991). 'Maturation of immature oocytes by coculture with granulosa cells', *Fertil. Steril.*, **55:** 95–9.

Das, K. et al. (1991). 'Direct positive effect of epidermal growth factor on the cytoplasmic maturation of mouse and human oocytes', *Fertil. Steril.*, **55:** 1000–1004.

Davis, J.S. et al. (1986). 'Luteinizing hormone stimulates the formation of inositol trisphosphate and cyclic AMP in rat granulosa cells: Evidence of phospholipase C generated second messengers in the action of luteinizing hormone', *Biochem J.*, **238:** 597–604.

Dekel, N. et al. (1981). 'Modulation of cell-to-cell communication in the cumulus-oocyte complex and regulation of oocyte maturation by LH', *Dev. Biol.*, **86:** 352–62.

______(1988). 'Dissociation between the inhibitory and the stimulatory action of cAMP on maturation of rat oocytes', *Mol. Cell. Endocrinol.*, **56:**115–21.

Deng, M.Q. et al. (1998). 'Spontaneous and fertilization-induced Ca oscillations in mouse immature germinal vesicle stage oocytes', *Biol. Reprod.*, **58:** 807–13.

De Pol et al. (1997). 'Apoptosis of germ cells during human prenatal oogenesis', *Hum. Reprod.*, **12:** 2235–41.

Donovan, P.J. (1994). 'Growth factor regulation of mouse primordial germ cell development', *Curr. Top. Dev. Biol.*, **29:** 189–225.

Downs, S.M. (1998). 'Precursors of the purine backbone augment the inhibitory action of hypoxanthine and dibutyryl cAMP on mouse oocyte maturation', *J. Exp. Zool.*, **282:** 376–84.

Downs, S.M. et al. (1985). 'Hypoxanthine is the principle inhibitor murine oocyte maturation in a low molecular weight fraction of porcine follicular fluid', *Proc. Natl. Acad. Sci.* USA, **82:** 454–8.

______(1986). 'Serum maintains the fertilizability of mouse oocytes matured *in vitro* by preventing the hardening of zona pellucida', *Gamete Res.*, **15:** 115–22.

______(1988). 'Induction of maturation in cumulus cell-enclosed mouse oocytes by follicle stimulating hormone and epidermal growth factor: Evidence for a positive stimulus of somatic cell origin', *J. Exp. Zool.*, **245:** 86-96.

Downs, S.M. and A.M. Mastropolo (1997). 'Culture conditions affect meiotic regulation in cumulus-cell enclosed mouse oocytes', *Mol. Reprod. Dev.*, **46:** 551–66.

Dunphy, W. et al. (1988). 'The xenopus cdc2 protein is a component of MPF, a cytoplasmic regulator of mitosis', *Cell*, **54:** 423–31.

Edwards, R.G. et al. (1965a). 'Maturation *in vitro* of mouse, sheep, cow, pig, rhesus monkey and human ovarian oocytes', *Nature*, **208:** 349–51.

______. (1965b). 'Maturation *in vitro* of human ovarian oocytes', *Lancet*, **ii:** 926–9.

______(1969). 'Early stages of fertilization *in vitro* of human oocytes matured *in vitro*', *Nature*, **221:** 632.

Eppig, J.J. and S.M. Downs (1984). 'Chemical signals that regulate mammalian oocyte maturation', *Biol. Reprod.*, **30:** 1–11.

Eppig, J. et al. (1996). 'Mammalian oocyte growth and development *in vitro*', *Mol. Reprod. Dev.*, **44:** 260–73.

Eppig, J.J. and A.C. Schroeder (1989). 'Capacity of mouse oocytes from preantral follicles to undergo embryogenesis and development to live young after growth, maturation and fertilization *in vitro*', *Biol. Reprod.*, **41:** 268–76.

Eppig, J.J. et al. (1985). 'Hypoxanthine and adenosine in murine ovarian follicular fluid: Concentrations and activity in maintaining oocyte meiotic arrest', *Biol. Reprod.*, **33:** 1041–49.

Evans T. et al. (1983). 'Cyclin: A protein specified by maternal mRNA in sea urchin eggs that is destroyed at cleavage division', *Cell*, **33:** 389–96.

Fulka, J. et al. (1998). 'Nuclear and cytoplasmic determinants involved in the regulation of mammalian oocyte maturation', *Mol. Hum. Reprod.*, **4:** 41–9.

Fukuda, Y. (1990). 'Birth of normal calves resulting from bovine oocytes matured, fertilized and cultured with cumulus cells *in vitro* up to the blastocyst stage', *Biol. Reprod.*, **42:** 114–9.

Funahashi, H. and B.N. Day (1993). 'Effects of different serum supplements in maturation medium on meiotic and cytoplasmic maturation of pig oocytes', *Theriogenology*, **39:** 965–73.

Gabrielli, B.G. et al. (1993). 'Requirement for Cdk2 in cytostatic factor-mediated metaphase II arrest', *Science*, **259:** 1766–69.

Gardner, D.K. and M. Lane (1998). 'Culture of viable human blastocysts in defined sequential serum-free media', *Hum. Reprod.*, **13: Suppl 3:** 148–59.

Gautier, J. et al. (1990). 'Cyclin is a component of maturation promoting factor from Xenopus', *Cell.*, **60:** 487–94.

______(1988). 'Purified maturation promoting factor contains a product of a Xenopus homolog of the fission yeast cell cycle control gene cdc2+', *Cell*, **54:** 433–9.

Ginsburg, M. et al. (1990). 'Primordial germ cells in the

mouse embryo during gastrulation', *Dev.*, **110:** 521–8.

Gomez, E. et al. (1993). 'Oocyte maturation in humans: The role of gonadotropins and growth factors', *Fertil. Steril.*, **60:** 40–46.

Gosden, R.G. (1995). 'Ovulation 1: Oocyte development throughout life', in J.G. Grudzinskas, J.L. Yovich (eds.), *Cambridge Reviews in Human Reproduction Gametes-The Oocyte*, Cambridge University Press, Cambridge.

Goto, K. et al. (1988). 'Pregnancies after co-culture of cumulus cells with bovine embryos derived from *in vitro* fertilization of *in vitro* mature follicular oocytes', *J. Reprod. Fertil.*, **83:** 753–8.

Goud, P.T. et al. (1998). '*In vitro* maturation of human germinal vesicle stage oocytes: Role of cumulus cells and epidermal growth factor in the culture medium', *Hum. Reprod.*, **13:** 1638–44.

______(1999). 'Presence and dynamic redistribution of type I inositol 1, 4, 5-trisphosphate receptors in human oocytes and embryos during *in vitro* maturation, fertilization and early cleavage divisions', *Mol. Hum. Reprod.*, In press.

Gwatkin, R.B.L. and O.F. Anderson (1976). 'Hamster oocyte maturation *in vitro*: Inhibition by follicular components', *Life Sci.*, **19:** 527–36.

Haghinat, N. and L.J. Van Winkle (1990). 'Developmental change in follicular cell-enhanced amino acid uptake into mouse oocytes that depends on intact gap junctions and transport system Gly', *J. Exp. Zool.*, **253:** 71–82.

Heikenheimo, O. et al. (1995). 'Cell-cycle genes c-mos and cyclin B1 are expressed in a specific pattern in human oocytes and pre-implantation embryos', *Hum. Reprod.*, **10:** 699–707.

Herbert, M. (1997). 'Development of calcium signalling mechanisms during maturation of human oocytes', *Mol. Hum. Reprod.*, **3:** 965–73.

Hirao, Y. et al. (1994). '*In vitro* growth and maturation of pig oocytes', *J. Reprod. Fertil.*, **100:** 333–9.

Homa, S.T. (1995). 'Calcium and meiotic maturation of the mammalian oocyte', *Mol. Reprod. Dev.*, **40:** 122–34.

Homa, S.T. and C.A. Brown (1992). 'Changes in linoleic acid during follicular development and inhibition of spontaneous breakdown of germinal vesicles in cumulus-free bovine oocytes', *J. Reprod. Fertil.*, **94:** 153–60.

Inoue, M. et al. (1995). 'Activation of mitogen-activated protein kinase during meiotic maturation of porcine oocytes', *Zygote*, **3:** 265–71.

Ishida, N. et al. (1993). 'Mos is degraded by the 26S proteasome in ubiquitin dependent pathway', *FEBS Lett.*, **324:** 345–8.

Ismail, R. et al. (1996). 'Hormonal regulation of the ligand for *c-kit* in the rat ovary and its effects on spontaneous oocyte meiotic maturation', *Mol. Reprod. Dev.*, **43:** 458–69.

Jaroudi, K.A. et al. (1997). 'Pregnancy after transfer of embryos which were generated from *in vitro* matured oocytes', *Hum. Reprod.*, **12:** 857–9.

Janssenswillen, C. et al. (1995). 'Maturation of human cumulus-free germinal vesicle-stage oocytes to metaphase II by co-culture with monolayer Vero cells', *Hum. Reprod.*, **10:** 375–6.

Kim, N.H. et al. (1998). 'Microtubule and microfilament organization in maturing human oocytes', *Hum. Reprod.*, **13:** 2217–22.

Kito, S. and B.D. Bavister (1997). 'Male pronuclear formation and early embryonic development of hamster oocytes matured *in vitro* with gonadotrophins, amino acids and cysteamine', *J. Reprod. Fertil.*, **110:** 35–46.

Kotsuji, F. et al. (1994). 'Effect of interactions between granulosa and thecal cells on meiotic arrest in bovine oocytes', *J. Reprod. Fertil.*, **100:** 151–6.

Larsen, W.J. et al. (1986). 'A dramatic loss of cumulus cell gap junctions is correlated with germinal vesicle breakdown in rat oocytes', *Dev. Biol.*, **113:** 517–21.

______(1987). 'Differential modulation of rat follicle cell gap junction population at ovulation', *Dev. Biol.*, **122:** 61–71.

Leese, H.J. and A.M. Barton (1985). 'Production of pyruvate by isolated mouse cumulus cells', *J. Exp. Zool.*, **234:** 231–6.

Lefèvre, B. et al. (1995). 'Cytoplasmic and nucleic calcium oscillations in immature mouse oocytes: Evidence of wave polarization by confocal imaging', *Exp. Cell Res.*, **218:** 166–73.

Liu, J., Compton, et al. (1997). 'Successful *in vitro* maturation of human oocytes not exposed to human chorionic gonadotropin during ovulation induction, resulting in pregnancy', *Fertil. Steril.*, **67:** 566–8.

Lorca, T. et al. (1993). 'Calmodulin-dependent protein kinase II mediates inactivation of MPF and CSF upon fertilization of xenopus eggs', *Nature*, **366:** 270–73.

Maruo, T. et al. (1993). 'Expression of epidermal growth factor and its receptor in the human ovary during follicular growth and regression', *Endocrinol.*, **132:** 924–31.

Masui, Y. and C. Markert (1971). 'Cytoplasmic control of nuclear behaviour during meiotic maturation of frog oocytes', *J. Exp. Zool.*, **177:** 129–46.

Mattioli, M. et al. (1989). 'Developmental competence of pig oocytes matured and fertilized *in vitro*', *Theriogenology.*, **31:** 1201–7.

______(1994). 'Concentration of cyclic AMP during the maturation of pig oocytes *in vivo* and *in vitro*', *J. Reprod. Fertil.*, **100:** 403–9.

______(1998). 'Calcium elevation in sheep cumulus-oocyte complexes after luteinising hormone stimulation', *Mol. Reprod. Dev.*, **50:** 361–69.

Mehlmann, L.M., and M. Terasaki et al. (1995). 'Reorganization of the endoplasmic reticulum during meiotic maturation of the mouse oocyte', *Dev. Biol.*, **170:** 607–15.

Mehlmann, L.M. et al. (1996). 'Redistribution and increase in cortical inositol 1, 4, 5 trisphosphate receptors after meiotic maturation of the mouse oocyte', *Dev. Biol.*, **180:** 489–98.

Minato, Y. and Y. Toyoda (1983). 'Development to normal young of mouse oocytes matured and fertilized *in vitro*', *Jpn. J. Zootechnol. Sci.*, **54:** 387–91.

Moor, R.M. and J.P. Heslop (1981). 'Cyclic AMP in mammalian follicle cells and oocytes during oocyte maturation', *J. Exp. Zool.*, **216:** 205–9.

Moor, R.M. et al. (1981). 'Selective effect of gonadotropins on cell coupling, nuclear maturation and protein synthesis in mammalian oocytes'.

Motilik, J. (1986). 'Changes in intercellular coupling between pig oocytes and cumulus cells during maturation *in vivo* and *in vitro*', *J. Reprod. Fertil.*, **76:** 31–7.

Motta, P.M. et al. (1994). 'Oocyte follicular cells association during development of human ovarian follicle: A study by high resolution scanning and transmission electron microscopy', *Arch. Histol. Cytol.*, **57:** 369–94.

Newton, H. (1998). 'The cryopreservation of ovarian tissue as a strategy for preserving the fertility of cancer patients', *Hum. Reprod. Update*, **4:** 237–47.

Nicolaidis, P. and M.B. Petersen (1998). 'Origin and mechanisms of non-disjunction in human autosomal trisomies', *Hum. Reprod.*, **13:** 313–9.

Ohsumi, K. and C. Katagiri (1991). 'Characterization of the ooplasmic factor inducing decondensation of and protamine removal from toad sperm nuclei: Involvement of nucleoplasmin', *Dev. Biol.*, **148:** 295–305.

O'Keefe, S.J. et al. (1991). 'The c-mos gene product is required for cyclin B accumulation during meiosis of mouse eggs', *Proc. Natl. Acad. Sci.* USA, **88:** 7869–72.

Pesce, M. et al., (1993). 'Stem cell factor and leukemia inhibitory factor promote primordial germ cell survival by suppressing programmed cell death (apoptosis)', *Dev.*, **118:** 1089–94.

Pesty, A. (1998). 'Nuclear calcium release by InsP3-receptor channels plays a role in meiosis reinitiation in the mouse oocyte', *Cell Calcium*, **24:** 239–51.

Pickering, S.J. et al. (1988). 'Cytoskeletal organization in fresh, aged and spontaneously activated human oocytes', *Hum. Reprod.*, **3:** 978–89.

Pincus, G. and E.V. Enzmann (1935). 'The comparative behaviour of mammalian eggs *in vivo* and *in vitro*. I. The activation of I-ovarian eggs', *J. Exp. Med.*, **62:** 665–75.

Prins, G.S. et al. (1987). 'Gonadotropins augment maturation and fertilization of human immature oocytes culture', *Fertil. Steril.*, **47:** 1035–7.

Racowsky, C. (1985). 'Effect of forskolin on the spontaneous maturation and cAMP content of hamster oocyte-cumulus complexes', *J. Exp. Zool.*, **234:** 87–96.

______. (1993). 'Follicular control of meiotic maturation in mammalian oocytes', in B.D. Bavister (ed.), *Preimplantation Embryo Development,* Springer-Verlag, New York, pp. 22–37.

Racowsky, C. and K.V. Baldwin (1989). '*In vitro* and *in vivo* studies reveal that hamster oocyte meiotic arrest is maintained only transiently by follicular fluid, but persistently by membrana/cumulus granulosa cell contact', *Dev. Biol.*, **134:** 297–306.

Racowsky, C. and R.A. Satterlie (1985). 'Metabolic, fluorescent dye and electrical coupling between hamster oocytes and cumulus cells during meiotic maturation *in vivo* and *in vitro*', *Dev. Biol.*, **108:** 191–202.

Resnick, J.L. et al. (1998). 'Role of fibroblast growth factors and their receptors in mouse primordial germ cell growth', *Biol. Reprod.*, **59:** 1224–9.

Roy, S.K. and P.J. Treacy (1993). 'Isolation and long term cultures of human preantral follicles', *Fertil. Steril.*, **59:** 783–90.

Russell, J.B. (1998). 'Immature oocyte retrieval combined with *in vitro* oocyte maturation', *Hum. Reprod.*, **13** Suppl 3: 63–75.

______(1997). 'Unstimulated immature oocyte retrieval: Early versus mid-follicular endometrial priming', *Fertil. Steril.*, **67:** 616–20.

Schramm, R.D. and B.D. Bavister (1995). 'Effects of granulosa cells and gonadotrophins on meiotic and developmental competence of oocytes *in vitro* in non-stimulated rhesus monkeys', *Hum. Reprod.*, 887–95.

Schroeder, A.C. and J.J. Eppig (1984). 'The developmental capacity of mouse oocytes that matured spontaneously *in vitro* is normal', *Dev. Biol.*, **102:** 493–7.

Schultz, R.M. et al. (1983). 'Regulation of mouse oocyte maturation: Implication of a decrease in oocyte cAMP and protein dephosphorylation in commitment to resume meiosis', *Dev. Biol.*, **97:** 264–73.

Shalgi, R. et al. (1979). 'The effect of LH on the fertilizability and developmental capacity of rat oocytes matured *in vitro*', *J. Reprod. Fertil.*, **55:** 429–35.

Shiraishi, K. et al. (1995). 'Developmental changes in the distribution of the endoplasmic reticulum and the inositol 1, 4, 5-trisphosphate receptors and spacial pattern of Ca^{2+} release during maturation of hamster oocytes', *Dev. Biol.*, **170:** 594–606.

Sirard, M.A. *et al.* (1988). 'The culture of bovine oocytes to obtain developmentally competent embryos', *Biol. Reprod.*, **39:** 546–52.

Spears, N. (1994). 'Mouse oocytes derived from *in vitro* grown primary ovarian follicles are fertile', *Hum. Reprod.*, **9:** 527–32.

Tanikawa, M. et al. (1998). 'Expression of c-kit messenger ribonucleic acid in human oocyte and presence of soluble c-kit in follicular fluid', *J. Clin. Endocrinol. Metab.*, **83:** 1239–42.

Tesarik, J. and C. Mendoza (1995). 'Nongenomic effects of 17 beta-estradiol on maturing human oocytes: Relationship to oocyte developmental potential', *J. Clin. Endocrinol. Metab.*, **80:** 1438–43

Trounson, A. et al. (1998). 'Oocyte maturation', *Hum. Reprod.*, **13** Suppl. 3: 52–62.

Trounson, A.O. et al. (1996). 'Maturation of human and bovine primary oocytes *in vitro* for fertilization and embryo production', *Singapore J. Obstet. Gynaecol.*, **27**: 78–84.

Trounson, A. (1994). '*In vitro* maturation and the fertilization and developmental competence of oocytes recovered from untreated polycystic ovarian patients', *Fertil. Steril.*, **62:** 353–62.

Tsafariri, A. et al. (1976). 'Inhibition of oocyte maturation by porcine follicular fluid: Partial characterization of the inhibitor', *Biol. Reprod.*, **14:** 511–6.

Vanderhyden, B.C. and D.T. Armstrong (1989). 'Role of cumulus cells and serum on the *in vitro* maturation, fertilization and subsequent development of rat oocytes', *Biol. Reprod.*, **40:** 720–28.

Verlhac, M.H. et al. (1994). 'Microtubule and chromatin behavior follow MAP kinase activity but not MPF activity during meiosis in mouse oocytes', *Development*, **120:** 1017–25.

______(1993). 'MAP kinase becomes stably activated at metaphase and is associated with microtubule-organizing centers during meiotic maturation of mouse oocytes', *Dev. Biol.*, **158:** 330–40.

Wakayama, T. et al. (1998). 'Full term development of mice from enucleated oocytes injected with cumulus cell nuclei', *Nature*, **394:** 369–74.

Wert, S.E. and W.J. Larsen (1990). 'Preendocytotic alterations in cumulus cell gap junctions precede meiotic resumption in rat cumulus-oocyte complex', *Tissue and Cell*, **22:** 827–51.

Wilmut, I. et al. (1997). 'Viable offspring derived from fetal and adult mammalian cells', *Nature*, **385:** 810–13.

Younis, A.I. et al. (1989). 'Influence of serum and hormones on bovine oocyte maturation and fertilization *in vitro*', *Gamete Res.*, **23:** 189–201.

Yoshida, M. et al. (1993). 'Glutathione concentration during maturation and after fertilization in pig oocytes: Relevance to the ability of the oocytes to form male pronucleus', *Biol. Reprod.*, **49:** 89–94.

Yoshimura, Y. et al. (1992). 'Induction of meiotic maturation of follicle-enclosed oocytes of rabbits by a transient increase followed by an abrupt decrease in cyclic AMP concentration', *J. Reprod. Fertil.*, **95:** 803–12.

Zhang, X. et al. (1993). 'Human menopausal gonadotropin during *in vitro* maturation of human oocytes retrieved from small follicles enhances *in vitro* fertilization and cleavage rates', *Fertil. Steril.*, **59:** 850–53.

6

Culturing Embryos and Gametes

Iqbal Khan

Early studies on mammalian embryo culture were predominantly restricted to the rabbit and the mouse. The culture media in these experiments were usually based upon various biological fluids. During the fifties and onwards, mouse embryos were developed in relatively simple defined media. However, preimplantation rabbit embryos needed more complex media to reach the blastocyst stage. By 1975, embryos of various other mammals, such as the sheep, ferret and rabbit, were routinely cultured from one cell to the blastocyst stage. Other species, including the cow, pig, rat and human embryos could be cultured partially (see review by Whittingham, 1977).

The birth of the first human *in vitro* baby girl on 25 July 1978 marks the beginning of a successful treatment for many infertile couples. It demonstrated that preimplantation human embryos could be cultured *in vitro* in a simple medium, and if transferred to the uterine cavity, they were capable of generating viable pregnancies. The culture medium used in this case was Earle's supplemented with pyruvate and 8% serum (Edwards, 1981).

It is fair to say that human *in vitro* fertilization and embryo transfer (IVF-ET) programmes utilized knowledge gained from animal studies, in particular on mice and hamsters. It is also very interesting that apart from human and non-human primates, most other species encounter a developmental block at some stage in their development *in vitro*. For example, in mice, this block is found at the one-cell stage, in hamsters at the 2- and 8-cell stages, and in bovine embryos at the 8-cell stage. Fortunately, the absence of a block in human embryos led to their development in various simple and complex culture media with comparative ease.

The primary aim of this chapter is to introduce recent developments in human preimplantation embryo culture, which has led to very high pregnancy and implantation rates.

PHYSICO-CHEMICAL FACTORS

TEMPERATURE

Although mouse embryos show remarkable tolerance to a brief exposure to room temperature, oocytes and embryos of other species may not be as resilient. Sheep oocytes, if exposed to a temperature of around 25°C–26°C for a brief period, show a retarded blastocyst formation *in vivo* (Moor and Crosby, 1985). Although very little data are available for human oocytes and embryos, it is reported that if human oocytes are exposed to room temperature for a brief period, it may cause irreversible disruption of the meiotic spindle (Pickering et al., 1990). Therefore, it is of the utmost importance to keep the human oocytes and embryos at an optimum temperature when they are outside the incubator. It is useful to use heated microscope stages and multiblock heaters to minimize temperature loss. Daily temperature checks are essential because overheating of these instruments would surely be lethal to the developing oocytes and embryos.

LIGHT

The use of fluorescent lights (short wavelength light) in the laboratory, especially in the laminar flow hoods, should be avoided. Hirao and Yanigamachi (1978) showed that if hamster oocytes were exposed briefly to fluorescent light, it was detrimental to fertilization. Similarly, rabbit embryos were adversely affected by short wavelength light (Daniel, 1964). Deterioration of the culture media and the formation of cytotoxic products have also been blamed on this source of light (MacMichael, 1986). It is prudent not to use fluorescent light in the lab. If it cannot be avoided, it should be covered with red filters. An alternative light source could be another solution.

Gas Phase

The type of gases and their composition in a culture system are of utmost importance, as they play a very important part in metabolism and pH control. The use of 5% CO_2 in air and, to a lesser extent, 5% CO_2, 5% O_2, 90% N_2 has become a standard gas phase for human embryo culture. However, several studies do point towards the deleterious nature of atmospheric oxygen (20%), or the beneficial nature of low oxygen tension on cell culture (Packer and Fuehr, 1977; Lim et al., 1999; Dumoulin et al., 1999). It seems logical to use 5% or less O_2 in the culture system as human oocytes and embryos reside and propagate *in vivo* in an atmosphere that is slightly away from blood capillaries. More recently, Gardner et al. (1999) showed that reduced oxygen in a culture system (G series) was responsible for increased blastocyst cell number, which led to high implantation rate (31% vs 64%).

pH

The culture media used for human oocyte and embryo development usually have a pH in the range of 7.35°–7.4°. There are two essential components which control the culture media pH: (1) 25mM HCO_3 and (2) 5% CO_2. The optimum pH for the development of human embryos is difficult to ascertain, as they seem to grow normally in a pH range of 7.2 to 7.5. However, certain culture media, such as P1, require a pH of 7.2 to 7.25 for optimum cell growth. This could be achieved by regulating the CO_2 in an incubator. Therefore, it is essential for each laboratory to find the exact pH of the particular media it is using, in order to achieve optimum embryo development. In our laboratory, the optimum pH range falls between 7.25–7.35 and it is very strictly controlled.

To summarize, human preimplantation embryos grow optimally at 37°C when they are placed in a culture medium with an osmotic pressure of around 280 mosm. The pH (7.25–7.35) of a medium is maintained by either 5% CO_2 in air, or 5% CO_2, and 5% O_2 in nitrogen. Recently, with the development of sequential culture media, these values are adjusted to accommodate optimal growth. For example, the P1 medium, which does not have glucose and phosphate but has taurine, requires a pH of 7.2. This has been achieved by increasing the incubator CO_2 concentration from the regular 5% to 6%. Similarly, in G1.2 media, the osmotic pressure is adjusted to 260 mosm instead of the usual 280 mosm. With the emphasis shifting to the transfer of embryos from the second or third day to day 5 (blastocyst), it is essential for embryologists to be aware of the exact culture conditions required for these media.

CULTURE MEDIA

There are two types of culture media available for human embryos.

1. Balanced salt solutions
2. Complex media

1. Balanced Salt Solutions-Based Media

These are simple media composed of a few essential salts and usually supplemented with an energy source, such as pyruvate, lactate or both, and a protein source, i.e., human serum albumin or bovine serum albumin. The most commonly used solution-based media in IVF are Earle's (Edwards,1981), T6 (Whittingham, 1971) and HTF (Quinn et al., 1985).

2. Complex Media

These media are composed of amino acids, vitamins, nucleic acid precursors and usual salts. They are also supplemented with serum or albumin. The most commonly used complex medium is Ham's F-10 (Ham, 1963). B1 and B2 (Menezo et al., 1984) and M3 (Medi-Cult) are also complex media, used mostly in France and the European countries.

Composition Of Culture Media

In vitro culture media are based on the following components:

1. Water
2. Inorganic ions
3. Essential metabolites
   a. Carbohydrates (energy source)
   b. Amino acids
   c. Vitamins
   d. Protein
   e. Buffer system

1. Water

Water is by far the single most important component of culture media. It constitutes around 99% of a medium. There are two sources of water: (1) ground water, and (2) surface water. Ground water comes from the clouds, while surface water comes from river reservoirs. Ground water usually contains significant concentrations of dissolved solids, but is low in colloidal organic particle content. This may be due to natural filtration through the soil.

Surface water usually has a higher content of organic and particle matter, but has a low concentration of dissolved solids. Both surface and ground water are usually contaminated with a variety of unwanted substances, for example, fertilizers and undissolved wastes.

Removal of contamination from water is essential before it can be used for culture media. In earlier studies in mice, Whittingham (1971) showed that when a culture medium was prepared with triple-distilled water instead of double-distilled water, the development of 2-cell embryos to blastocysts was faster and better. Distillation of water has been abandoned in favour of reverse osmosis since it was demonstrated that possible leaching of ions from glass and the accumulation of pyrogen have a deleterious effect on growing embryos. At present, Millipore reverse osmosis (RO) and the Milli-Q system, or a similar purification system, are utilized for the preparation of culture media. This water is pyrogen-free and has a resistivity of above 18 megahom.

Before setting up a filtration system, analysis of the feed water source is very important. The tests will reveal the extent of contamination in the water—the chlorine, silica, pH, iron, bacteria, as well as water residues. For complete details on water quality control, and management for culture media grade water, please refer to the excellent review article by Weimer et al. (1998).

2. Inorganic Ions

All mammalian embryos require inorganic ions, in addition to those involved in the regulation of osmotic pressure and hydrogen ion concentration. In most cases, the ions required are sodium, potassium, calcium, magnesium, iron, carbonate, phosphate, and probably sulphate. Mammalian embryos, including human, can be developed in a variety of media with different ionic compositions, e.g., Earle's (Edwards, 1981 & 1985); T6 (Whittingham, 1971); HTF (Quinn et al., 1985); Ham's F-10 (Ham, 1963); B1 and B2 (Menezo et al., 1984) and the recently formulated P1 (Pool et al., 1998); Blastocyst media (Behr et al., 1997); BIX (Quinn, 1995); and G-series (Gardner et al., 1998a). Wales (1970) has reported ranges of ionic concentration which support the growth of 2-cell mouse embryos to blastocyst *in vitro*: the potassium concentration ranged from 0.4 to 48 mM, the magnesium concentration from 0 to 9.6 mM, and the phosphate concentration 0 to 7.2 mM.

It seems that oviduct fluid from humans and mice has high potassium and chloride ion concentration (Gardner and Leese., 1990). There are conflicting reports regarding the effects of high potassium ion concentration on culture media. Roblero et al. (1990) reported that it stimulates the fertilizing capacity of sperm and enhances embryo development. However, others reported a negative effect on embryo cleavage (Gardner and Sakkas,1993).

The osmotic pressure of most mammalian fluids is usually due to sodium chloride. However, the glucose concentration is also responsible for a significant part of the osmotic pressure of the medium. If the glucose concentration is raised, it may affect the osmotic pressure. Although the prescribed osmolality for the human *in vitro* culture media is around 280 mosm, mouse embryo development showed enhancement when the osmolality was reduced (Lawitts and Biggers, 1991; Bavister and McKiernan, 1992).

3. Essential Metabolites

a. Carbohydrates: A carbohydrate source seems to be essential for developing embryos. The most commonly available source is glucose, although pyruvate is utilized in the early stages. As embryo development reaches beyond the 4-cell stage, more and more glucose is utilized (Whitten and Biggers, 1968; Lawitts and Biggers, 1991). There are several recent *in vitro* studies which implicate glucose in early cleavage arrest in the mouse and hamster (see review article by Gardner and Lane, 1993a). These data suggest that early embryos, including human, do not use glycolysis as their pathway prior to the blastocyst stage.

b. Amino Acids: Although human preimplantation embryos have been grown from zygotes to blastocysts in simple salt solutions that lack amino acids, vitamins, etc., recent studies suggest that their inclusion in a culture medium significantly increases both pregnancy and implantation rates (Gardner et al., 1998a, b). It has been established for quite a while that animal cells have a specific requirement for amino acids. Mammalian oocytes and embryos are no exception in this regard. Furthermore, the female reproductive tract of the mouse (Gardner and Leese, 1990) and rabbit (Miller and Schultz, 1987) contains substantial levels of free amino acids. Gardner and Lane (1993) reported a significant increase in the rates of cleavage, blastocyst formation and hatching when mouse zygotes were exposed to amino acids that were present in high levels *in vivo*. Furthermore, amino acids that had low levels in oviductal fluid caused a significant reduction in cleavage and hatching rates.

c. Vitamins: Although the vitamin B group is important in amino acid and carbohydrate metabolism, its specific role is unclear. There are many mammalian species, including humans, which can develop from zygotes to blastocysts without vitamins.

d. Protein: In the early period of IVF, 5%–15% maternal serum was used in the embryo culture medium by the majority of clinics. At present, few IVF centres still use either the patient's serum or donor cord serum. The majority of IVF laboratories have switched to human serum albumin (HSA) or synthetic serum substitute (SSS, supplied by Irvine Scientific, CA), for both culture and embryo transfer. It is advisable to quality-control the HSA as batch-to-batch differences in its ability to support embryo development are not uncommon.

Culture Media: Past and Present

In the eighties and early nineties, most IVF centres in Europe and Australia were using simple salt solution-based media, while in the United States, Ham's F-10, a complex medium containing amino acids and vitamins, was used most extensively. These media were supplemented with maternal or cord serum as a protein source. Due to variability in growth and development of embryos caused by patient-to-patient differences in serum quality, as well as the time-consuming preparation technique, serum was replaced in culture media by human serum albumin (Staessen et al., 1990; Khan et al., 1991).

Simple salt solution-based media were originally designed for the development of mouse embryos (Whitten and Biggers, 1968). These media, with very little modification, are still in use for human IVF, i.e., Earle's (Edwards, 1981; Khan et al., 1991); T6 (Whittingham, 1971), and Hams F-10 (Ham, 1963). These early media were effective in fertilization and the development of zygotes to 4 to 8-cell-stage embryos. At those stages, they were put back either into the uterine cavity or the fallopian tubes of the patient. The main criticism levelled against these media was that too few embryos reached full-term pregnancy after their transfer. Furthermore, if left in culture, fewer embryos reached the blastocyst stage. There was very little difference in the ability of these media to grow human embryos. A study of four different media, i.e., modified Whitten's, Hams F-10, T6 and

Earle's, has found no significant difference in fertilization, cleavage and pregnancy rates (Mohr et al., 1983).

There is no doubt that an improvement in culture conditions, especially in the culture medium, is required. The low pregnancy rates or low rate of blastocyst formation could be the result of the existing suboptimal culture media. To that effect, Quinn et al. (1985) were the first to design a culture medium that was based on the ionic composition of the human oviduct. In continuation of this trend, various *in vivo* studies have indicated that the lumen of the oviduct has no static environment, and the changes in the concentration of metabolites, amino acids and vitamins take place according to the time of the cycle and region of the oviduct (Gardner and Lane, 1996). Gardner and Lane (1993) showed that mouse embryo development was enhanced in a culture medium containing amino acids. Furthermore, studies by the same authors (Gardner and Lane, 1996) showed that Eagle's non-essential amino acids, with glutamine and EDTA, can bypass the 2-cell block in CFI mouse embryos in culture and subsequently lead to a high rate of blastocyst development.

These studies point towards a requirement for a sequential *in vitro* culture medium which can fulfil not only the nutritional needs of a developing embryo, but also avoid the unnecessary cell stress caused by high levels of certain substances present in some culture media. For example, the exposure of embryos to simple salt solution-based media such as Earle's or HTF, which contain high levels of glucose and phosphate, was deleterious to developing embryos (Conaghan et al., 1993). This observation and similar others led to the new formulation of culture media based on modified HTF, which did not have glucose and phosphate, e.g., the P1 medium (Pool et al., 1998) and B IX medium (Quinn, 1995). These media, supplemented with 10% HSA or SSS, were very successful in culturing zygotes to 4 to 8-cell-stage embryos. Transfer of such embryos led to significantly higher pregnancy and implantation rates, compared to embryos cultured in the regular HTF. Furthermore, when P1-grown 8-cell-stage embryos were placed in the Blastocyst medium (Irvine Scientific) supplemented with 10%–15% SSS, blastocyst formation increased to 53.5% (Behr et al., 1997 & 1999).

However, Gardner and Lane (1993; 1996) and Gardner et al. (1998a) proposed another alternative with similar high implantation rates, as reported above, with the P1 and Blastocyst media. Their sequential media (G1 & G2) were the result of their extensive animal studies. They kept a low concentration of glucose in their G1 medium, which also had Eagle's non-essential amino acids, taurine and EDTA. The addition of a low concentration of glucose in the G1 medium and a slightly higher concentration in the G2 medium was in line with the observation that both oviductal fluid and the uterine cavity contain glucose in that proportion. Furthermore, the deleterious nature of glucose in the early developmental stages, observed by many, could be offset by the presence of amino acids and EDTA in these media (Gardner and Lane, 1993; Gardner et al., 1998a). Recently, G1 and G2 media have been replaced with a new 'improved' version, G1.2 and G2.2 media, available commercially through IVF Scandinavia.

Comparative studies with G1 and G2 media on day-3 (8-cell-stage) versus day-5 (blastocyst) transfer show a significantly higher implantation rate in the latter (30% vs 51%) (Gardner et al., 1998a, b). Similarly, Behr et al. (1999) achieved 53.5% blastocyst formation by using P1 and Blastocyst media. They reported a 50% implantation rate when 3 fresh blastocysts were transferred.

In conclusion, although the transfer of only one or two blastocysts could reduce the occurrence of multiple gestation, one must make a change in their culture system with utmost caution. Laboratories, which were geared to transfer embryos at the 4- or 8-cell stage, should first achieve an acceptable blastocyst formation rate in their patient's supernumerary embryos before attempting a blastocyst transfer. Furthermore, the results summarized above should be viewed in proper context. The patients who would gain maximum benefit from two or three blastocyst transfers are those who are young and at high risk for multiple gestation. At present, it is not clear how patients of advanced maternal age (with few oocytes) would fare under this new blastocyst transfer policy (Behr et al., 1999).

REFERENCES

Bavister, B.D. and S.H. McKiernan (1992). 'Regulation of hamster embryo development *in vitro* by amino acids', in B.D. Bavister (ed.), *Preimplantation Embryo Development*, Plenum Press, New York.

Behr, B., et al. (1997). 'Human blastocyst development *in vitro* without co-culture using a sequential culture system', *Poc. Am. Soc. Rep. Med.*, p. 81.

______(1999). 'Preliminary clinical experience with human blastocyst development *in vitro* without co-culture', *Hum. Reprod.*, **14**: 454–7.

Conaghan, J. et al. (1993). 'Effect of pyruvate and glucose on the development of human preimplantation embryos *in vitro*', *J. Reprod. Fertil.*, **99**: 87–95.

Daniel, J.C. (1964). 'Cleavage of mammalian ova inhibited by visible light', *Exp. Cell. Res.*, **29**: 515.

Dumoulin, J.C.M. et al. (1999). 'Effect of oxygen concentration on human *in vitro* fertilization and embryo culture', *Hum. Reprod.*, **14**: 465–9.

Edwards, R.G. (1981). 'Test-tube babies', *Nature*, **293**: 253.

Edwards, R.G. (1985). '*In vitro* fertilization and embryo replacement: Opening lecture', *Ann. N.Y. Acad. Sci.*, **442**: 1–22.

Gardner, D.K. and H.J. Leese (1990). 'Concentration of nutrients in mouse oviduct fluid and their effect on embryo development and metabolism *in vitro*', *J. Reprod. Fertil.*, **88**: 361.

Gardner, D.K. and D. Sakkas (1993). 'Mouse embryo cleavage, metabolism and viability: Role of medium composition', *Hum. Reprod.*, **8**: 288–95.

Gardner, D.K. and M. Lane (1993). 'Embryo culture systems', in A Trounson and D.K. Gardner (eds.), *Handbook of in vitro fertilization.*, CRC Press, Boca Raton, FL, USA, pp. 85–114.

______(1996). 'Alleviation of the '2-cell block' and development to the blastocyst of CFI mouse embryos: Role of amino acids, EDTA and physical factors', *Hum. Reprod.*, **11**: 2703–12.

Gardner, D.K. et al. (1998a). 'Culture and transfer of human blastocysts increases implantation rates and reduces the need for multiple embryo transfers', *Fertil. Steril.*, **69**: 84–8.

______(1998b). 'A prospective randomized trial of blastocyst culture and transfer in human *in vitro* fertilization', *Hum. Reprod.*, **13**: 3434–40.

______(1999). 'Reduced oxygen tension increases blastocyst development, differentiation and viability', Abstract in: ASRM/CFS Conjoint Annual Meeting in Toronto, Ontario, Canada, September, pp. 25–30, S30–S31.

Ham, R.G. (1963). 'An improved nutrient solution for diploid Chinese hamster and human cell lines', *Exp. Cell. Res.*, **29**: 515–26.

Hirao, Y. and R. Yanagimachi (1978). 'Detrimental effect of visible light on meiosis of mammalian eggs *in vitro*', *J. Exp. Zool.*, **206**: 365–70.

Khan, I. et al. (1991). 'Human serum albumin versus serum: A comparative study on embryo transfer medium', *Fertil. Steril.*, **56**: 98.

Lawitts, J.A., and J.D. Biggers (1991). 'Overcoming the 2-cell block by modifying the standard components in a mouse embryo culture medium', *Biol. Reprod.*, **45**: 245.

Lim, J.M. et al. (1999). 'Development of *in vitro*-derived bovine embryos cultured in 5% CO_2 in air or in 5% O_2, 5% CO_2 and 90% N_2', *Hum. Reprod.*, **14**: 458–64.

MacMichael, G. (1986). 'The adverse effect of UV and short-wavelength visible radiation on tissue culture', *Amer. Biotechnol. Laboratory*, **4**: 30–31.

Menezo, Y.J.R. et al. (1984). 'Serum is not necessary in human *in vitro* fertilization, early embryo culture, and transfer', *Fertil. Steril.*, **58**: 479.

Miller, J.G.D. and G.A. Schultz (1987). 'Amino acid content of preimplantation rabbit embryos and fluids of the reproductive tract', *Biol. Reprod.*, **36**: 125.

Mohr, L.R. et al. (1983). 'Evaluation of human egg *in vitro*', in H.M. Beier, H.R. Linden (eds.), *Fertilization of the Human Egg in vitro*, Springer-Verlag, Berlin, p. 211.

Moor, J.G.O. and I.M. Crosby (1985). 'Temperature-induced abnormalities in sheep oocytes during maturation', *J. Reprod. Fertil.*, **75**: 467–73.

Packer, L. and K. Fuehr (1977). 'Low oxygen concentration extends the lifespan of cultured human diploid cells', *Nature* (London), **267**: 423–5.

Pickering, S.J. et al. (1990). 'Transient cooling to room temperature can cause irreversible disruption of the meiotic spindle in the human oocyte', *Fertil. Steril.*, **54**: 102–8.

Pool, T.B. et al. (1998). 'Oocyte and embryo culture, basic concepts and recent advances', *Infertil. Reprod. Med. Clin. N. Am.*, **9**: 181–203.

Quinn, P. et al. (1985). 'Improved pregnancy rate in human *in vitro* fertilization with the use of medium based on the composition of human tubal fluid', *Fertil. Steril.*, **44**: 493–8.

Quinn, P. (1995). 'Enhanced results in mouse and human embryo culture using a modified human tubal fluid medium lacking glucose and phosphate', *J. Assist. Reprod. Genet.*, **12**: 97–105.

Roblero, L.S. et al. (1990). 'High potassium concentration and the cumulus corona oocyte complex stimulate the fertilizing capacity of human spermatozoa', *Fertil. Steril.*, **54**: 328.

Staessen, C. et al. (1990). 'Comparison between human serum and albuminar-20 (TM) supplement for *in vitro* fertilization', *Hum. Reprod.*, **5**: 336.

Wales, R.G. (1970). 'Effects of ions on development of the preimplantation mouse embryo *in vitro*', *Aust. J. Biol.*, **23**: 421.

Weimer, K.E. et al. (1998). 'The importance of water quality for media preparation', in Brian Dale (ed.), *Development of the Human Embryo in vitro*, Oxford University Press, vol. 13, suppl. 4, pp. 166–72.

Whitten, W.K. and J.D. Biggers (1968). 'Complete development *in vitro* of the preimplantation stages of the mouse in a simple chemically defined medium', *J. Reprod. Fertil.*, **17**: 399.

Whittingham, D.G. (1971). 'Culture of mouse ova', *J. Reprod. Fertil. Suppl.*, **14**: 7.

______(1975). 'Fertilization, early development and storage of mammalian ova *in vitro*', in M. Balls and A.E. Wild (eds.), *The Early Development of Mammals*, Cambridge University Press, Cambridge, pp. 1–24.

7

Assisted Reproduction in Women with Polycystic Ovaries

K. Joo Thong and David T. Baird

INTRODUCTION

Polycystic ovarian syndrome (PCOS) is the commonest cause of oligomenorrhoea, recurrent miscarriage (Sagle et al., 1998), anovulatory infertility (Hull, 1987) and hirsutism (Adams et al., 1986). First described by Stein and Leventhal in 1935, the aetiology remains the subject of speculation. This heterogeneous disorder ranges from findings of polycystic ovarian morphology, as detected by pelvic ultrasound, to the other end of the spectrum with accompanying obesity, menstrual irregularity and hyperandrogenism, which may occur alone or in combination.

INCIDENCE OF PCOS

Using ultrasound as the criterion for diagnosis, Adams et al. (1986) found that 57% of women with anovulation and 92% with idiopathic hirsutism had PCOS. Interestingly, Polson et al. (1988) reported findings of polycystic ovaries in 22% of 149 'normal' female volunteers. In this study, a majority of the women with a diagnosis of polycystic ovaries on pelvic scan had menstrual irregularity, and a quarter had elevated luteinizing hormone (LH) on a single random blood test.

The ultrasonic appearance of polycystic ovaries was reported in 92% of families of women with PCOS (Hague et al., 1988). It is likely that the mode of inheritance is similar to that of non-insulin-dependent diabetes mellitus (Alcolado and Alcolado, 1991).

AETIOLOGY

The importance of genetic and environmental factors in the aetiology of PCOS is not known. Although inherited enzyme abnormalities, such as deficiencies of 21-hydroxylase and 3β-hydroxysteroid dehydrogenase, can result in a clinical and ovarian phenotype that is similar to PCOS, it is likely that these disorders account for a small proportion of PCOS. The high prevalence of polycystic ovaries in families of affected individuals is suggestive of a genetic component to the disease (Hague et al., 1988; Carey et al., 1993). A single base change in the promoter region of CYP17 (gene encoding P450c17α) is associated with the PCOS phenotype, but this is not the main causative gene in families with PCOS (Carey et al., 1993). A recent study of 150 families screened for 37 candidate genes demonstrated that follistatin (5p14), the binding protein for activin, was most closely linked to hyperandrogenism and menstrual irregularity (Urman et al., 1999).

PCOS is associated with or may be the result of dysregulated activity of 17α-hydroxylase/17–20 lyase in the ovary (Rosenfield et al., 1990). The available evidence suggests that more than one gene is involved, with environmental factors having a major influence on the clinical and biochemical expression of the syndrome.

The importance of environmental factors was demonstrated in a study of twins, which demonstrated discordance between twin pairs in assessment of ovarian morphology based on pelvic ultrasound (Jahanfar, 1995). A concordance of some biochemical markers, e.g., sex hormone binding globulin (SHBG), was reported. The criticisms of this study were: the selection bias at recruitment and the high prevalence of PCO, i.e. 50%, which was higher than in the normal population.

DIAGNOSIS

At present, there is no consensus definition of PCOS or polycystic ovary on ultrasound appearance. The diagnosis of PCOS is made on the basis of the clinical presentation and ultrasound findings. Using high-resolution ultrasound, it is relatively easy to identify the polycystic ovaries. Polycystic ovaries are described as containing 10 or more cysts, 2–8 mm in diameter, arranged around a dense stroma or scattered throughout the increased stroma (Adams et al., 1985). These findings can be distinguished from multifollicular ovaries, which are found in weight loss-related amenorrhoea and during puberty. There is no increase in the ovarian stroma and the cysts are larger in multifollicular ovaries (Adams et al., 1985).

The appearance of polycystic ovaries can be identified from the age of 6 years (Bridges et al., 1993) and it is difficult to establish at what age they first appear on the pelvic ultrasound. For practising clinicians, it is important to distinguish between PCOS and polycystic ovaries. In PCOS, the definition is applicable to women with menstrual irregularity, hyperandrogenism (acne, seborrhoea, hirsutism) or obesity, and these are found in association with polycystic ovaries.

The endocrinological abnormalities found in PCOS are varied, and are often associated with elevated LH, prolactin, androgens (e.g., testosterone, androstenedione) and oestrogens. Raised plasma LH concentration is found in 40% of women (Balen et al., 1995), and moderate hyperprolactinaemia (between 600–2000 mU/l) is reported. In PCOS, the acyclical oestrogen production may stimulate the pituitary lactotrophs, resulting in hyperprolactinaemia (Franks et al., 1985). The high oestrogen level found in women with PCOS results from the extraovarian conversion of androstenedione, which largely takes place in the adipose tissue.

In a recent study of ovarian morphology using a 3-dimensional ultrasound, it was found that the main reason for the increase in ovarian volume was the increased stroma (Kyei-Mensah et al., 1998). In addition, colour and pulsed Doppler ultrasound demonstrated that the stroma of polycystic ovaries has a very high blood flow (Zaidi et al., 1995). This is consistent with histological studies showing an increased stromal vascularity (Goldzeiher et al., 1962) and large amounts of vascular endothelial growth factor (VEGF) in the thecal cells of the polycystic ovary.

PRETREATMENT COUNSELLING PRIOR TO *IN VITRO* FERTILIZATION (IVF)

Women with PCOS seeking infertility treatment may have anovulation as the cause of infertility or any other causes of infertility. If anovulation is the cause of infertility, anti-oestrogens such as clomiphene citrate or tamoxifen should be prescribed to induce ovulation. In clomiphene-resistant cases, gonadotrophin treatment is next in the line of treatment. IVF should be offered only after 4–6 cycles of unsuccessful gonadotrophin therapy. Women with PCOS may sometimes respond poorly to ovarian stimulation during the IVF treatment and this should form part of the initial counselling.

The pretreatment counselling should include an explanation of the drugs to be administered and advice as to the potential complications, such as ovarian hyperstimulation syndrome (OHSS) and multiple pregnancies. At this appointment, it is important to stress to obese women that optimal weight loss is essential prior to the commencement of assisted conception.

The two main features of the pretreatment counselling are—(1) the likelihood of women with PCOS overstimulating due to the multiple antral follicles of the polycystic ovaries, and (2) the endocrine and metabolic disorder(s) in women with PCOS. The hyperandrogenism and hyperinsulinism in PCOS may complicate pregnancy. Hyperinsulinaemia may result in obesity associated with gestational diabetes, hypertension and pre-eclampsia (MacGillvray, 1983; Treharne, 1984). Advising obese women to go on a diet in order to achieve an ideal weight may reduce the risk of pre-eclampsia.

Women with PCOS should be counselled with respect to the increased rate of miscarriage as a result of an abnormal endocrine milieu and elevated LH, possibly affecting oocyte maturation or endometrial receptivity (Sagle et al., 1988; Regan et al., 1990). To date, there is no evidence of an increased risk of congenital anomalies in women with PCOS.

DOWNREGULATION IN ASSISTED CONCEPTION

Currently, the gonadotrophin-releasing hormone (GnRH)-agonist is routinely used prior to stimulation of the ovaries, using human menopausal gonadotrophin (hMG) or recombinant gonadotrophins. Pituitary desensitization suppresses the raised LH and androgen levels in women with PCOS. The long protocol is widely used as it reduces the necessity of cancelling IVF cycles and, therefore, the clinical pregnancy rate per cycle started is increased (Hughes et al., 1992; Antoine et al., 1996). However, women with PCOS are more likely to hyperstimulate on the long protocol (Salat-Baroux et al., 1990).

In clinical practice, the short or the long protocol using GnRH-agonist for downregulation results in the retrieval of significantly more oocytes from women with polycystic ovaries than normal ovaries (Jacobs et al., 1987). It has been demonstrated that prolonged downregulation of up to 30 days reduces the androgen levels, but does not increase the pregnancy rate (Salat Baroux et al., 1988).

The GnRH-antagonist, Cetrorelix, was recently marketed in the United Kingdom for downregulation in assisted conception. The efficacy of the combination of Cetrorelix and human menopausal gonadotrophins for IVF was reported (Diedrich et al., 1994; Felberbaum et al., 1995; Olivennes et al., 1995). However, there are no data on the efficacy of Cetrorelix and hMG or recombinant FSH for the specific treatment of women with PCOS. Further randomized studies will be required to investigate the efficacy of GnRH-antagonist versus GnRH-agonist for pituitary desensitization in women with PCOS.

CONTROLLED OVARIAN STIMULATION (COS)

The main aim of COS is to enable multifollicular development, resulting in collection of mature oocytes and avoiding ovarian hyperstimulation syndrome. Before the use of GnRH-agonist for downregulation, ovarian stimulation was carried out using clomiphene citrate, with or without hMG or FSH, or using high-dose gonadotrophins alone. The main disadvantages of this form of ovarian stimulation were a premature LH surge with ovulation prior to oocyte recovery, or premature luteinization, resulting in poor-quality oocytes.

In women with PCOS, usually a large number of oocytes are retrieved, but there is poor fertilization and implantation (Dor et al., 1990; Aboulghar et al., 1997). Overall, the pregnancy rate is similar to that of a control group of women, but there is a higher miscarriage rate (Dor et al., 1990). Recent reports suggested that the poor fertilization rate may be due to the poor quality of oocytes in women with PCOS (Cano et al., 1997; Aboulghar et al., 1997).

TYPES OF GONADOTROPHINS

There is some debate on the optimal agent, hMG or FSH alone, for superovulation for women with PCOS. For years, hMG, which is extracted from the urine of menopausal women, has been used for ovarian stimulation. It contains a mixture of LH and FSH, with urinary contaminants. LH is necessary for the stimulation of thecal androgen production, but the amount of LH required for follicular development and steroidogenesis is minimal. Women with PCOS may have elevated LH and there are theoretical grounds for the administration of FSH alone to minimize the circulating LH levels. To date, most studies found no benefit of FSH alone over hMG in IVF treatment (Tanbo et al., 1990; Salat Baroux et al., 1988; Larsen et al., 1990). When hMG is administered to women at a pharmacological dosage, it will result only in a slight elevation of the serum LH level and this is the likely explanation for the above findings.

Daya (1995), in a metanalysis of eight randomized studies, found a higher pregnancy rate in women given FSH alone in comparison to hMG. This metanalysis should be interpreted with caution as it included small studies, and women with normal and polycystic ovaries were included.

RECOMBINANT VERSUS PURIFIED URINARY FSH

Highly purified FSH used for COS contains urinary contaminants. Recombinant gonadotrophins (Gonal-F[R] and Puregon) are commercially available and are virtually free of proteins (Loumaye et al., 1995; Mannaerts et al., 1996). The efficacy and safety of recombinant FSH (r-FSH) has been demonstrated in clinical trials (Bergh et al., 1997; Out et al., 1996). In a large randomized study carried out by Organon, comparing r-FSH (Puregon) with Metrodin (Serono), significantly more oocytes were retrieved in the r-FSH group. The pregnancy rate was higher if pregnancy resulting from frozen embryo replacement was included (Out et al., 1996). However, there are no randomized studies comparing r-FSH with urinary gonadotrophins for women with PCOS undergoing assisted conception treatment. It is likely that r-FSH has a higher bioactivity (Mannaerts et al., 1996), and it is prudent to consider starting women under 35 years with PCOS at 100–150 IU of recombinant FSH for COS.

REDUCING THE RISK OF OHSS

In women undergoing assisted conception treatment, the responsiveness of the PCO ovaries to gonadotrophin stimulation is monitored using transvaginal ultrasound alone or in combination with serum oestradiol. Women who are at risk of OHSS are those who are less than 35 years, having more than 20 follicles on the day of hCG and whose serum oestradiol is more than 8000 pmol/L on the day of hCG. Currently, serum oestradiol is the only widely used biochemical predictor in women at risk of OHSS. Although the threshold for withholding hCG to trigger ovulation will vary from different centres—and this has ranged from 800 pg/mL to 4000 pg/mL (2900 to 14,500 pml/L) (Schenker, 1993; Haning et al., 1983)—it is important to remember that in one study, 38% of women with severe OHSS had a serum oestradiol of 22,000 pmol/L on the day of hCG (Asch et al., 1991). Withholding hCG to trigger ovulation is the most widely used method to prevent OHSS in women deemed at risk of developing the syndrome. Following this, it would be prudent to advise the woman to continue with pituitary downregulation for a further two weeks, or for a shorter period if she has her menses within two weeks. Therefore, the treatment for each woman should be individualized.

In women at risk of OHSS, reports have suggested that delaying hCG or 'coasting' (Urman et al., 1992; Sher et al., 1993) may reduce the risk of OHSS and reduce a cancellation of cycles. The serum oestradiol in these 'at-risk' women is measured serially until it drops to 10,000 pmol/L. Despite prolonged 'coasting', severe OHSS has been reported (Waldenstrom et al., 1999) and couples should be informed of this risk if prolonged 'coasting' is offered as a choice of treatment.

Regular and careful transvaginal scanning, together with serum oestradiol monitoring are recommended to reduce the occurrence of severe OHSS in women with PCOS. In its severe form, OHSS is associated with ascites, pleural effusion, ovarian enlargement with cyst formation and electrolyte imbalance (Golan et al., 1989). Disseminated intravascular coagulation, oliguria and fatalities have been reported in women with severe OHSS.

LUTEAL SUPPORT

There is no uniform approach to luteal-phase support (Seppala, 1985). Centres either use progesterone and its derivatives, hCG, a combination of both, or no luteal support. Following downregulation with GnRH-agonist, the effect of these agents on the corpora lutea may result in luteal-phase insufficiency if luteal-phase progesterone is omitted (Smitz et al., 1988). With the recent introduction of GnRH-antagonist in clinical practice and in the absence of data which does not demonstrate the absence of luteal-phase insufficiency, clinicians should continue luteal phase support in these women.

The administration of hCG for luteal support is known to increase the incidence of OHSS (Golan et al., 1988). As there is no convincing data that the administration of hCG will result in a higher pregnancy rate, many centres now administer progesterone derivatives, either in the form of pessaries, gel or intramuscular injection.

CONCLUSION

The management of women with PCOS undergoing assisted conception is challenging to clinicians. The accompanying metabolic and endocrine disorder in women with PCOS requires a follow-up of these women following treatment. The evidence suggests that assisted conception treatment is an effective therapy for PCOS women who are refractory to ovulation induction *in vivo,* or who have co-existing infertility disorders.

REFERENCES

Aboulghar, M.A. et al. (1997). 'Oocyte quality in patients with severe ovaraian hyperstimulation syndrome', *Fertil. Steril.*, **68**: 1017–21.

Adams, J. et al. (1985). 'Multifollicular ovaries: Clinical and endocrine features and response to pulsatile gonadotrophin releasing hormone', *Lancet*, **2**: 1375–8.

Adams, J., D.W. Polson, S. Franks (1986). 'Prevalence of polycystic ovaries in women with anovulation and idiopathic hirsutism', *Br. Med. J.*, **293**: 355–9.

Alcolado, J.C., R. Alcolado (1991). 'Importance of maternal history of non-insulin dependent diabetic patients', *Br. Med. J.*, **302**: 1178–80.

Antoine, J.M. et al. (1996). 'Ovarian stimulation using human menopausal gonadotrophins with or without LHRH analogues in a long protocol for *in vitro* fertilisation: A prospective randomised comparison', *Hum. Reprod.*, **5**: 565–9.

Asch, R.H. et al. (1991). 'Severe ovarian hyperstimulation syndrome in assisted reproductive technology: Definition of high risk groups', *Hum. Reprod.*, **61**: 1395–9.

Balen, A.H. et al. (1995). 'Polycystic ovary syndrome: The spectrum of the disorder in 1741 patients', *Hum. Reprod.*, **8**: 2107–11.

Bergh, C. et al. (1997). 'Recombinant human follicle stimulating hormone (r-hFSH; Gonal-F) versus highly purified urinary FSH (Metrodin HP): Results of a randomized comparative study in women undergoing assisted reproductive techniques', *Hum. Reprod.*, **12**: 2133–9.

Bridges, N.A. et al. (1993). 'Standards for ovarian volume in childhood and puberty', *Fertil Steril.*, **60**: 456–60.

Cano, F. et al. (1997). 'Oocyte quality in polycystic ovaries revisted: Identification of a particular subgroup of women', *J. Ass. Reprd. Genet.*, **14**: 254–61.

Carey, A.H. et al. (1993). 'Evidence for a single gene defect in polycystic ovaries and male pattern baldness', *Clin. Endocrinol.*, **38**: 653–8.

Daya, S. (1995). 'Follicle stimulating hormone versus human menopausal gonadotrophin for *in vitro* fertilization: Results of a meta-analysis', *Horm. Res.*, **43**: 224–9.

Diedrich, K. et al. (1994). 'Suppression of the endogenous luteinizing hormone surge by the gonadotrophin-releasing hormone antagonist Cetrorelix during ovarian stimulation', *Hum. Reprod.*, **9**: 788–91.

Dor, J. et al. (1990). 'The treatment of patients with polycystic ovary syndrome by *in vitro* fertilization: A comparison of results with those patients with tubal infertility', *Hum. Reprod.*, **5**: 816–8.

Felberbaum, R.E. et al. (1995). 'Preserved pituitary response under ovarian stimulation with hMG and GnRH antagonists (Cetrorelix) in women with tubal infertility', *Eur. J. Obstet. Gynecol. Reprod. Biol.*, **61**: 151–5.

Franks, S. et al. (1985). 'Ovulatory disorders in women with polycystic ovary syndrome', in H.S. Jacobs (ed.), *Reproductive Endocrinology. Clin. Obstet. Gynaecol.*, **12**: 605–32.

Golan A. et al. (1988). 'Ovarian hyperstimulation syndrome following D-Try-6 luteinising hormone-releasing hormone microcapsules and menotrophin for *in vitro* fertilisation', *Fertil. Steril.*, **50**: 912–6.

———(1989). 'Ovarian hyperstimulation syndrome: an update review', *Obstet. Gynecol. Surv.*, **44**: 430–40.

Goldzieher, J.W. and J.A. Green (1962). 'The polycystic ovary. I. clinical and histological features', *J. Clin. Endocrinol. Metab.*, **22**: 325–38.

Hague, W. et al. (1988). 'Familial polycystic ovaries: A genetic disease?', *Clin. Endocrinol.*, **29**: 593–606.

Haning, R.V. Jr. et al. (1983). 'Plasma estradiol is superior to ultrasound and urinary oestriol glucuronide as a predictor of ovarian hyperstimulation during induction of ovulation with menotropins', *Fertil. Steril.*, **40**: 31–6.

Hughes, E.G. et al. (1992). 'The routine use of gonadotrophin-releasing hormone agonists prior to *in vitro* fertilization and gamete intrafallopian transfer: A meta-analysis of randomised control trials', *Fertil. Steril.*, **58**: 888–96.

Hull, M.G.R. (1987). 'Epidemiology of infertility and polycystic ovarian disease: Endocrinological and demographic studies', *Gynecol. Endocrinol.*, **1**: 235–45.

Jacobs, H.S. et al. (1987). 'Profertility uses of luteinising hormone agonist analogues', in B.M. Vickery, J.J. Neston (eds.), *LHRH and Its Analogues*, MTP Press, Lancester, pp. 303–22.

Jahanfar, S. et al. (1995). 'A twin study of polycystic ovary syndrome', *Fertil. Steril.*, **63**: 478–86.

Kyei-Mensah, A.A. et al. (1998). 'Relationship of ovarian stromal volume to serum androgen concentrations in patients with polycystic ovary syndrome', *Hum. Reprod.*, **13**: 1437–41.

Larsen T. (1990). 'Comparison of human urinary follicle stimulating hormone and hMG for ovarian stimulation in polycystic ovary syndrome', *Fertil. Steril.*, **53**: 426–31.

Loumaye, E. et al. (1995). 'Human follicle-stimulating hormone produced by recombinant DNA technology: A review for clinicians', *Hum. Reprod. Update*, **12**: 294–7.

MacGillivray, I. (1983). *'Pre-eclampsia—The hypertensive disease of pregancy'*, WB Saunders, London, pp. 44–5, 227–8.

Mannaerts, B.M.J.L. et al. (1996). 'Clinical profiling of recombinant follicle stimulating hormone (r-FSH: Puregon): Relationship between serum FSH and efficacy', *Hum. Reprod. Update*, **2**: 153–61.

Olivennes, F. et al. (1995). 'Scheduled administration of a gonadotrophin-releasing hormone antagonist (Cetrorelix) on day 8 of *in vitro* fertilization cycles: A pilot study', *Hum. Reprod.*, **10**: 1382–6.

Out, H.J. et al. (1996). 'Recombinant follicle stimulating hormone (r-FSH: Puregon) in assisted reproduction: More oocytes, more pregnancies', *Human Reprod. Update*, **2**: 162–71.

Polson, D.W. et al. (1988). 'Polycystic ovaries—a common finding in normal women', *Lancet*, **I**: 870–72.

Regan, L. et al. (1990). 'Hypersecretion of luteinising hormone, infertility and miscarriage', *Lancet*, **336**: 1141–4.

Rosenfield, R.L. et al. (1990). 'Dysregualtion of cytochrome P450c 17α as the cause of polycystic ovarian syndrome', *Fertil. Steril.*, **53**: 785–91.

Sagle, M. et al. (1988). 'Recurrent early miscarriage and polycystic ovaries', *Br. Med. J.*, **297**: 1027–8.

Salat-Baroux, J. et al. (1988). 'Comparison between long and short protocols of luteinising hormone releasing hormone agonist in the treatment of PCOD by *in vitro* fertilization', *Hum. Reprod.*, **3**: 535–9.

Salat-Baroux, J. and J.M. Antoine (1990). 'Accidental hyperstimulation during ovulation induction', in P.G. Crosignani (ed.), *Ovulation Induction. Bailliere's Clin. Obstet. Gynaecol.*, **4**: 627–37.

Schenker, J. (1993). 'Prevention and treatment of ovarian hyperstimulation', *Hum. Reprod.*, **8**: 653–9.

Seppala M. (1985). 'The World Collaborative Report on *in vitro* Fertilization and Embryo Replacement: Current State of the Art in January 1984', *Ann NY Acad. Sci.*, **442**: 558–63.

Sher, G. et al. (1993). 'Eliminating the risks of life-endangering complications following overstimulation with menotropin fertility agent: A report on women undergoing *in vitro* fertilization and embryo transfer', *Obstet. Gynaecol.*, **81**: 1009–11.

Smitz, J. et al. (1988). 'The luteal-phase and early pregnancy after combined GnRH-agonist / hCG treatment for superovulation in IVF and GIFT', *Hum. Reprod.*, **3**: 585–90.

Tanbo, T. et al. (1990). 'Stimulation with hMG versus follicle stimulating hormone after pituitary suppression in polycystic ovary syndrome', *Fertil. Steril.*, **53**: 798–803.

Treharne, I. (1984). 'Obesity in pregnancy', in J. Studd, (ed.), *Progress in Obstetrics and Gynaecology*, vol. 4, Churchill Livingstone, Edinburgh, pp. 127–38.

Urman, B. et al. (1992). 'Management of overstimulated gonadotrophin cycles with a controlled drift period', *Hum. Reprod.*, **7**: 213–17.

Waldenstrom, U. et al. (1999). 'High pregnancy rates and successful prevention of severe ovarian hyperstimulation syndrome by "prolonged coasting" of very hyperstimulated patients: A multicentre study', *Hum. Reprod.*, **14**: 294–7.

Zaidi, J. et al. (1995). 'Ovarian stromal blood flow in women with polycystic ovaries: A possible new marker for diagnosis', *Hum. Reprod.*, **10**: 1992–6.

8

Genital Tuberculosis and Assisted Reproduction

Sadhana K. Desai

Tuberculosis is endemic in India even though there is widespread use of vaccination for its prevention, as well as ready availability of multidrug therapy for control of the disease. It is reported that 50% of the Indian population suffers from tuberculosis at some point in their lifetime (WHO, 1996). The disease is rare in developed countries. However, in recent years, the incidence of this disease is rising in the Western world due to increasing migration from the Asian subcontinent, as well as due to the emergence of strains of Mycobacterium tuberculosis which are resistant to multidrug therapy (Ashurst, 1996). When tuberculosis affects the genital organs in a woman, it produces devastating effects, resulting in infertility which is difficult to treat.

INCIDENCE

Genital tuberculosis is still rare in the United States as well as in European countries (Klein et al., 1976). In a very large series from the European countries, the incidence of genital tuberculosis in infertile women was reported to be only 5% (Schaefer, 1964), and from 47 Swedish hospitals, only 187 cases of genital TB were reported in a ten-year period from 1968 to 1977 (Falk et al., 1980). In a survey conducted in France in 1985, it was found that genital TB was seen in only 6% of French infertile women, while it was detected in 33% of North African immigrant women (Adrai J. et al., 1985). The incidence of genital TB is high in developing countries, especially in India, where the incidence is reported to be 10% to 15% among women subjected to endometrial biopsy for primary infertility (Gupta, 1957), and 14.7% in infertile women undergoing diagnostic laparoscopy (Merchant, 1989). Genital TB is a major pelvic factor causing tubal infertility in Indian women (Parikh et al., 1997). We also found genital TB to be a major factor causing irreparably blocked tubes in 38% of women with tubal factor of infertility (see Desai, 1995).

SOURCE

Tuberculosis is a disseminated disease and genital tuberculosis is always secondary to TB elsewhere in the body. The usual source is the respiratory tract (Aka et al., 1997). In a study of 448 cases of genital tuberculosis with infertility, we found the primary sites to be the lungs and pleura, peritoneal cavity, intestines, bones, spine, meninges, urinary tract, and the cervical and inguinal lymph nodes (Desai, 1995). There is a long latent phase between the involvement of the primary site and the appearance of the clinical symptoms. Therefore, the primary site is already healed and is difficult to find by the time the diagnosis of genital TB is made.

DIAGNOSIS

The fallopian tube is the initial site of involvement, with a secondary extension to the endometrium in 50% to 90% of cases (Sutherland, 1979; Schaefer, 1976). The infection usually occurs via the haematogenous and lymphatic routes, as well as by direct spread from the peritoneal cavity. Most women hardly have any symptoms and infertility is the only presenting symptom in them. Diagnosis of early TB is difficult. Histological examination of the endometrium or a surgical biopsy from the genital organs for granulomatomas is the most useful means of a establishing diagnosis.

A culture of the menstrual secretion or of the endometrium is another method of establishing an early diagnosis; especially a repeat sample will offer a higher yield and establish the diagnosis after histological examination of the endometrium has been negative for genital TB (Oosthuizen et al., 1990). Laparoscopy is also an important way to establish the diagnosis of genital tuberculosis. Various types of lesions are described, such as a tubo-ovarian mass with tuberculous granulomas or caseating nodules on the tubes or the peritoneum, miliary tubercles on the inflamed oedematous tubes, salpingitis isthmica nodosa with multiple nodularity of the tubes, and frozen pelvis with tubercles in the peritoneal cavity (Yang et al., 1996).

Hysterosalpingography also helps in detecting the disease. Blocked tubes with obstruction at the ampullary end, isthmic block with thinning of the fallopian tubes, beaded appearance due to multiple obstructions and blocked tubes with obliteration of the uterine cavity, and filling defects in the uterus due to intrauterine adhesions in the absence of a history of curettage or abortion are all sequelae of genital TB (Charles, 1980).

In recent years, the introduction of Gas Liquid Chromatography Mass Spectrometry (GLC-MS), which facilitates a direct analysis of the presence of tuberculesiearic acid (TBSA), a structural component of *Mycobacterium*, and the gene probe amplified Mycobacterium TB direct test have resulted in rapid detection of TB (Gaby et al., 1996). TB IgA, TB IgG and TBIgM levels and the Mantoux test are useful indirect tests for the detection of active TB (Rattan et al., 1993; Srivastava et al., 1997).

GENITAL TB AND INFERTILITY

A majority of patients with genital TB are cases of primary infertility. The main cause of infertility is damage to the fallopian tubes. The fallopian tubes need not always be blocked, but the ovum pick-up function of the tubes is always affected, especially if the damage occurs to the muscular coat of the tube or to the endosalpinx. Distortion of the tubo-ovarian anatomy can also lead to infertility. These tubes are usually not amenable to surgical correction unless the disease is diagnosed very early. The result of microsurgery tuboplasty is poor and chances of ectopic pregnancy are high (Durukan et al., 1990). When the endometrium is involved, implantation failure occurs, leading to infertility, and if conception occurs, the chances of abortion are high (Saracoqlu et al., 1992). When the endometrium is extensively damaged, it may cause intrauterine adhesions or extensive fibrosis, leading to scanty menstruation or amenorrhoea. Intrauterine adhesions may be surgically corrected, but fibrosis of the endometrium due to atrophy up to the basal layer is difficult to treat by hormone therapy or by surgery. When the ovaries are involved in the disease process, ovarian function may get affected. Oligomenorrhoea may occur and destruction of the ovaries may cause diminished ovarian reserve, raising the basal FSH and oestradiol levels (Gurgan et al., 1996).

ROLE OF ASSISTED REPRODUCTION

Since an early diagnosis of genital tuberculosis is difficult, by the time the patient presents as a case of infertility, irreparable damage to the fallopian tubes has already occurred.The fallopian tubes are usually blocked and even if they are not blocked, the tubal function is generally affected; therefore, pregnancies following medical and surgical treatment of genital TB are rare. Most pregnancies end up as ectopic pregnancies (Durukan et al., 1990), or abortions (Saracolqlu et al., 1992). Falk et al. (1980) retrospectively studied cases of genital TB during a 10-year period between 1968 and 1977, and found no intrauterine pregnancy and four ectopic pregnancies (three of which occurred in one patient). Schaefer reviewed the post-therapy fertility of 7,000 cases with genital TB from the literature and found 125 extrauterine pregnancies, 67 abortions and only 31 term pregnancies (Schaefer, 1964). De Vynck et al. (1990) reported 13 pregnancies in 34 patients, following a full course of anti-TB chemotherapy.

The results of the tuboplasty operation in this group of women are also not encouraging. Tuboplasty, either macrosurgical or microsurgical, can very rarely lead to term pregnancy and may increase the chance of tubal pregnancy, or may even flare up pelvic TB (Gomel, 1983; Ballon, 1975). Winston et al. (1991) treated 5 patients with genital TB and found two new pregnancies, while Tumarov et al. (1990) advocated the selective use of microsurgical techniques and achieved a 9% improvement in the pregnancy rate. Sutherland reported the results of 206 patients treated with antikoch's therapy. Nineteen patients required surgery because of the failure of medical treatment. Forty-five pregnancies occurred subsequently in 26 patients, 11 abortions, and 11 etopic and 23 live births (Sutherland, 1977). Leblanc (1959) performed 51 salpingostomies in patients of genital TB. Post-operative tubal patency was present in 25%. There was one extra-uterine pregnancy and no term pregnancy. Frydman et al. (1985) also found no pregnancies in eight patients who underwent microsurgical tubal operations. However, the very same women conceived after they were subjected to IVF-ET at a later date. Frydman was the first to demonstrate the usefulness of *in vitro* fertilization in the management of the tubal factor of infertility due to TB in 1985. Out of 12 women with a history of blocked tubes due to genital TB, 6 pregnancies were reported following IVF-ET. Varma (1991) from UK also suggested ART as a treatment of choice in selected cases of genital TB, stating that medical, surgical or conservative treatment are associated with a poor fertility outcome.

We have performed IVF-ET on 83 cases of damaged fallopian tubes due to genital TB. In all, 125 ovum pick-ups were done on these patients, resulting in 21 clinical pregnancies, i.e. a pregnancy rate of 20% per OPU and 25% per patient. This pregnancy rate is comparable to other indications for IVF-ET in our clinic, where 13 singleton, 3 twin and 1 triplet pregnancies occurred. There were 3 abortions and 1 ectopic pregnancy, suggesting that even after IVF-ET, the incidence of ectopic pregnancy and abortion rates was higher (see Desai, 1995).

We believe that IVF treatment probably represents the most successful treatment for patients with genital TB. Marcus et al. (1994) have also reported a 40% pregnancy rate in 10 patients treated with IVF-ET. Gurgan et al. (1996) reported a 16.3% clinical pregnancy rate in 44 cases treated with IVF-ET. These authors found less oocytes, a poor pregnancy rate and a higher abortion rate in cases with genital TB. They also observed that these patients required a higher hMG dose, suggesting a diminished ovarian reserve in patients of genital TB. According to Gurgan, they represent a less favourable subset among other tubal factors of infertility in patients undergoing IVF-ET. However, in our study of 83 cases of genital TB undergoing IVF-ET, we found no such difference.

SPECIAL PRECAUTIONS TO BE OBSERVED IN PATIENTS UNDERGOING IVF-ET

Although IVF gives women with genital TB the best chance of becoming pregnant, a systematic work-up is necessary prior to commencing IVF treatment. When the indication for IVF is a tubal factor of infertility, it is important to find out whether the aetiological factor is genital TB or not. It was observed by Winston that when IVF-ET is performed in the presence of active disease, patients are not likely to conceive (Soussis et al., 1998), and in case they do, the disease may flare up and may also cause life-threatening complications (Gull et al., 1995). Unfortunately, the diagnosis of the latent form of TB is not easy and requires a study of the disease, history of the case, endometrial biopsy, culture of menstrual blood, laparoscopy, subcutaneous 50 IU tuberculin test and Elisa test for anti-TB antibodies (Kolachevskaia et al., 1994). In the presence of active or latent disease, a full course of multidrug chemotherapy must be given prior to the commencement of treatment. In case of doubt, especially in patients with a history of a full course of anti-TB chemotherapy in the past, we recommend at least three months of anti-TB chemotherapy prior to the IVF-ET treatment.

Genital TB affects not only the tubes but also the endometrium in 50% of cases. It is, therefore, important that patients undergoing IVF-ET for the tubal factor of infertility due to genital TB are properly evaluated for endometrial function by hysterosalpingography, hysteroscopy and ultrasound examination.

It is extremely important to fully assess the uterine cavity. This is best done by pre-IVF evaluation of the uterine cavity by hysteroscopy (Bordt et al., 1984; Goldenberg et al., 1991). If intrauterine adhesions are present, they can be divided prior to IVF-ET (Schenker, 1996). The cavity must be reasonably good, both anatomically as well as functionally. In particular, there should be no adhesions at the fundus of the uterus. Frydman et al. (1985) did laparoscopy and hysteroscopy procedures on seven of his patients who had failed to conceive after IVF-ET and found that the cause of the failure of IVF-ET was intrauterine adhesions in all the cases. We routinely do hysteroscopy prior to IVF-ET, in women with a tubal factor of infertility due to genital TB. Endometrial biopsy should be taken at that time to exclude active tuberculosis.

A transvaginal scan of the endometrium in the periovular period to assess endometrial thickness, as well as a colour Doppler study of the endometrium at that time, are useful parameters to assess the physiological function of the endometrium. Campbell has studied the function of the endometrium by colour Doppler study in women undergoing IVF-ET (see Steer et al., 1992). We use this parameter routinely in our patients undergoing IVF-ET. In our opinion, in patients of genital TB, when the endometrium fails to respond to hormonal therapy and the endometrial thickness remains less than 7 mm at the time of ovum pick-up, there is hardly any chance of pregnancy.

Gurgan et al. (1996) have divided the endometrium of patients with genital TB into two types: atropic and tropic endometrium. These authors have found a poor pregnancy rate when an atropic endometrium is detected. Since the disease sometimes destroys the ovaries and affects ovarian function, it is also advisable to do basal FSH and E2 levels on day 2 or 3 of menses, prior to the commencement of IVF-ET.

CONCLUSION

In conclusion, we would like to state that assisted reproduction seems to offer the best chance for women with genital tuberculosis to conceive. However, a proper systematic work up prior to commencing the treatment should be done. It is important that women should receive a full course of anti TB chemotherapy and not have any active disease prior to treatment of infertility by ART.

REFERENCES

Adrai, J. et al. (1985). 'La sterilite de la femme nordafricaine immigree', *Rev. Fr. Gynecol Obstet.*, **80** (10): 733–6.

Aka, N. and E.Z. Vural (1997). 'Evaluation of patients with active pulmonary tuberculosis for genital involvement', *J. Obstet. Gynaecol. Res.*, **23**: 4, 337–40.

Ashurst, M. (1996). 'News—multidrug resistant tuberculosis will spread', *Br. Med. Journal.*, **12**: 614.

Ballon, S. (1975). 'Reactivation of silent pelvic tuberculosis by reconstructive surgery', *A.M. J. of Obstet. Gynaecol*, **122**: 911–13.

Bordt, J. et al. (1984). 'Diagnostic hysteroscopy in an IVF programme, WHO report', Abstract of 3rd World Congress of IVF-ET, Helsinki.

Charles, David (1980). *Infections in Obstetrics and Gynaecology*, W B Saunders Company, Philadelphia. pp. 243–52.

Desai, S. K. (1995). *Infertility and Transvaginal Sonography Current Concepts*, J. P. Brothers Medical Publishers, New Delhi.

De-Vynck, W.E. et al. (1990). 'Genital tuberculosis associated with female infertility in the Western Cape', *S. Afr. Med. J.*, 77 (12): 630–31.

Durukan, T. et al. (1990). 'Abdominal pregnancy 10 years after treatment of pelvic TB', *Am. J. Obstet. Gynecol.*, **163**: 594–5.

Falk, V. et al. (1980). 'Genital tuberculosis in women: Analysis of 187 newly diagnosed cases from 47 Swedish hospitals during the ten-year period 1968 to 1977', *Am. J. Obstet Gynecol.*, **138**: 974–7.

Frydman, R. et al. (1985). '*In vitro* fertilization in tuberculous infertility', *J. In Vitro Fert. Embryo., Transfer*, **4**: 184–9.

Gaby E. Pfyffer, et al. (1996). 'Diagnostic performance of amplified mycobacterium tuberculosis direct test with CSF, other non-respiratory and respiratory specimens', *J. of Clinical Microbiology.*, 834–41.

Goldenberg, M. et al. (1991). 'Hysteroscopy in a program *in vitro* fertilization', *Journal of In Vitro Fertilization and Embryo Transfer*, **8**: 336–8.

Gomel, V. (1983). *Microsurgery in Female Infertility*, Little Brown Co., Boston, pp. 129–30.

Gull, I. (1995). 'The effect of an *in vitro* fertilization pregnancy on a woman with genital T.B.', *Hum. Reprod.*, **10**: 3052–4.

Gupta, S. (1957). 'Pelvic tuberculosis in women', *J. Obstet. Gynecol. India*, 7: 181.

Gurgan, T. et al. (1996). 'Results of *in vitro* fertilization and embryo transfer in women with infertility due to genital tuberculosis', *Fertil. Steril.*, **65**: 367–70.

Klein, T.A. et al. (1976). 'Pelvic T.B.', *Obstet. Gynecol.*, **48**: 99–104.

Kolachevskaia, E.N. et al. (1994). 'Clinical course and diagnosis of female genital tuberculosis', *Probl. Tuberk.*, pp. 26–9.

Leblanc, E.J. (1959). 'Technique and results of salpingostomies', *Fertil. Steril.*, **10**: 412–3.

Marcus, S.F. et al. (1994).'Tuberculous infertility and *in vitro* fertilization', *Am. J. Obstet. Gynecol.*, **171**: 1593–6.

Merchant, R. (1989) 'Endoscopy in the diagnosis of genital tuberculosis', *J. Reprod. Med.*, **34**(7): 468–74.

Oosthuizen, A.P. et al. (1990). 'Tuberculosis of the female genital tract in patients attending an infertility clinic', *S. Afr. Med. J.*, 77(11): 562–4.

Parikh, F.R. et al. (1997). 'Genital tuberculosis—a major pelvic factor causing infertility in Indian women', *Fertil. Steril.*, **67**: 3,497–500.

Rattan, A. et al. (1993). 'Detection of antigens of mycobacterium tuberculosis in patients of infertility by monoclonal antibody-based sandwiched enzyme linked immunosorbent assay (ELISA)', *Tuber lung dis.*, **74**(3): 200–203.

Saracoqlu, O.F. et al. (1992). 'Pelvic tuberculosis', *Int. J. Gynaecol. Obstet.*, **37**(2): 115–20.

Schaefer, G. (1976). 'Female genital tuberculosis', *Clin. Obstet. Gynecol.*, **19**: 223–34.

Schenker, J.G. (1996). 'Etiology of and therapeutic approach to synechia uteri', *Eur. J. Obstet. Gynecol. Reprod. Biol.*, **65**: 109–13.

Soussis, I. et al. (1998). '*In vitro* fertilization treatment in genital tuberculosis', *J. Assist. Reprod. Genet.*, **15**: 6, 378–80.

Srivastava, N. et al. (1997). 'Role of ELISA (enzyme-linked immunosorbent assay) in genital tuberculosis', *Int. J. Gynaecol. Obstet.*, **57**: 205–6.

Steer, C.V. et al. (1992). 'The use of transvaginal colour flow imaging after *in vitro* fertilization to identify optimum uterine condition before embryo transfer', *Fertil. Steril.*, **57**: 372–6.

Sutherland, A. M. (1977). 'Twenty-five years of experience of the drug treatment of tuberculosis of the female genital tract', *Br. J. Obstet. Gynecol.*, **84**: 881–6.

______(1979). 'Gynaecological TB', *Br. J. Hospital Med.*, **2**: 569–74.

Tumarov I.P. and M.N. Kochorova (1990). 'Use of microsurgical technics in the treatment of tubal infertility of tuberculous etiology', *Probl. Tuberk.*, **2**: 6–8.

Varma, T.R. (1991). 'Genital tuberculosis and subsequent fertility', *Int. J. Gynaecol. Obstet.*, **35**(1): 1–11.

WHO report, 24 March 1996.

Winston, R.M.L. and R.A. Margara (1991). 'Microsurgical salpingostomy is not an obsolete procedure', *Br. J. Obstetrics. Gynaecol.*, 637–42.

Yang Y. et al. (1996). 'Laparoscopic diagnosis of tubal infertility and fallopian tube lesions', *Chung Hua Fu Chan Ko Tsa Chih*, **31**(6): 327–9.

9

Imaging in Assisted Conception

Chander P. Lulla

INTRODUCTION

Pelvic imaging and the management of infertility are linked in several ways. An abnormality disclosed by an image of a pelvic structure can be the cause of infertility. Alternatively, an abnormal image can be the sign of a physiological disturbance that is causing both the infertility and the image. When an infertile couple visits the clinic, the initial emphasis should be on an accurate diagnosis of the condition that is inhibiting their ability to conceive.

Ultrasonography (USG) is an imaging technique that has assumed a major role in both the diagnosis and treatment of infertility. There has been rapid evolution of endovaginal sonography and its application in infertility since 1984, such that it was embraced for monitoring follicle development, and along with the biopsy needle, oocyte retrieval was made possible. Non-invasive imaging, especially by ultrasound, can also be used to guide an endoscopic procedure for both diagnosis and treatment. Lately, Duplex Color Doppler imaging allows the determination of the velocity and impedance of blood flow in a given vessel, and thus permits an anatomical and physiological assessment of the uterus and ovaries to provide a better seed and soil status in an infertility management programme.

Three-dimensional USG now provides new insights into congenital fusional defects of the uterus. This would facilitate prior correction and improved fertility outcomes.

The last decade has seen a transformation in the approach to treating infertility. The developments in IVF have so improved the capacity for overcoming this disability that we have had to overhaul our ideas on the causes of infertility. The more substantial the pathology, the stronger the case for treating the pathology and expecting this pathology-based treatment to resolve the infertility. On the other hand, the weaker the pathology diagnosed—and especially in cases of unexplained infertility—the more we rely on the duration of the infertility to give a maximum estimate of the intrinsic fecundability.

IMAGING IN INFERTILITY

The scope of this chapter includes the following: a working knowledge of the normal and abnormal menstrual cycle; the nature and the causes of infertility, and how the imaged female pelvis reflects pathology within as a direct cause of infertility. It also evaluates newer imaging modalities for evaluation of the infertility patient, while discussing how to perform image-guided interventional procedures; how to manage the complications of infertility treatment; how to evaluate the male factor of infertility; and the biological hazards of ultrasonography.

NORMAL AND ABNORMAL MENSTRUAL CYCLE

THE OVARIAN CYCLE

Follicle growth has been described as a continuum. Peters (1975) and Hackeloer (1979) were the first to demonstrate with ultrasound the sequential events in the normal menstrual cycle. Since then, ultrasound has enjoyed an expanding role in follicular monitoring, with broadened indications for its use.

An eight-stage process for follicular growth and maturation, taking 85 days, had been proposed by Gougeon in 1986. By day 5 of the menstrual cycle, several recruited follicles can be observed on transvaginal sonography (TVS), with a diameter of 2–3mm, compared with 5mm by transabdominal sonography (TAS). The internal ovarian hormonal struggle results in one follicle (sometimes two or three) achieving dominance by the end of the first week of the cycle, and the remaining follicles get suppressed and undergo atresia. (Pache TD et al., Mendelson, 1990). The follicles reach a diameter of 10mm approximately 5–6 days before ovulation. The rate of growth of the dominant follicle is linear from day 5 to ovulation (see Fig. 9.1), averaging 2–2.5 mm per day, until a mean diameter of 2 cm is reached (Rossasvik, 1985). At midcycle, when the dominant follicle is mature, a surge of LH from the pituitary gland initiates the process of ovulation.

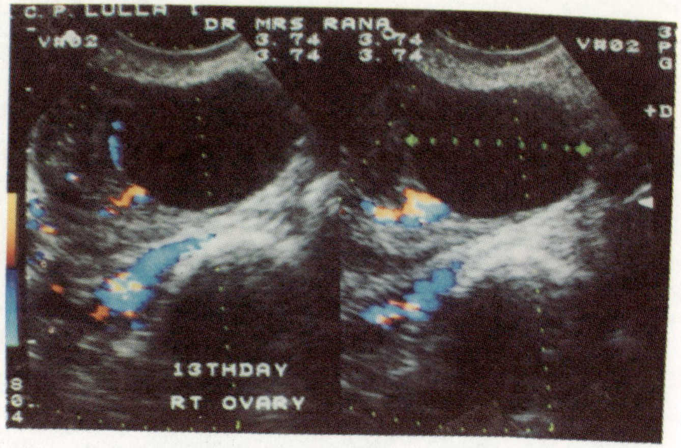

Fig. 9.1. Midcycle, well-sized 2-cm follicle with perifollicular vascularity

A few anatomical structures must be differentiated from ovarian follicles. These include: (1) the cross-section of the internal iliac artery and the vein; (2) bowel; (3) hydrosalpinx; and (4) ovarian cysts.

Prediction of Ovulation

By means of imaging (see Fig. 9.2), the following indicators may give evidence of ovulation:

(1) Before ovulation, the granulosa cell layer separates from the hypervascular and oedematous thecal layer. This may be seen ultrasonographically 24 hours before ovulation as a line of decreased echogenicity around the follicle.

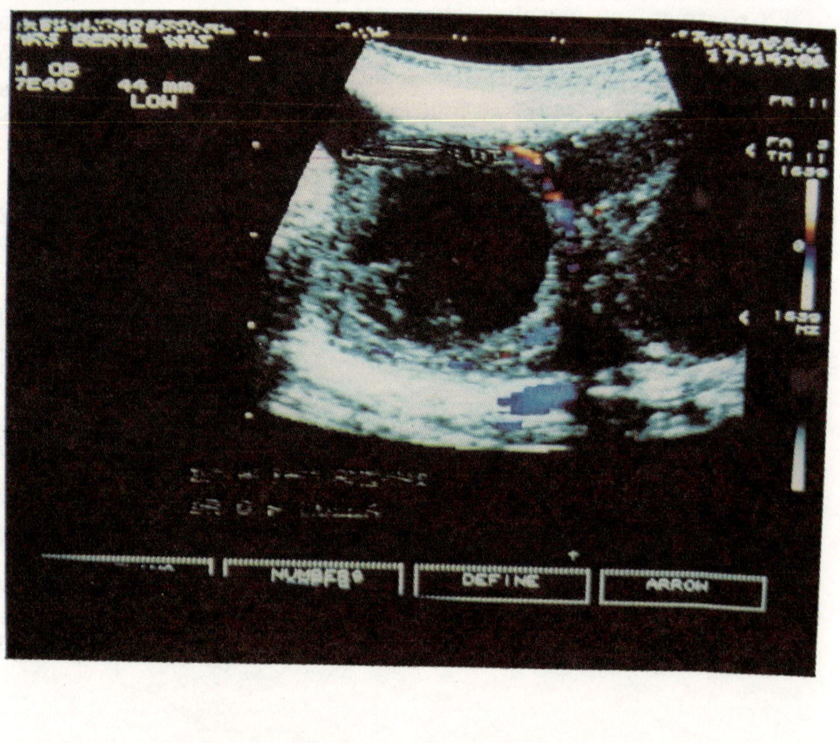

Fig. 9.2. The cumulus oophorus is seen projecting into the follicle-suggesting impending ovulation

(2) In a majority of cases, the ovarian size is increased (70% to 100%), as is the surface area.
(3) A hypoechoic ovary, with a thickened 'irregular contour', may be seen.
(4) Folding and separation of the granulosa layer has a crenated appearance, seen 6 to 8 hours before ovulation.
(5) The cumulus oophorus may be seen projecting into the follicle.
(6) Visualization of fluid around the ovary is occasionally seen.

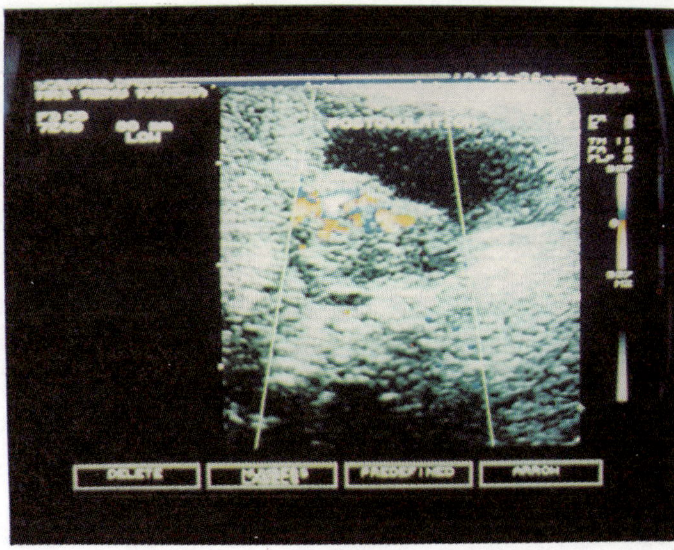

Fig. 9.3B. Post-ovulation periovulatory fluid seen

Evidence of ovulation

Follicular rupture results in the formation of a corpus heamorrhagicum, which evolves between 1 hour to several days after ovulation. The follicle at this time is very echogenic because of the blood in its lumen. It is also of diminished size when compared with its preovulatory dimension (see 9.3A and 9.3B and 9.4). Over the next 4 to 5 days, it may increase in size but ultimately, its dimension diminishes. Evidence of ovulation can be seen in about 80% of cycles. Although fluid in the pouch of Douglas may be seen in 25% of patients who have ovulated, the volume of fluid has been determined to be greater than that attributable to the release of fluid from the follicle itself (Herlitty).

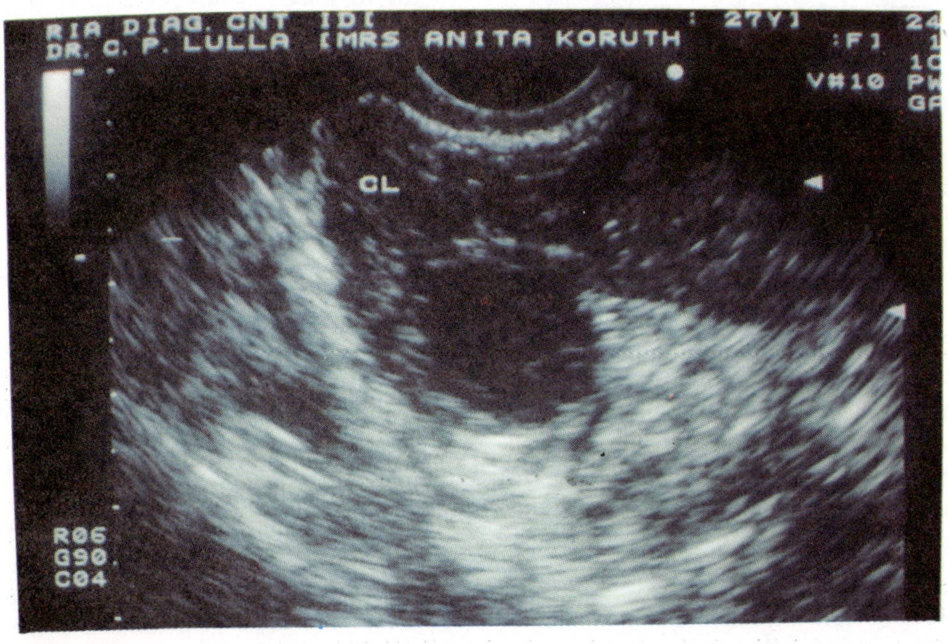

Fig. 9.3A. Corpus haemorrhagicum indicating rupture of follicle. The follicle appears crenated with internal echoes.

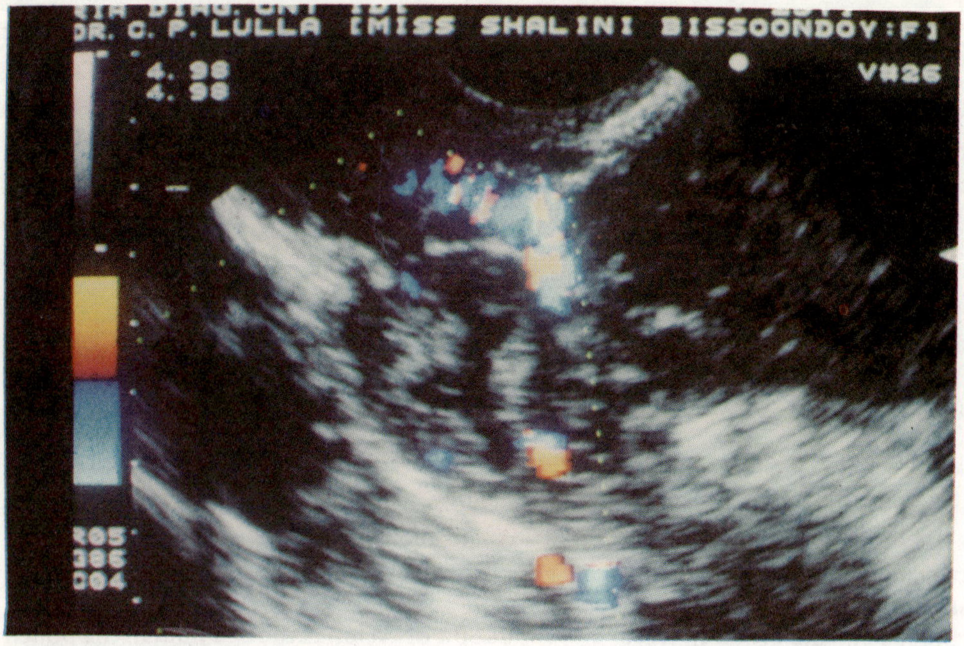

Fig. 9.4. Corpus luteum revealing triradiate, collapsed appearance

Endometrial Changes

The endometrium, an end organ for circulating oestrogens/progesterones, can also be examined, with alterations reflecting the changes in the circulating hormonal milieu. Ovarian stimulation with FSH thickens the endometrium in 24% of women, who during a preceding natural cycle, had a thin endometrium (Sher, 1993).

Some authors have suggested that pregnancy is more common in patients whose endometrium appears thicker or grows faster (Giotlandio; Rabinowitz). These original studies have been followed by many reports from several institutions that have characterized the importance of endometrial thickness in prognosticating the probability of implantation and pregnancy. (Bergh, 1992; Dickey, 1993; Glissant; Gonen; Randall; Sher; Shoham). Currently, adequate data are available to define the role of endometrial thickness measurement and to assist the physician in counselling patients regarding their chances of conception.

Endometrial thickness in the post-menstrual early follicular phase, before any stimulation, is typically 5mm or less. Endometrial growth is slow during the first few days of ovulation induction protocols, but then increases rapidly at a rate of 1 to 2 mm per day in the final 2 to 3 days before ovulation (Rabinowitz; Shoham). Mean pre-ovulatory endometrial thickness measurements vary according to the stimulation protocol used for the ovulation induction cycles; however, the measurements are about 8mm in spontaneous cycles, 9 to 10mm in clomiphene citrate-stimulated cycles, and about 12mm in cycles stimulated with exogenous gonadotrophins (Dickey, 1993).

An obvious increase in endometrial thickness is associated with the more aggressive stimulation protocols, presumably due to their associated higher peak oestradiol levels. However, within a given stimulation protocol, most authors could not demonstrate a significant correlation between endometrial thickness and the peak oestradiol level. (Bergh; Dickey, 1992; Dickey, 1993; Glissant; Gonen; Randall; Shoham; Fleischer). Many of the studies correlating endometrial thickness with the ensuing pregnancy rates were done by comparing the mean endometrial thickness measurements in patients who conceived with the measurements of those who did not (Giotlandio; Rabinowitz; Gonen; Randall). In several early series, using lower frequency transabdominal transducers, researchers could not demonstrate any differences in the maximal endometrial thickness attained in women who did or did not become pregnant (Fleischc, 1986). However, with the use of the more accurate high-frequency transvaginal transducer in the late 1980s, investigators, in a series of reports, were able to demonstrate higher mean endometrial thickness measurements in women who conceived (Dickey, 1992; 1993; Gonon; Sher; Shoham). Endometrial thicknesses were equivalent in the early follicular phase, and differences became apparent only on the day of human chronic gonadotrophin (hCG) administration. Gonon and co-workers 1986 reported that the average thickness of endometria in women who did and did not conceive in assisted reproduction cycles were 7.8+/-2.0 mm and 6.3+/-2.2 mm, respectively (P<. 005). The difference in endometrial thickness seemed particularly important, because the number of follicles that developed, the peak oestradiol level achieved, the number of oocytes retrieved, and the number of embryos transferred were equivalent in women who did and did not become pregnant. These types of differences were also apparent in pure ovulation induction cycles. Shoham and co-workers reported that women who conceived had an average endometrial thickness of 10.4+2.4mm, as compared to a mean thickness of 8.9+2.0 mm for those who failed to conceive.

The practical application of these findings for individual patients is problematic. The type of stimulation protocol used greatly influences endometrial thickness and thus, the value of a series of measurements. The mean endometrial thickness of the patients who conceived in the Gonon and co-workers' study (stimulation with clomiphene citrate plus human menopausal gonadotrophins) was lower than that found in the women who failed to conceive in the Shoham and co-workers' study (stimulation with human menopausal gonadotrophins only.) General stimulation protocols, which, include clomiphene citrate, produce an endometrial thickness that is about 2 mm smaller than that produced with exogenous gonadotrophins alone.

The significant overlap in endometrial thickness measurements between patients who do and do not become pregnant does not mean that endometrial thickness is of no value in clinical care. Endometrial receptivity is one of many factors that may limit the success rates of a given stimulation cycle. Many of the patients who did not conceive may have failed due to some other factor. Therefore, many authors evaluated their data to determine if there was a critical threshold below which conception was unlikely to occur under virtually any circumstances. It was determined that the type of stimulation protocol had a profound effect on the probability of successful implantation. During ovulation induction cycles, Shoham and co-workers found that no pregnancies occurred in women whose maximal endometrial thickness was less than or equal to 7mm. Similarly, Gonon and co-workers found that all pregnancies occurred in women whose endometrial thickness exceeded 6 mm. In an extensive review of this area, Dickey and co-workers evaluated their own data from four different stimulation protocols to determine if a threshold existed below which conception was unlikely to occur. No pregnancies resulted from cycles in which the peak endometrial thickness was less than 6mm, independent of the stimulation protocols. They further determined that pregnancies were common in spontaneous and clomiphene citrate-stimulated cycles with an endometrial thickness of 6mm or more. Based on these reports, a thickness of 6 mm appears to represent a critical threshold. There was no detectable improvement in the pregnancy rates when the endometrial thickness exceeded 6mm. A similar effect was found in cycles stimulated with exogenous gonadotrophins; the threshold value was 8mm (Dickey, 1992).

The results of several longitudinal studies of endometrial developments in natural and stimulated cycles have demonstrated that not only does endometrial thickness increase, but a distinctive multilayer pattern also normally develops by the completion of the follicular phase. The ultrasonographic appearance, commonly described as a triple-line pattern, is seen in most patients (Forrest; Sher; Smith; Welker).The normal appearance of the endometrium in the late follicular phase has three distinct hyperechoic lines, separated by two hypoechoic areas. The outermost hyperechoic line on each side represents the junction between the innermost portion of the myometrium and the

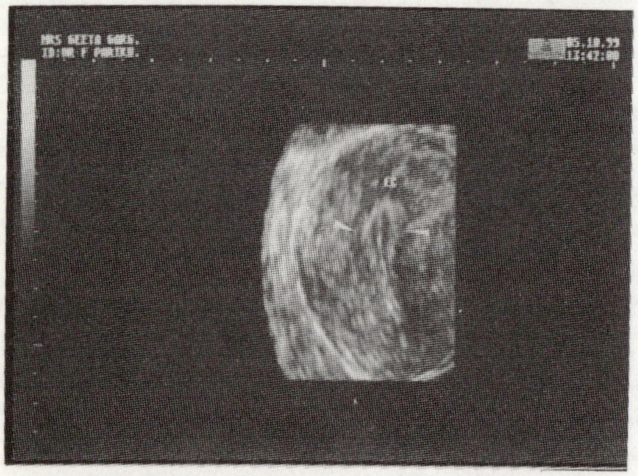

Fig. 9.5. Triple-layer endometrium in late follicular phase

vascular stratum basale. The central hyperechoic lines represent the plane where the luminal endometrial epithelia from the two walls of the endometrial cavity meet. The endometrial cavity is a potential space in the non-gravid non-menstrual state and is not visible between the two walls of the cavity. For this reason, the luminal epithelium from each side of the endometrium appears as only a single hyperechoic line. However, some investigators noted that some women did not develop this characteristic appearance. These observations led to several studies that correlated pregnancy and implantation rates with the presence or absence of this tripe-line pattern. It was demonstrated in these studies, that a relationship does exist between an absence of this endometrial pattern and a substantially lower chance of a successful pregnancy.

Most of the literature describes the different ultrasonographic images as falling into one of three categories (Check; Gonen Grunfeld; Rogers; Sakamoto; Ueno). Different authors have categorized the patterns using the different names; however, the three patterns could be described as the following. The normal patterns (termed a C pattern by Genon and Casper) have a clear delineation of three hyperechoic lines, separated by clearly hypoechogenic areas. The abnormal patterns (termed an A pattern by Genon and Casper) provide an entirely hyperechoic endometrium, with no hypoechoic areas being visible. An intermediate pattern (termed a B pattern by Genon and Casper) shows hypoechoic areas between the outer hyperechoic line and the central hyperechoic line, but the demarcation is less distinct. The more recent literature may be interpreted to mean that there may be no differences in reproductive performance between the classic triple-line pattern and the intermediate triple-line pattern. Genon and Casper reported that about 75% of the patients

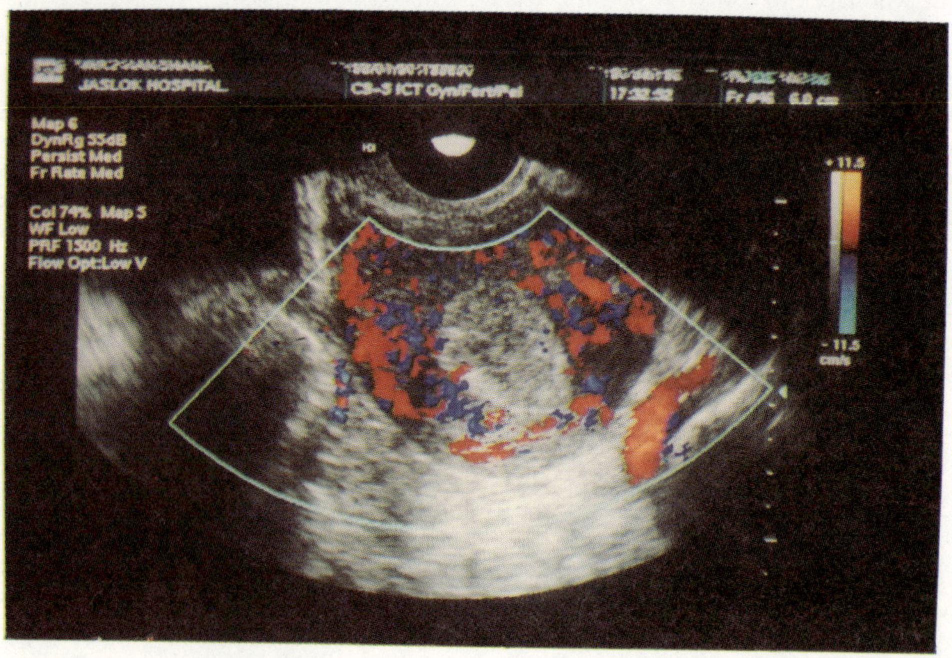

Fig. 9.6. Echogenic abnormal endometrium

who became pregnant had a triple-line pattern, whereas less than 60% of the patients who failed to conceive developed a triple-line pattern during the stimulation cycle.

Several reports detail the ability of the pattern of endometrial development to prognosticate pregnancy rates. Since patients with a normal development may have a number of other factors contributing to their failure to implant, the emphasis has been appropriately placed on those women with abnormal hyperechoic patterns of development. Ueno and co-workers described no pregnancies in 12 patients with an abnormal endometrial pattern and a pregnancy rate of 43.5% in women who developed a triple-line pattern. Several other authors have also found that the implantation rates in patients with the abnormal hyperechoic endometrial patterns are substantially lower than in those with a triple-line appearance (Check; Genon; Grunfeld; Rogers; Ueno).

The data on their patients reported by Ueno and co-workers and Dickey and co-workers were further divided into groups with either clear triple-line patterns or the intermediate, less clear triple-line patterns. Both investigators found that pregnancy and implantation rates were identical in the two groups, and suggested that a simpler and equally useful classification scheme would be to divide patients into those with any type of triple-line pattern and those with a uniform hyperechoic appearance of the endometrium. Therefore, many investigators and clinicians have abandoned the older three-category system in favour of a normal (triple-line) or abnormal (hyperechoic) classification.

Relatively few data are available to characterize the impact of the type of stimulation protocol on the pattern of endometrial developments. Limited investigations comparing natural cycles to exogenous gonadotrophin-stimulated cycles, and comparing clomiphene citrate-stimulated cycles to exogenous gonadotrophin-stimulated cycles have not demonstrated differences in the relative proportion of patients who develop the different patterns. It is apparent that, unlike the data on endometrial thickness, the higher peak oestradiol levels associated with some stimulation protocols do not affect pattern of development (Shoham).

Baseline Ultrasound

It is useful to carry out baseline TVS of the pelvis before commencing expensive and time-consuming IVF treatment. Endometrial polyps, submucous fibroids or hydrosalpinx can be diagnosed by ultrasound. At the time of the baseline ultrasound, it is useful to establish whether the ovaries are accessible for retrieval, and the position of the uterus for the embryo transfer.

Follicle Tracking

Follicular tracking with ultrasound can be accomplished either transvaginally or transabdominally, with or without a Colour Doppler imaging of pelvic blood flow. Follicles are measured in three dimensions (antero-posterior, cephalo-caudal and transverse). Changes in the leading follicle morphology, size and internal echo texture, and the appearance of free fluid in the cul-de-sac are documented. In a normal cycle, a scan on days 11, 12, 13, 14, and 15 should suffice. Cost constraints and logistics problems may dictate that the number and timing of scans be changed. The ultrasound prediction of attainment of follicular maturity can be compounded with hormonal assays. The aim of the stimulation is to achieve a lead follicle of at least 1.7 cm, with at least three or four follicles whose diameter is 1.4cm or more, with an oestradiol level of approximately 740pmol/mL for each such follicle. When this point is reached, HCG 5-10,000 U is administered to induce the final maturation of the follicle and its oocyte by initiating the ovulation process, with the precise timing of the injection being determined by subtracting 36 hours from the scheduled time of intended oocyte retrieval.

Endometrial Tracking

The measurement of endometrial thickness is best accomplished by scanning the endometrium in the longitudinal axis of the uterus. The measurement extends from the junction of the stratum basale, which is highly echogenic, and the inner myometrium, which is less echogenic, on the anterior side of the endometrium to the same plane on the posterior side of the endometrium. Although some early reports measured the distance from the myometrial-endometrial junction to the endometrial cavity, the most frequently used measurement encompasses the entire width (both sides) of the endometrium.

The ultrasonographic pattern of the endometrial is determined by scanning the midline of the uterus along its longitudinal axis. The assignment of a specific pattern is subjective and not based on any quantitative measurements.

DIAGNOSIS OF CONDITIONS THAT MAY RESULT IN INFERTILITY

OVARIAN FACTORS

Diagnosis of Anovulation

Transvaginal ultrasonography (TVS) allows for a diagnosis of the empty follicle syndrome, an unruptured luteinized follicle, dysfunctional cyst formation and polycystic ovarian (PCO) syndrome.

In an **anovulatory cycle**, serial ultrasounds will reveal the following (see Fig. 9.7A):

(1) A lack of any follicular development or with a few nonovulatory(10 mm) follicles. The follicle may not develop more than 16 mm in size suggestive of the same.

(2) The absence of sonographic luteal phase-endometrium.

(3) Endometrial hyperplasia is seen in long-standing cases.

(4) Lack of development of a mature corpus luteum.

Empty Follicle Syndrome

This was first described in 1986 by Coulam, who found that some aspirated follicles, with a normal USG appearance did not contain any oocyte. It is correlated with an increased E2 to progesterone ratio and increased androtenedione levels, suggestive of dysfunctional follicular development. Most patients usually have mild endometriosis.

Luteinized Unruptured Follicles/Cyst

Jewelewicz in 1975 described the concept of pseudo-ovulation with luteinization of an unruptured follicle. In patients with LUF, the follicle does not rupture on the expected day and achieves a size much larger than the normal preovulatory size of 2 cm. USG revealed a thin-walled cyst with essentially clear contents. Some of these follicles may develop irregular intrafollicular echoes. The plasma

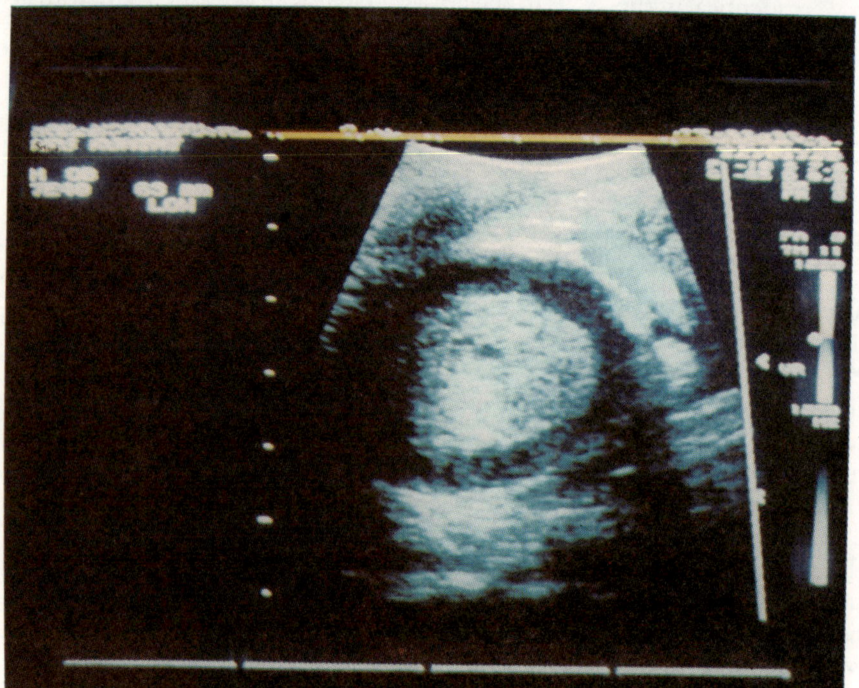

Fig. 9.7A. Ovarian cystic lesion with hyperechogenic contents, indicating dermoid cyst resulting in anovulation

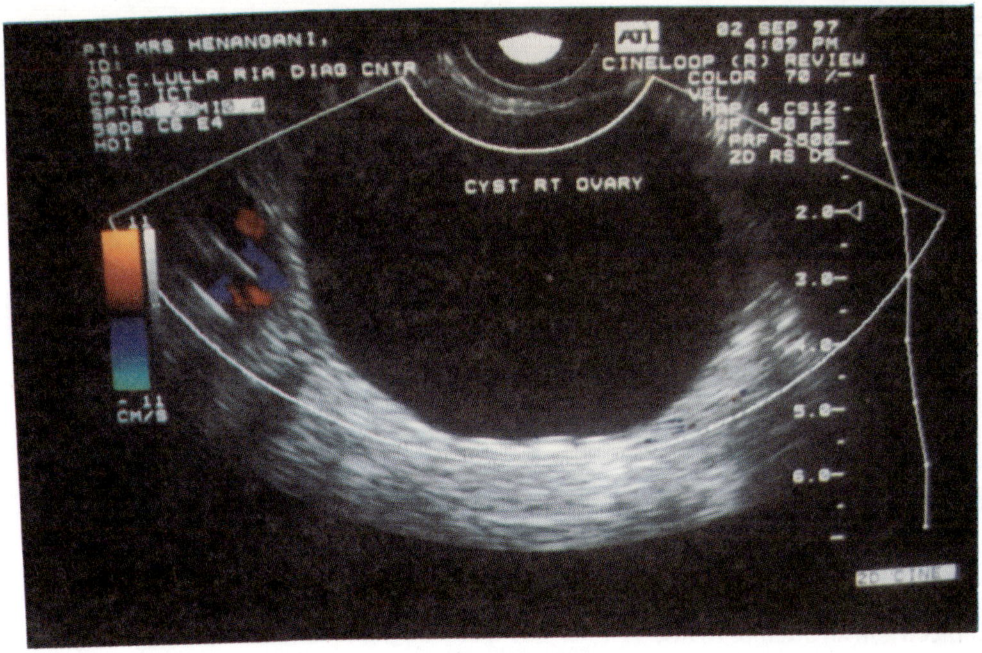

Fig. 9.7B. Luteinized unruptured follicle. Large cyst with thin walls and clear contents

progesterone levels, basal body temperature and endometrial biopsy indicated that ovulation had occurred. However, laparoscopic assessment failed to demonstrate the stigma of recent ovulation, suggesting that the oocyte was trapped in the luteinized follicle. The body temperature and hormonal assessment indicate ovulation.

The syndrome affects both ovaries, which may attain a volume of two to five times that of normal ovaries. Multiple peripherally placed, small follicles (8–9 mm in size) are present in 40% to 80% of cases with hyperechogenic central stroma. The ovaries in PCOS are heavy because of the multiple cysts and thick stroma, and may be situated

Polycystic Ovarian Syndrome (PCOS)

The ultrasound examination may have variable results. In a majority of cases, the ovarian size is increased (70% to 100%), as is the surface area.

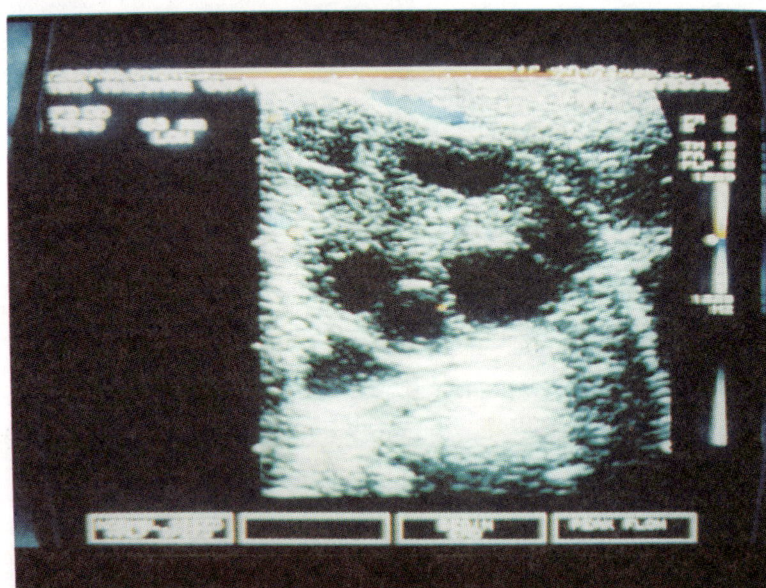

Fig. 9.8. Polycystic ovary showing echogenic stroma with multiple small-sized, peripherally placed follicles

deep in the cul-de-sac, in close apposition, giving rise to the characteristic 'Kissing Ovaries'.

Orsini and co-workers described four characteristic ultrasonographic appearances of PCOS: large and cystic ovaries, normal-sized ovaries with cystic features, and normal-sized and hyperechogenic solid ovaries. There is very little correlation between ultrasound findings and the symptoms or their duration. Treatment for PCO may be initiated with trial of clomiphene citrate (CC). Ultrasound is often performed near the expected midcycle (after a progesterone-induced withdrawal bleed), in an attempt to document ovulation in the patient so treated.

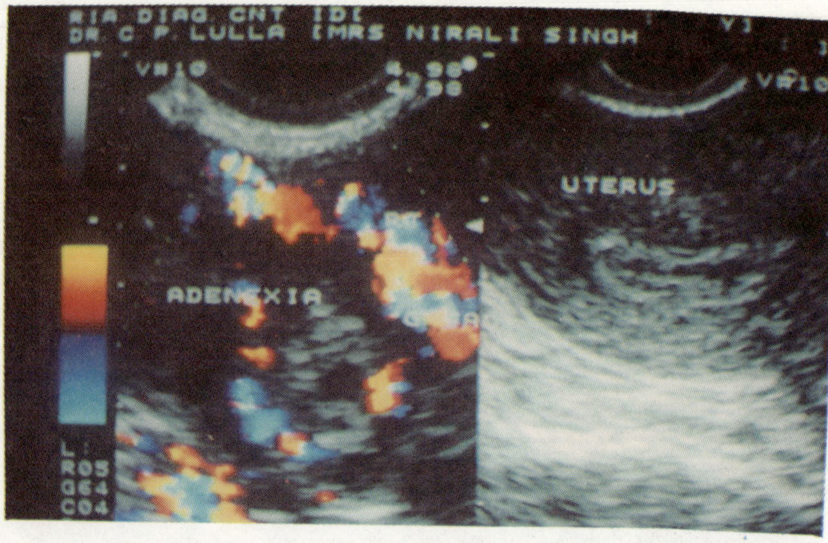

Fig. 9.9A: Ectopic pregnancy. On the right side, adnexial ring-like mass lesion with increased circumferential vascularity and on the left side, uterine endometrial cavity appears empty

Tubal Factors

The incidence of tubal factors in infertility still remains about 20%. Tubal obstruction may result from an ectopic pregnancy, pelvic inflammatory disease or endometriosis.

Ectopic Pregnancy

With the development of endovaginal scanning techniques, the reliability and role of ultrasound in the diagnosis of this entity have been clearly established. The triad of an empty uterus, free fluid, and an adexnal mass, coupled with a positive pregnancy test, should always alert one to the possibility of an ectopic pregnancy (Fig. 9.9A, B). This combination of findings is accurate in 95% of cases. Colour flow imaging allows for an assessment of the viability of the chronic tissue. In 10% of cases, a definitive diagnosis can be made by the demonstration of a live ectopic pregnancy. Of current interest is the recent demonstration of

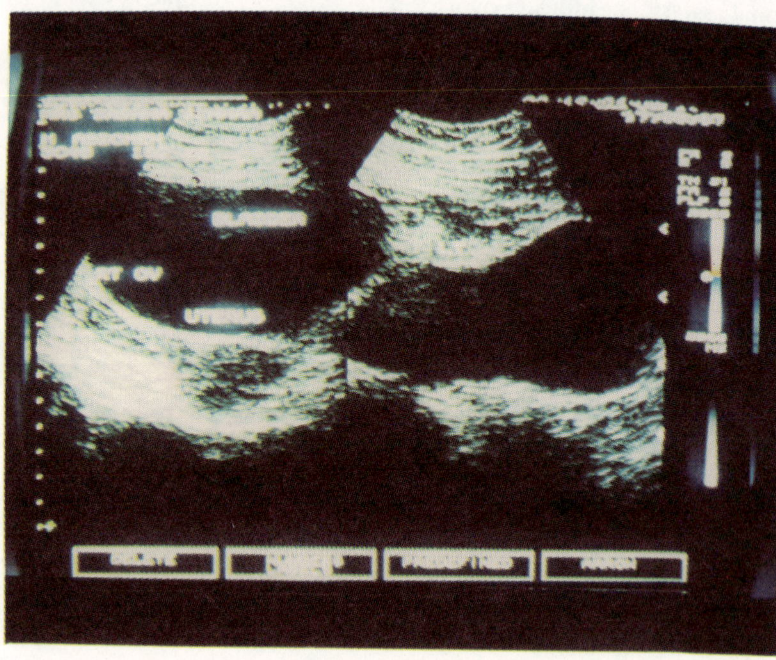

Fig. 9.9B: Tubular cystic mass of hydrosalpinx on left side

conservation and 'semi-invasive' management strategies, including non-surgical treatment of selected patients, by injection of the fetus with potassium chloride and or methotrexate (Pouly; Feichtinger; Timor-Tritsch).

Pelvic Inflammatory Disease (PID)

Clinically, the diagnosis of pelvic inflammatory disease should be suspected in patients with lower abdominal pain, purulent discharge and fever. The ultrasound findings are often nonspecific. Initially, the uterus may be enlarged, with indistinct margins. In the early phase of the illness, there may be mild adexnal enlargement, with loss of tissue plane definition. As the process becomes more severe, ill-defined areas of decreased echogenecity may be seen. These may be purely cystic or solid in appearance, and may be associated with the fluid in the cul-de-sac. The fluid accumulation often extends posterior to the uterus. Ultimately, frank abscess may develop. The differential diagnosis from haematoma, ectopic pregnancy and endometriosis may be extremely difficult. Tubal obstruction and hydrosalpinx may result from this process.

Endometriosis

It is in the demonstration of adnexal masses from endometriosis that ultrasound plays its greatest role. The presence of a well-defined hypoechoic mass with internal echoes may suggest the diagnosis. Although the classic endometrioma may be demonstrated, there is evidence that more diffuse forms of endometriosis may often go undetected on ultrasound. Firedman, using ultrasound, demonstrated the presence of endometriosis in only 4 of 37 patients (10.8%). It has been suggested that ovulatory disorders may be the cause of the infertility in endometriosis, but Matson et al. did not find differences in oocyte retrieval rates between grade I and IV endometriosis, despite their findings that pregnancy rates were progressively lower the more severe the grade of endometriosis.

It is uncommon to visualize the normal fallopian tube by ultrasonography (expect by passage of agitated saline or ultrasound contrast material). The abnormal dilated hydrosalpinx, however, can be well diagnosed with ultrasonography.

Tubal patency testing is possible with the use of salpingography (see Fig. 9.11). The uterus is distended with saline while scanning transabdominally or transvaginally (Richman). In addition, uterine pathologies, such as septa, polyps and submucous myomata, can also be demonstrated. In Randolphy's study, ultrasonic results agreed in 53 out of 54 cases with hyteroscopic assessment. No patient with obstructed tubes showed fluid in the cul-de-sac, and 5 of 56 patients with one tube proven to be patent did not accumulate fluid giving a sensitivity of 100% and a specificity of 91%. Side-specific patency could be established with nearly the same accuracy in 76 out of 112 patients.

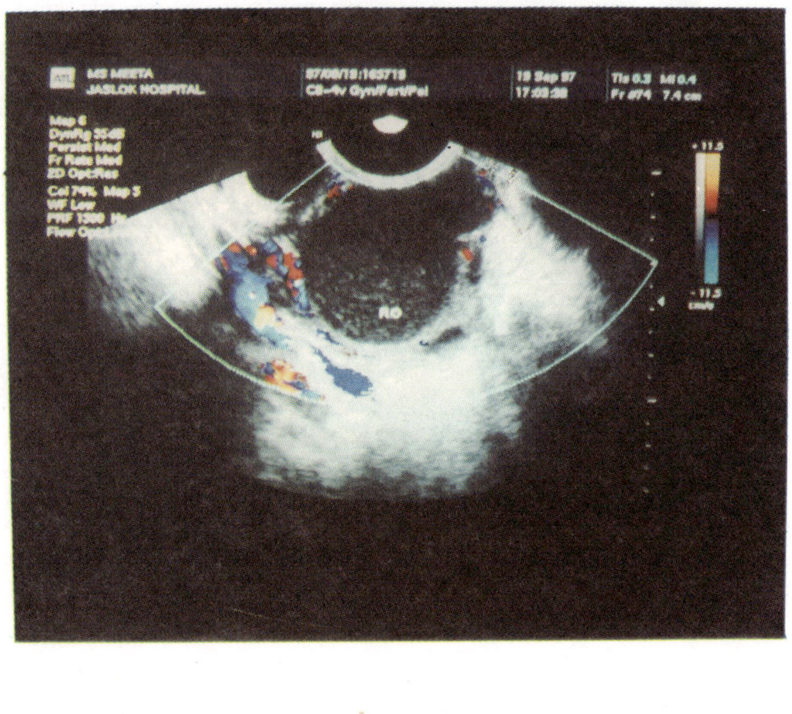

Fig. 9.10. Endometrioma. Cyst with low-level internal echoes

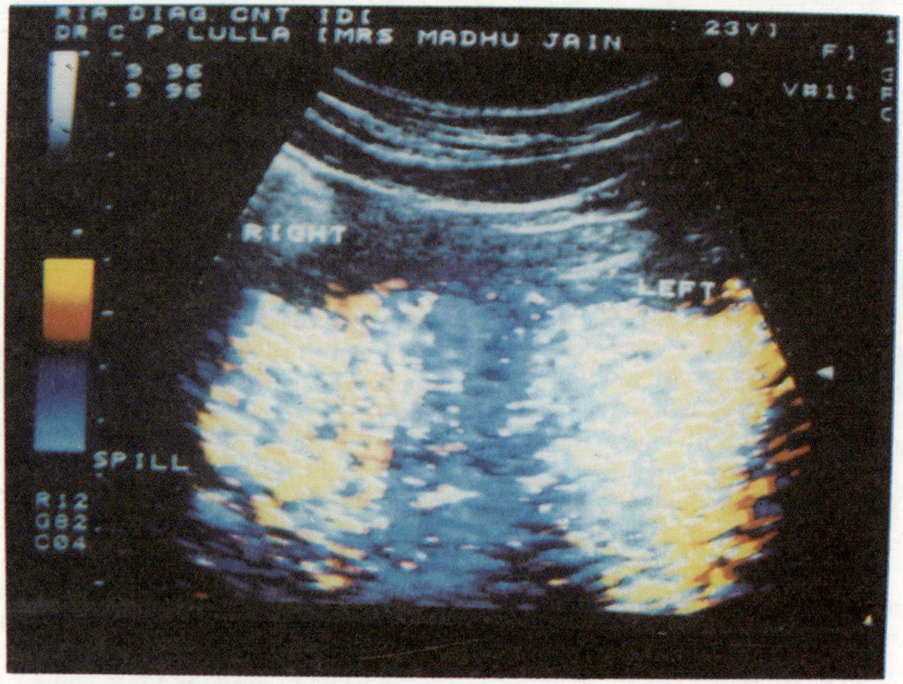

Fig. 9.11. Colour sonosalpingography. Colour Doppler signals are used to outline the passage of saline in the fallopian tubes. Bilateral spillage of colour signals (waterfall sign) is seen, indicating tubal patency

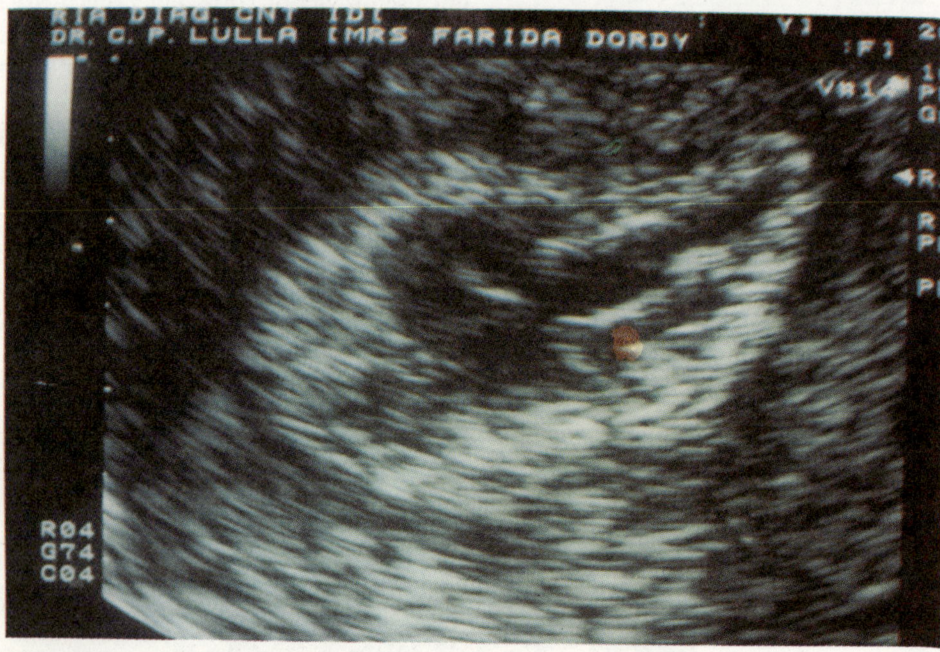

Fig. 9.12A. Sonohysterography outlining endometrial cavitary septae formation

In Richman's study, unilateral tubal patency was established correctly in 24 of 25 patients and bilateral obstruction was correctly diagnosed in 9 out of 9 patients.

UTERINE FACTORS

This may lead to an inability to conceive or cause repetitive early pregnancy loss. These abnormalities include:

1. Congenital anomalies and abnormalities associated with cervical incompetence.
2. Uterine fibroid or other acquired uterine abnormalities.
3. Endometrial cavity pathology and/implantation failure.

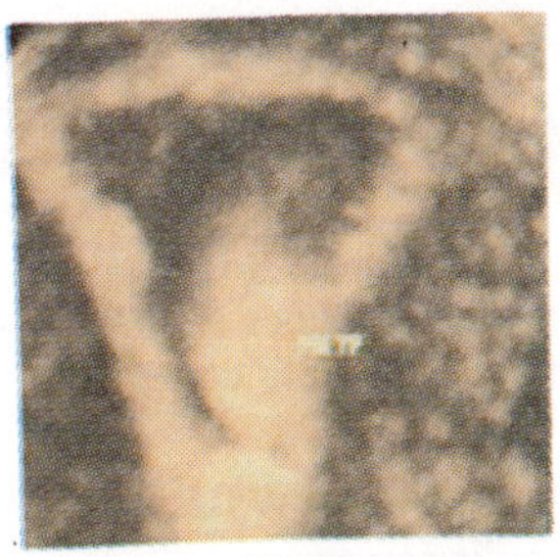

Fig. 9.12B. Sonohysterography outlining endometrial polyp

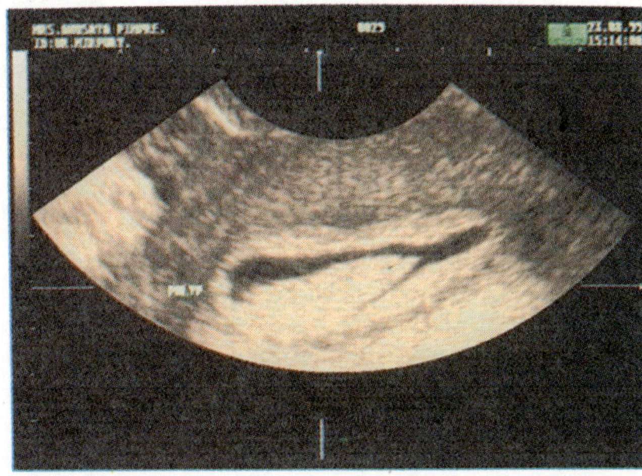

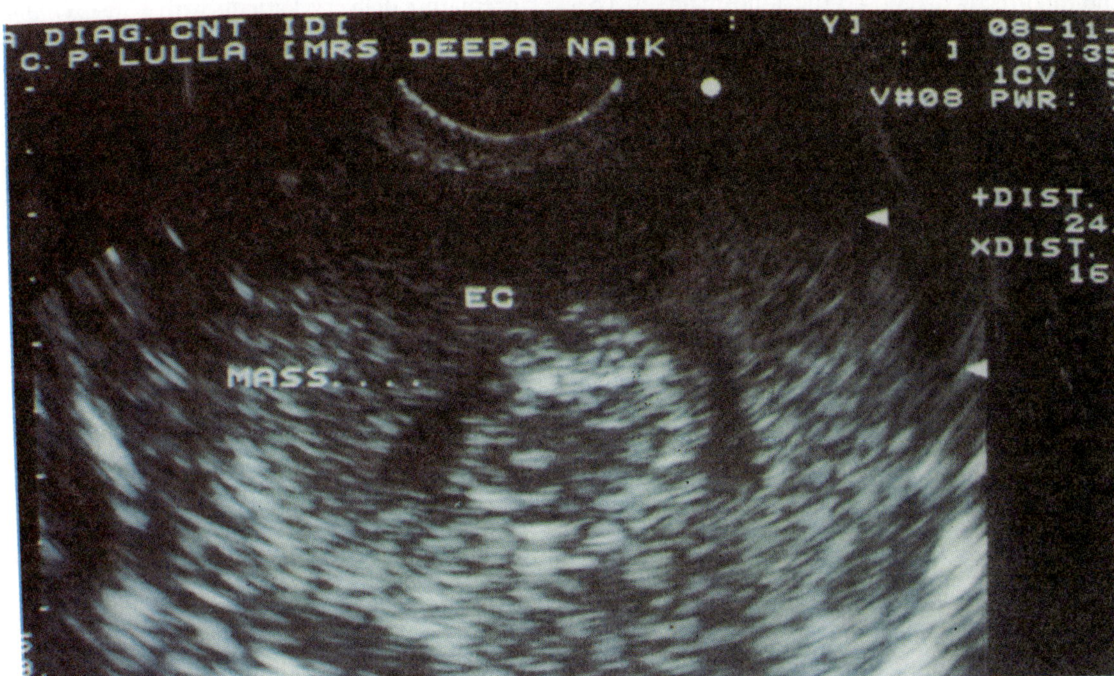

Fig. 9.12C. Sonohysterography outlining submucous fibroid

Congenital Abnormalities

Congenital abnormalities of the uterus are common in the population of patients with early fetal wastage. The uterus must be carefully examined in both the sagittal and transverse planes (slow transverse scanning will reveal two endometrial cavities). Care must be taken not to confuse a dual transverse endometrial echo created by the rectus artifact. In all cases where duplication of the uterus is suspected, evaluation of the urinary tract is suggested as there is a high association of concurrent abnormalities (see Fig. 9.13 A and B). In Malini's study of 68 patients, the patients were divided into five groups. Class I included segmental mullerian agenesis involving the vagina, cervix and uterus to various degrees; class II involved patients described as having 'peculiar-appearing uterus'; class III, uterus didelphys; class IV, bicornuate/septate uterus; and class V, obstructed lower genital tract with a normal upper tract. Ultrasound was diagnostic of the abnormality in 50% of cases and confirmatory in 37% of cases, and incorrectly diagnosed the abnormality in 13% of cases. Of the 50 patients examined, 9 had at least one absent kidney. Uterine hypoplasia, secondary to mullerian agencies, can cause infertility, while those with unicornuate or rudimentary horn may have problems of spontaneous abortion or premature delivery. Patients with a uterus didelphy, i.e. a completely split uterus and cervix, are often

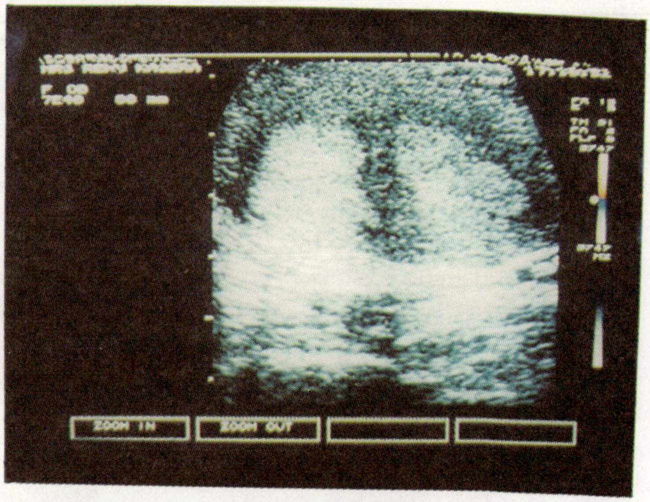

Fig. 9.13A. Bicornuate uterus. In the late secretory phase, splitting of endometrial echoes is seen. This needs to be differentiated from subseptate uterus

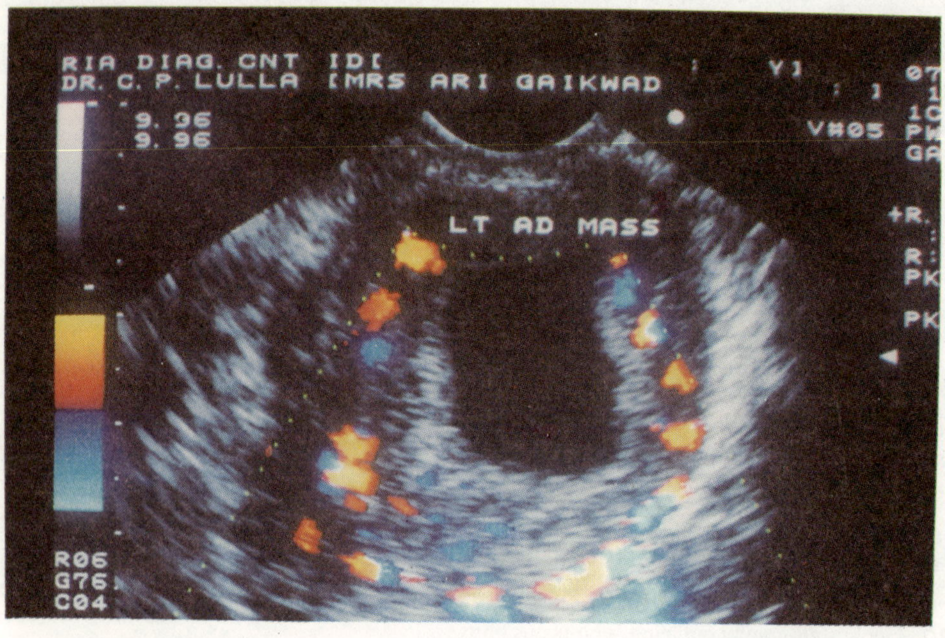

Fig. 9.13B. Rudimentary horn of uterus with haematometra presenting as left adnexial cystic mass lesion with thick wall (uterine myometrium)

fertile, requiring ultrasound assistance to determine the side on which ovulation is taking place. The bicornuate uterus (two horns and a single cervix) may be complete, partial, or accurate; however, this rarely causes fetal wastage. Patients with a septate uterus are often infertile or suffer from early fetal wastage.

Fibroids

Submucous and occasionally intramural uterine fibroids have been associated with infertility and early fetal loss (Butterman). Uterine contour irregularity was the commonest ultrasound finding according to Gross et al., as compared to a focal mass, either hypoechoic or hyperechoic, seen in about 75% of patients. Here, oestrogen is important in the development of fibroids, a finding that is confirmed by their apparent enlargement during reproductive life and regression during menopause. Recently, GnRH-agonists have been used in the treatment of patients with fibroids (Firedman). These agents cause a decrease in the size of the uterine fibroids as oestrogen circulating in the blood is diminished. The expected progressive diminution in uterine size occurs over several months of the required treatment and should be monitored with ultrasound. In seven studies covering 57 patients in total, the mean volume of uterine size reduction was 50% after 3 to 6 months of therapy. The fibroid size will often return to the pretreatment size after cessation of treatment. It is suggested that this form of management be used before planned myomectomy. Some have suggested that if the fibroid causes cornual obstruction, treatment with GnRH-agonists may alleviate this and permit conception.

Endometrial Cavity Pathology and Implantation Failure

Endometrial atrophy, either due to endometrial adhesions after trauma (Asherman syndrome) (Yaffe) or from chronic inflammation, as in tuberculous endometriosis (Bazaz-Malik), can lead to infertility. The endometrium on USG would appear as thin as a line or not well defined.

Pregnancy sometimes becomes established despite a very restricted amount of endometrium, but with untreated intracavity adhesions, there is a high prevalence of spontaneous miscarriage and premature delivery.

Endometrial space-occupying lesions, such as an endometrial or submucous fibroid, prevents the anterior and posterior endometrium from pressing effectively upon the hatching blastocyst. There can also be secondary endometriosis, comparable to the presence in the cavity of an intrauterine device.

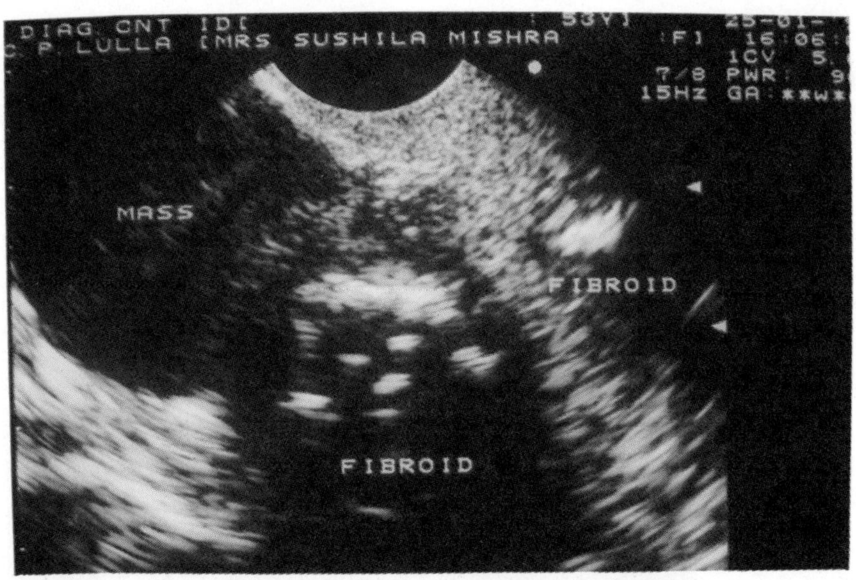

Fig. 9.14. Fibroids. Multiple intramural, partially calcified fibroids distorting the endometrial cavity

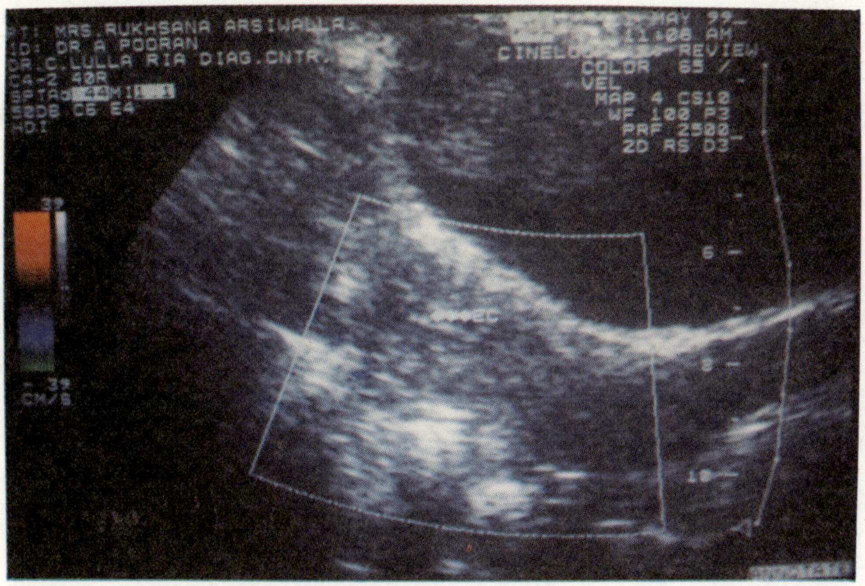

Fig. 9.15A. Endometrial atrophy due to endometrial adhesions after trauma (Asherman syndrome) or from chronic inflammation, as in tuberculous endometriosis. A poor, ill-defined endometrial cavity is seen

HSG is the best tool for revealing the location of adhesions as well, whereas ultrasound is the best for indicating the amount of residual endometrial mucosa. Ultrasound findings in adhesions and polyps can be equivocal, unless considered carefully in relation to endometrial appearances that are normal for the particular stage of the endometrial cycle. Atrophy and adhesions might be inferred only by showing patchy endometrial development, despite late-follicular-phase activity in an ovary. Endometrial polyps should be suspected ultrasonographically when there is focal or general echogenecity of the endometrium at times in the folliculate phase of the cycle, when the endometrium is ordinarily relatively lucent.

PHYSIOLOGY OF UTERINE CIRCULATION

The uterine arteries originate from the anterior division of the internal iliac arteries. On reaching the uterus, they divide into ascending and descending branches. After penetrating the myometrium, the arteries divide further into arcuate arteries that course within the uterine walls.

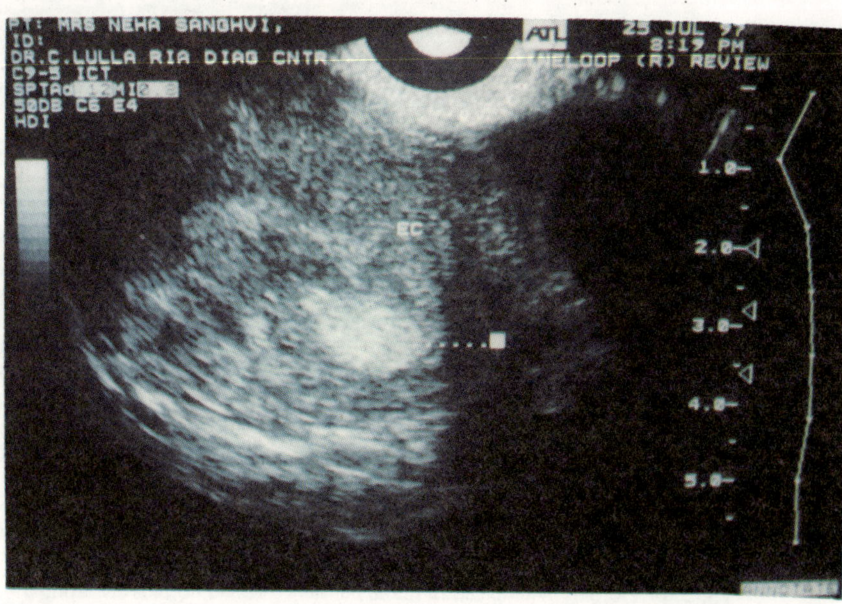

Fig. 9.15B. Endometrial polyp. Focal hyperechogenicity is seen in the thickened endometrial cavity

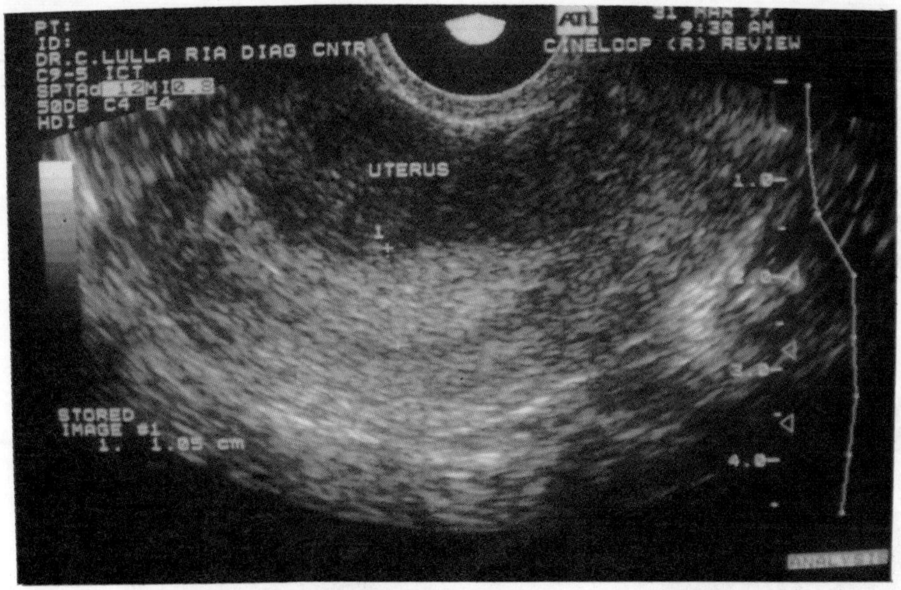

Fig. 9.15C. Endometrial polyp. Diffuse endometrial thickening is seen

In the arcuate arteries, blood flows in a direction parallel to the surface. The radial arteries arise perpendicular to the arcuate arteries and are, therefore, directed towards the uterine cavity. Radial arteries give rise to basal and spiral arteries. Uterine blood flow is regulated by many factors, essentially by the levels of the reproductively active steroid hormones. Oestrogens cause vasodilatation and increased blood flow to the uterus, whereas progesterone has the opposite effect (Williams).

Goswamy and Steptoe had used a modified systolic/diastolic ratio (S/D) and modified resistance index (RI) to characterize uterine perfusion and the changes thereof during the menstrual cycle. They demonstrated that the RI and the S/D ratio fell with the rise in the oestrogen level during the early follicular phase, then rose in the periovulatory period, parallel to the preovulatory progesterone levels. These changes indicated an increased uterine perfusion periovulatory period. A secondary increase in the luteal phase was also closely related to changes in the hormone levels (de Zielger).The changes in the impedance of uterine arterial vessels during the ovarian and menstrual cycles have been further detailed. *The pulsatility index* (as a measurement of downstream resistance) was found to fall from a mean of 3.8 in the early follicular phase to 3.0 in late follicular phase. A further decrease to 2.5 was observed in the luteal phase (Steer). Several possible criteria could be evaluated (Taylor).

1. The presence or absence of blood flow, or determination of its direction.
2. Quantification of blood flow and characterization of downstream impedance.
3. Quantification of changes associated with hormonal modifications during the menstrual cycle.
4. Actual blood flow rate analysis. Taylor and coworkers demonstrated that different vessels have specific waveform (vessel signatures) (Taylor). Doppler signals can be obtained from several areas of the uterus, but are optimal in the main uterine arteries lateral to the cervix and the lower uterine segment, that is, roughly at the level of the internal os.

Goswamy and co-workers described decreased uterine perfusion as a possible cause of infertility. Other investigators have shown that improved pregnancy rates seem to be correlated with an enchanced blood flow in the uterine vessels (Steer). Changes in the uterine blood flow are not completely related to hormone levels and some IVF patients with high levels of oestrogen do not have adequate uterine flow indices. Among 20 IVF patients studied with transvaginal Doppler ultrasonography, the worst factors in terms of

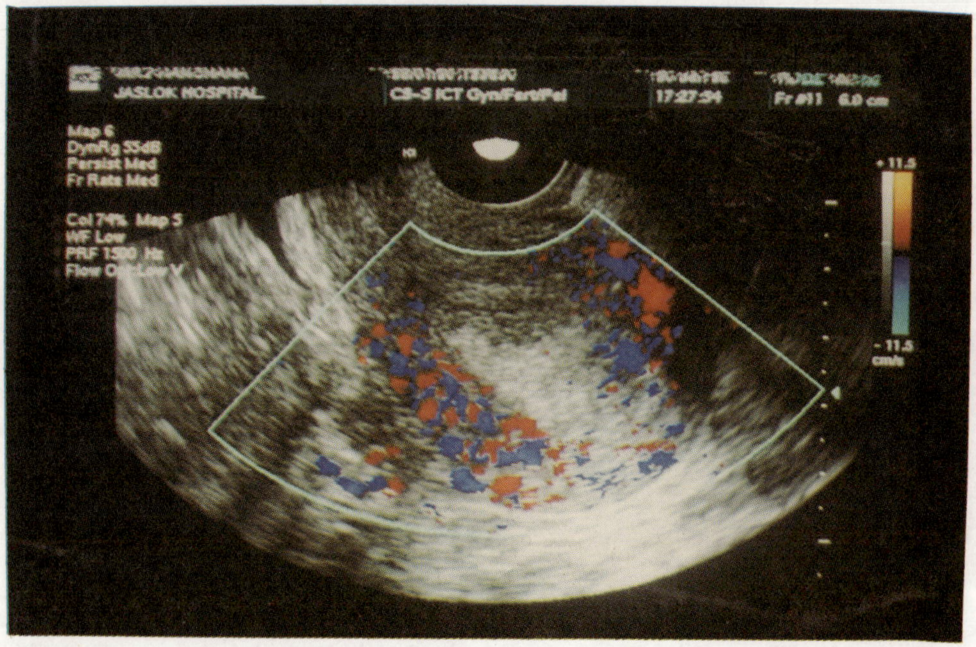

Fig. 9.16. Colour Doppler reveals normal morphological periendometrial blood flow in the midcycle

pregnancy rate, not unexpectedly, were low oestradiol levels and a lack of increase in the blood flow between the beginning of the cycle and the day of embryo transfer (Abramowicz). Contrary to what has been shown in the ovarian arteries, i.e. differences between the ovulatory and contralateral side, flow indices in both uterine arteries behave similarly during the cycle, regardless of the location of the luteal gland (Setti).

Women with blood flow characteristics indicative of a better-than-expected uterine environment may be at higher risk of implantation of all transferred embryos and, therefore, at higher risk of a multiple pregnancy. In a study of 82 patients, uterine receptivity was examined by the pulsatility index as a measure of uterine blood flow impedance (lower impedance = better flow, better receptivity). The ideal values of the pulsatility index were between 2.00 and 2.99, with a pregnancy rate of 47% (17 of 36 patients), but a high multiple pregnancy rate of 47% (8 to 17 patients) (Steer).

Ovarian Circulation

Both ovarian arteries take origin from the aorta and reach the ovaries through the infundibulopelvic ligaments. After giving off small branches that penetrate the ovarian stroma, they anastomose with distal vessels of the ascending branches of the uterine arteries. The clearest Doppler signals can be obtained in the ovarian artery just before it reaches the ovarian hilus. This vascular position also corresponds most closely to the general ovarian impedance. The flow can also be elucidated from within the ovarian tissues.

Differences in ovarian blood flow between the ovulatory and nonovulatory sides can be recognized early in the cycle. Deutinger's longitudinal study of 14 patients suggested that increased blood flow occurs early in the cycle in the ovary destined to become the ovulatory one, before other signs are recognized (Deutinger).

Newer Imaging Modalities

Colour Doppler Ultrasound in Infertility

Colour flow mapping has been used to describe changes that occur in the follicle at or around the time of the luteinizing hormone surge and peak (Bourne, Persion). Angiogenesis takes place in the ovary following ovulation, as a part of luteogenesis (Koos, Tanaka).

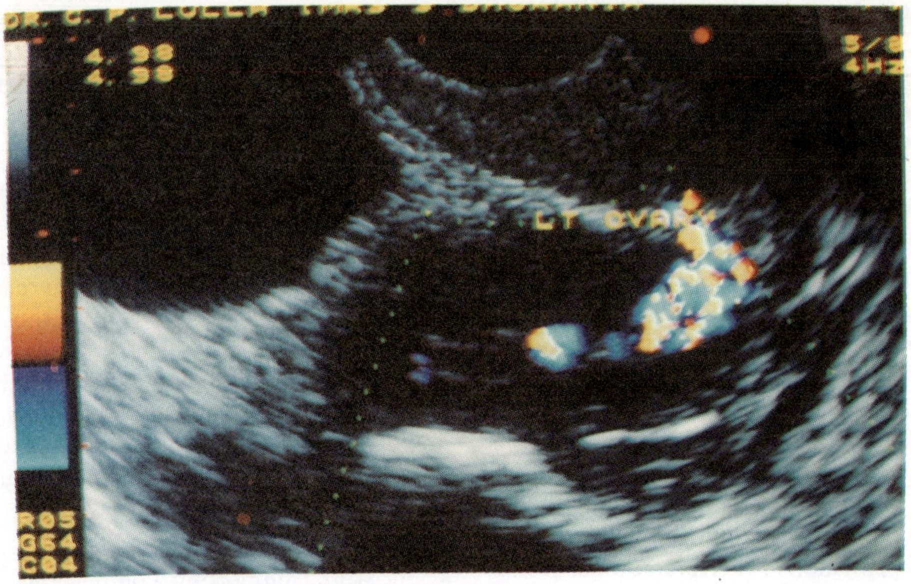

Fig. 9.17. Normal ovarian artery in ovarian stroma

Prediction of the probability of success in assisted reproductive procedures was the first clinical demonstration of the importance of Doppler flow studies in pelvic vessels (Mcsweeney). Cyclical changes are demonstrated by transvaginal Doppler ultrasonography in both uterine and ovarian arteries with better forward flows (i.e. less resistance) in IVF cycles.

The RI measured in the uterine artery is relatively low in patients before gonadotrophin stimulation; there is a gradual increase in the indices until the day of follicle aspiration and a subsequent rapid decline throughout the luteal phase (Thaler). The mean RI in the uterine artery is 0.88 in the proliferative phase, and decreases to a nadir of 0.84 6 days after ovulation. In the same study, flow rates were the lowest on the day of follicle aspiration (about 65mL/min) and rapidly increased thereafter, to a maximum of 96mL/min, 12 days into the luteal phase.

Deutinger and co-workers studied 38 patients from their IVF programme. All patients were treated with GnRH-agonists to suppress ovarian function before follicular stimulation with human menopausal gonadotrophin. Ovulation was then induced by the administration of hCG in accordance with standard ovulation induction protocols. Doppler measurements were performed daily on both ovarian arteries. A marked increase in diastolic flow velocity was observed towards follicular puncture for ovum harvesting. Decreased pulsatility indices, a sign of decreased resistances to flow, continued after follicle puncture. Resistances to flow were significantly lower in patients defined as high responders i.e. those with oestradiol levels higher than 200 pg. per follicle greater than 15 mm on the day of HCG administration, than in those defined as low responders (Duetinger). Fleischer reported that stimulated ovaries exhibit higher flow velocities, and the pulsatility index and RI depend on the number of follicles induced in each cycle.

Some investigators maintain that the vascular indices in the uterine arteries differ between patients who become pregnant in an IVF programme versus those who do not; however, the indices of the ovarian vessels do not have predictive values (Sterzik). Sixty-five patients in an assisted reproductive technology programme were followed by transvaginal Doppler evaluation of the ovaries beginning 3 days after embryo transfer, or 5 days after GIFT. The scans continued weekly until pregnancy was diagnosed or menses ensued. The difference between the RI of those who became pregnant and those who did not was significant. Higher blood flow velocities (less resistance) were present in the patients who became pregnant. No patient with an RI of above 0.5 became pregnant (Baber). The conclusion was that transvaginal Doppler interrogation of the ovarian vasculature permits early prediction of treatment failure and may be indicative of corpus luteum inadequacy.

Despite improvements in fertilization rates and stimulation regimens, the probability of implantation per embryo transferred remains low in the assisted conception programme (10% to 15%) (Abramowicz, 1992). The most promising application of colour Doppler could be in this field. Changes in the ovarian and uterine perfusion can be measured with colour Doppler, and it may be that embryo replacement could be better timed to improve implantation rates (Abramowicz, 1992: 317–27).

Three-Dimensional Ultrasound of the Uterus

Despite many recent technical improvements, there are still important limitations to the accuracy of ultrasound diagnosis in gynaecology. An important problem is caused by the pelvic anatomy, which severely restricts the movement of the transducer during the scan. This results in a very limited number of scanning planes available for examination.

The examination of the uterus is usually limited to transverse and longitudinal sections, which give an incomplete view of the uterine fundus. For this reason, conventional two-dimensional (2D) sonography is not adequate for the definite diagnosis of congenital fusion defects of the uterus.

The three-dimensional (3D) ultrasound technique overcomes some of the limitations of 2D sonography mentioned above. The major advantages are the ability to obtain ultrasound sections, which are impossible to see on a routine scan, and the ability to perform accurate volume measurements. In addition, 3D anatomical reconstruction of the organs of interest is possible.

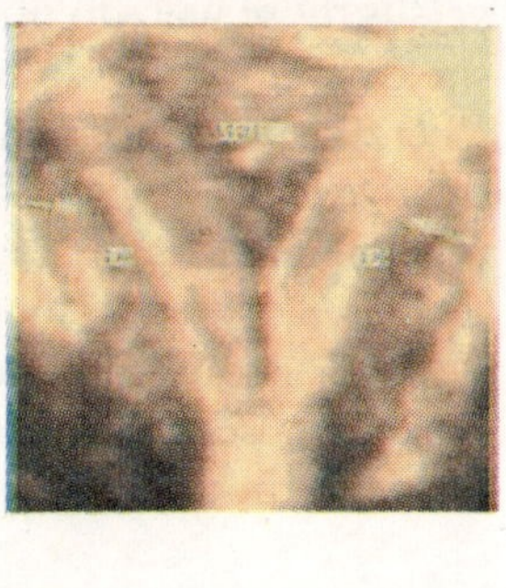

Fig. 9.18. 3D image of the endometrium reveals separation of endometrial echo, with no indentation of the fundal myometrium, indicating subseptate uterus rather than bicornuate uterus

Three perpendicular planes are simultaneously shown on the screen, thus facilitating easier understanding of uterine anatomy. The number and orientation of reformatted planes are not limited, thus providing sections through the uterus that could not be obtained on a routine scan. The most useful plane is a coronal section through the whole length of the uterus, from the fundus to the cervix. This plane, being perpendicular to the direction of the ultrasound beam spread, cannot be seen on a conventional transvaginal scan.

Volume measurements can also be performed using stored ultrasound volumes. We have been mostly interested in the measurement of endometrial volume. Three perpendicular reformatted sections are displayed on the screen and a longitudinal plane is chosen for volume measurements. The other two planes are used to ensure that the whole of the uterine cavity has been included in the measurement. The actual measurement is performed by delineating the whole of the uterine cavity in a number of parallel longitudinal sections 1–2 mm apart. The endometrial volume is then calculated automatically by the in-built computer software programme. The normal endometrial volume is 2 to 5mL.

Three-Dimensional Ultrasound for the Detection of Congenital Uterine Anomalies

The prevalence and clinical significance of congenital uterine anomalies are uncertain. They appear to be associated with an increased risk of miscarriage, premature birth, fetal loss, malpresentations and Caesarean sections (Harger, Rock). The diagnosis of congenital uterine anomaly is usually made in patients with previous pregnancy loss. Its prevalence in the general population is largely unknown. This is partly due to the lack of a simple and accurate diagnostic test which can be used in low-risk patients.

Hysterosalpingography is widely accepted as a

standard method for diagnosis of congenital uterine anomalies. It is an invasive test, which requires the use of contrast medium and exposure to radiation. Although HSG provides a good outline of the uterine cavity, it gives no information about the outer uterine contour. Therefore, distinction between different types of lateral fusion disorders is often impossible (White-House; Randolph). In these cases, laparoscopy or laparotomy may be necessary to achieve a final diagnosis. Although recent reports have indicated high accuracy of magnetic resonance imaging (MRI) for the diagnosis of congenital uterine defects (Pellerito), the technique remains very expensive and is rarely used for this indication. Due to the limitations of the current diagnostic methods, the final diagnosis is usually achieved only by combining the results of two or more tests.

The important advantages of ultrasound over other imaging methods are its noninvasiveness, safety and simplicity. Unfortunately, efforts to characterize congenital uterine anomalies by 2D B-mode ultrasound were not successful.

When used as a screening test, transvaginal sonography has provided sensitivity rates of up to 100%. However, the distinction between the different types of anomalies is often impossible (Valdes; Fedel). Ultrasound is operator-dependent and hardcopy images can be difficult for a third party to interpret. Therefore, other diagnostic methods are usually required to complete the diagnostic evaluation, particularly in those patients who are scheduled for corrective surgery.

The American Fertility Society Classification of Mullerian Anomalies (The American Fertility Society) was used to describe uterine defects. The criteria for the diagnosis of an arcuate uterus were a normal appearance of the cervix and myometrium, the absence of a fundal cleft, and a rounded, concave appearance of the fundal portion of the uterine cavity. In the case of a subseptate uterus, the proximal part of the uterine cavity was partially divided by a septum. The myometrium appeared normal. However, if a fundal indentation is present, it has to be less than 1cm in depth to allow for classification as a subseptate uterus. The diagnosis of bicornuate uterus is made when divergent, well-founded cornua are seen, separated by a large fundal cleft.

The sensitivity and specificity and the positive and negative predictive values of 2D and 3D ultrasound for the diagnosis of a normal uterus and congenital uterine anomalies were calculated in 58 patients with technically acceptable 3D volumes. All cases of congenital anomalies were detected by both 2D and 3D scans. Five false-positive diagnoses of arcuate uterus and three of major uterine anomalies had decreased specificity and positive predictive values of 2D in comparison to 3D scans. There were no false-positive of false-negative diagnoses of congenital uterine anomalies with 3D ultrasound 1995 (Jurkovic). The results indicate that 3D ultrasound may become an important method of assessment of the uterine anatomy and diagnosis of congenital uterine anomalies. In most patients, 3D ultrasound has made possible a clear visualization of the uterine cavity and the diagnosis of congenital anomalies. The images are easier to obtain in the luteal phase of the cycle, due to the increased thickness and the echogenicity of the endometrium.

Oocyte Retrieval

Most ART programmes routinely use one or a number of ovarian stimulation protocols to achieve multifollicular development; pregnancy rates improve as the number of transferred embryos is increased.

Lenz had first described ultrasound-guided follicle puncture in 1981(Lenz). Ultrasound- guided techniques have now replaced the earlier laparoscopic procedures. Oocyte retrieval is generally performed in a surgical suite or near equivalent under intravenous sedation, although in certain circumstances, a general anaesthesia may be required because of the patient's extreme discomfort.

The transvaginal approach is now most commonly employed worldwide (Hartz), offering relatively painless access to the ovary. The needle tip or an automated puncture device is now used to direct a 30-cm 16- or 18-gauge needle through the vaginal wall into each individual follicle. All follicles in excess of 1.0 cm are punctured and aspirated. Occasionally, flushing of the curette with the culture medium is required, in order to dislodge the cumulus and oocyte from the follicle wall. The follicular fluid is transported immediately at body temperature to a laboratory, where a gametologist examines it for the presence of oocytes. After the retrieval procedure, the pelvis is evaluated generally for fluid leakage, an invariable accompaniment of the procedure. This should not cause alarm unless it is excessive and fluid becomes visible in the flanks.

Inadvertent puncture of a pelvic vein or adherent bowel may occur, most often without serious sequel. Complications associated with transvaginal oocyte retrieval are infrequent. In a consecutive series of 3,656 procedures, Dicker and co-workers reported 9 (0.24%) tubo-ovarian abscesses or pelvic abscesses and 3 (0.08%) with severe intra-abdominal bleeding (Dicker).

Embryo Transfer

Transfer of the early embryo to the uterus is a critical last step in the ART treatment cycle. This technique involves replacement of the embryo within the uterus. TVS-guided intrauterine transfer of the embryo not only ensures that the tip of the catheter is appropriately positioned, but also assists the operator when submucous myomas or uterine anomalies make anatomically correct embryo transfer difficult (Husley). Three-dimensional transvaginal scanning has recently been used to confirm the 'landing site' of transferred embryos (Feichtinger).

COMPLICATIONS—DIAGNOSIS AND MANAGEMENT

The complications of ovulation induction include ovarian hyperstimulation syndrome (OHS) and multiple pregnancy.

Ovarian Hyperstimulation Syndrome (OHS)

This syndrome includes the presence of enlarged cystic ovaries, increased capillary permeability resulting in a variable degree of ascites, pleural effusion and possibly, thromboembolic states, which at worst, can result in shock and death. It has been described in low- or normal-oestrogen states, thus limiting the value of oestrogen monitoring in the prevention of OHS. TVS can detect those patients prone to developing hyperstimulation (Figs. 9.19 and 9.20) during the follicular phase of superovulatory cycles. Blankstein et al. had noted an increase in intermediate-sized follicles (9–15

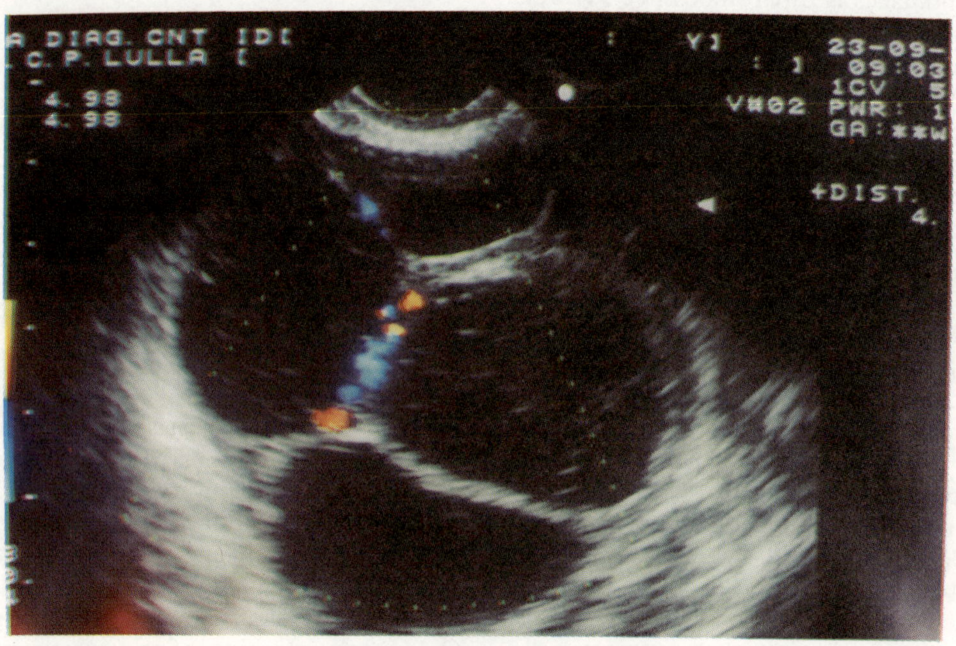

Fig. 9.19. Ovarian hyperstimulation. Enlarged ovaries with multiple cysts are seen

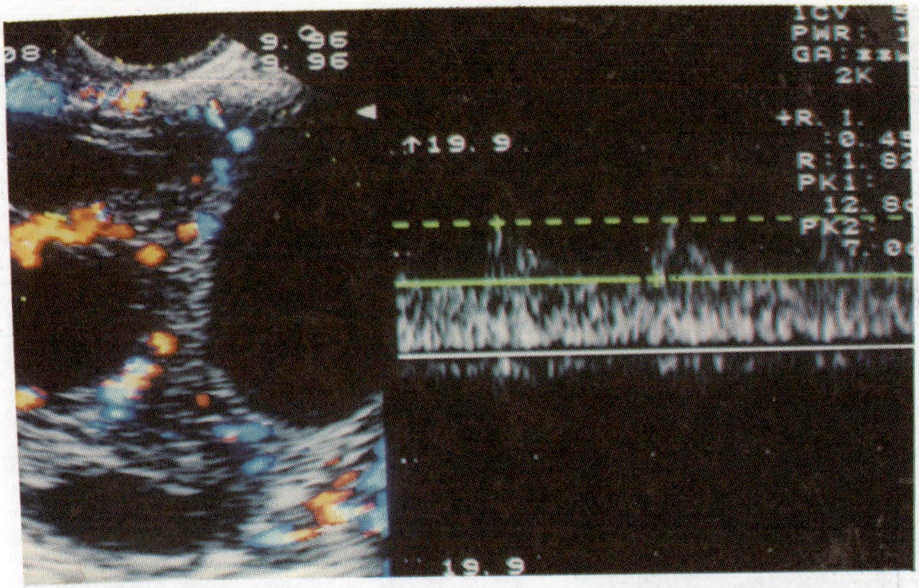

Fig. 9.20. Ovarian hyperstimulation. Premature low-resistance pattern (high diastolic flow) of vascularity is seen, suggesting fall in resistance and subsequent development of OHS

mm) with mild hyperstimulation, and a predominance of smaller follicles (under 9 mm) in women in whom severe hyperstimulation developed subsequently (Blankstein). A premature fall in ovarian resistance indices may also be a marker for the subsequent development of OHS.

Multiple Pregnancy

A second significant complication of ovulation induction is the development of multiple pregnancy. Patients stimulated with clomiphene citrate developed multiple follicles in 35% to 60% of cases, and up to 80% in hMG cycles. It remains very difficult to predict or control the incidence of multiple pregnancy, but patients should always be informed about this possibility in cycles in which multiple follicles in excess of 15 mm are identified on the day of planned hCG administration.

IMAGING OF MALE FACTOR INFERTILITY

Up to 50% of the defects causing infertility occur in the male partner. These defects account for a reduction in the quantity and quality of sperm in the ejaculate. The causes of male infertility are broadly classified as potentially correctable or non-correctable lesions, although abnormalities that cause testicular failure and impaired spermatogenesis cannot be corrected. Obstruction can occur at any level of the urogenital tract—proximal (e.g., affecting the epidermis) or distal (e.g., affecting the ejaculatory duct). Stenosis, obstruction or abnormalities of the distal sperm transport system result in a diminished semen volume and blockage of the flow of sperm into the ejaculate. Transrectal and testicular ultrasonography are now the primary methods of imaging for male factor infertility.

Transrectal Ultrasonography (TRUS)

Seminal Vesicles

The seminal vesicle is formed as a saccular dilatation of the vas deferens (distal mesonephric duct), near its junction with the urogenital sinus. Congenital anomalies in the seminal vesicles as well as obstructive lesions result in a diminished semen volume, low pH and low fructose levels.

Seminal vesicle abnormalities are reported to occur in a majority of patients with agenesis of the vas deferens.

Congenital unilateral absence of the vas deferens is present in 1 to 7 men per 1,000 individuals in the normal male population. Congenital bilateral absences of the vas deferens occur in approximately

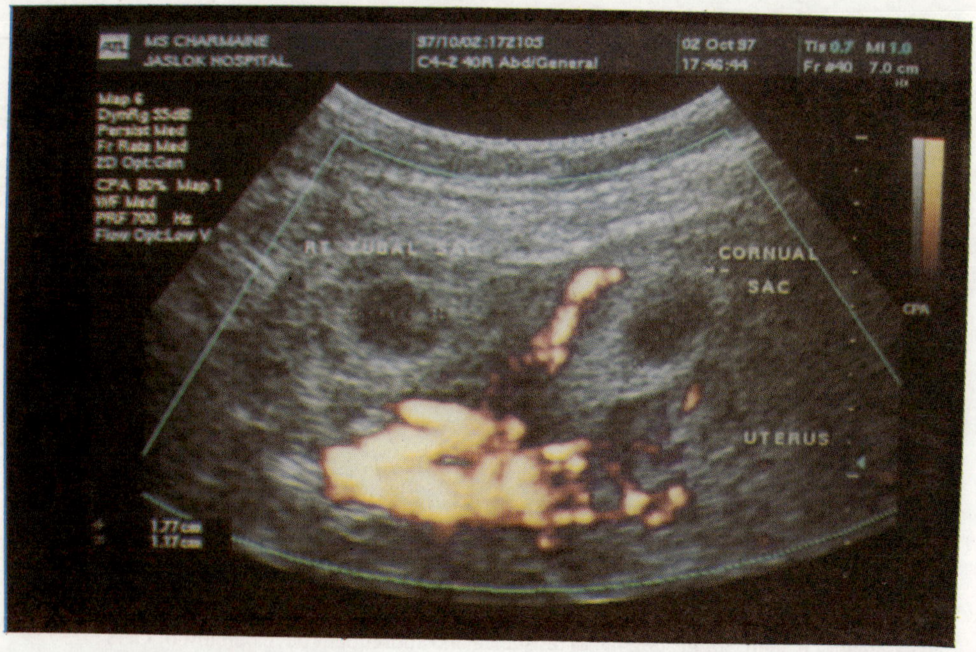

Fig. 9.21. Multiple pregnancy following ART. Heterotropic pregnancy is seen with intrauterine and right-sided tubal pregnancy.

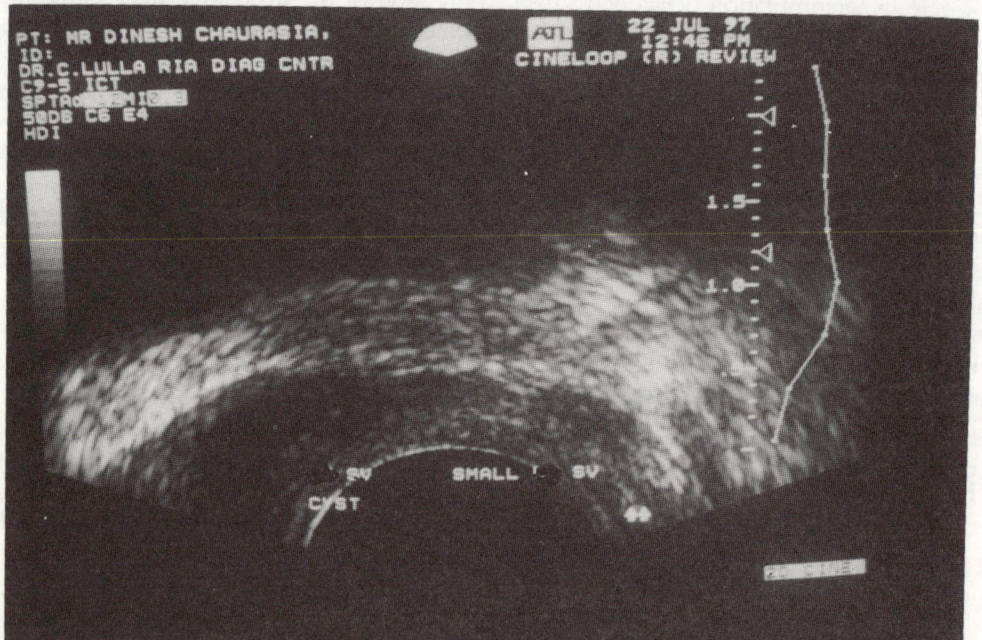

Fig. 9.22. Congenital seminal vesicle cyst seen on the right side and atrophy of seminal vesicle seen on the left side.

1% of infertile men and account for 4% to 17% of patients with azoospermia. Sixteen per cent to 43% of patients with bilateral agenesis of the vas deferens also have renal anomalies, such as renal agenesis, crossed renal ectopia, or an ectopic pelvic kidney, usually on the left side (Charny; Kaneti; Kenney; Rubin; Trigauz).

Seminal vesicle cysts may be either congenital or acquired, in association with obstructive lesions. Congenital seminal vesicle cysts are rare. They are usually associated with an ectopic ureter draining into the seminal vesicle from a dysplastic kidney, with unilateral renal agenesis or with other genitourinary anomalies (Heaney; Walls).

When an infection involves the seminal vesicles, fibrotic changes may produce cystic dilatation, obliteration, or stricture of the lumen. The seminal vesicles can then be identified as an-echogenic, nonhomogeneous structures, lacking normal convoluted ductal architecture. Chronic inflammation may decrease seminal function and causes infertility.

Stone Formation is Another Sequel of Infection

TRUS readily demonstrates stones as echogenic foci with acoustic shadowing in the seminal vesicles in the distal portion of the vas deferens, or in the ampullary region (Asch; Malatinsky).

Ejaculatory Ducts

TRUS is useful in detecting the various anatomical abnormalities associated with complete and partial ejaculatory duct obstruction or stenosis. The confluence of the seminal vesicles and the terminal ampullary region of the vas deferens in the prostate form the ejaculatory duct; therefore, an occlusion of the ejaculatory duct results in a diminished semen volume.

In midline cysts, which are variably referred to as ejaculatory duct cysts, mullerian duct cysts, or urogenital sinus cysts, the orifices of the ejaculatory duct enter the cysts. These cysts contain sperm and may obstruct the free flow of seminal fluid during ejaculation (Hamilton). Stone formation is an inflammation of the ejaculatory duct. In these cases, TRUS demonstrates echogenic foci with acoustic shadowing in the ejaculatory duct (Littrup).

Prostate

Obstruction within the prostate may be produced by cysts or by the sequel of infections, for instance, prostatitis. Acute infections in the prostate, with

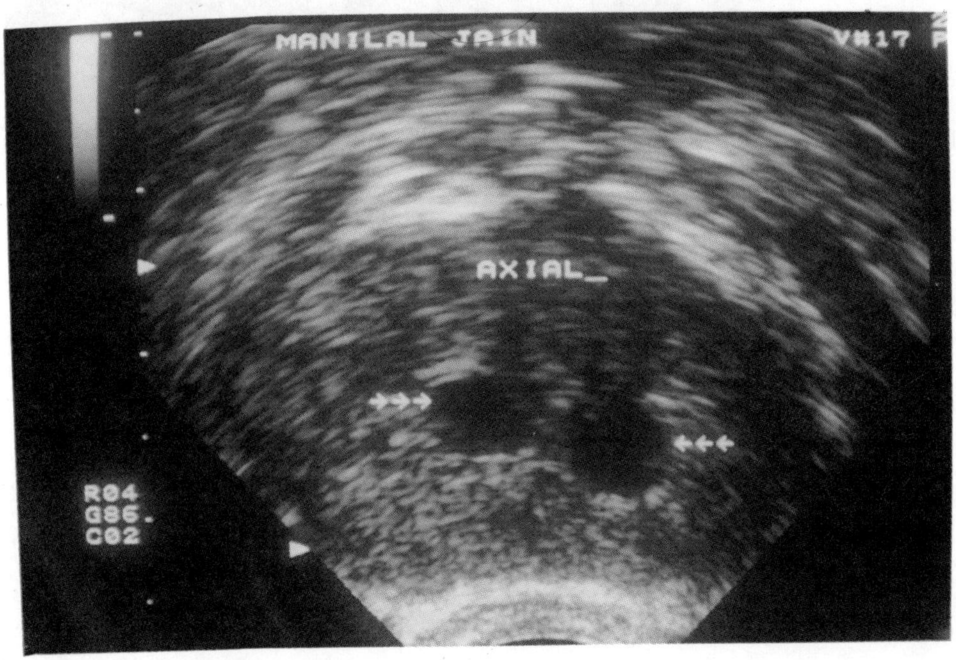

Fig. 9.23A. Ejaculatory duct cysts seen at the mouth of the ejaculatory ducts in the prostate on TRUS imaging

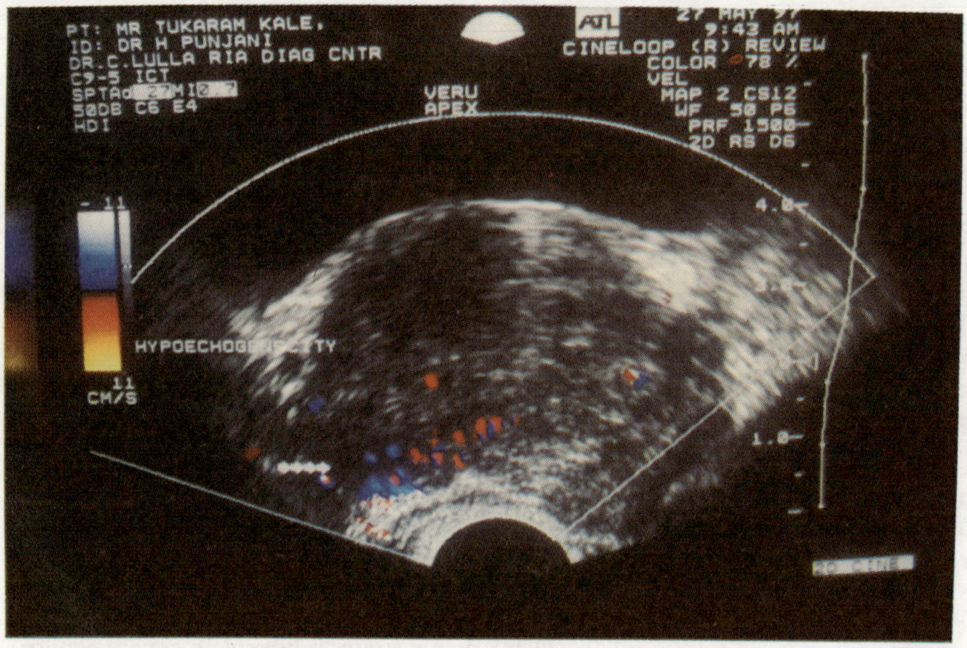

Fig. 9.23B. TRUS reveals a large hypoechoic abscess in the right side of the prostate gland

or without abscess formation, may produce chronic inflammatory changes. These changes are recognized by the disorganization of the normal anatomy produced by scarring of prostatic tissues, and by occasional stone formation. These changes may produce obstructions to the semen flow and infertility. TRUS can identify anatomical obstructive abnormalities that may contribute to the causes of the infertility.

Testicular Ultrasonography And Colour Doppler

Varicocele is the most common surgically correctable cause of male infertility. Colour Doppler study is a simple non-invasive method for varicocele detection and can be used in the office setting. It also combines noninvasive simultaneous B-mode imaging for testicular pathologies and evaluation of the vascularity of the scrotum. Since the concept of subclinical varicocele was introduced, the use of colour Doppler (see Fig. 9.24) has become commonplace. Accordingly, there has been a significant increase in the number of patients diagnosed with varicoceles. With the current use of diagnostic colour doppler for varicocele detection, the incidence of bilateral varicocele in infertile men is reportedly as high as 70% (McClure).

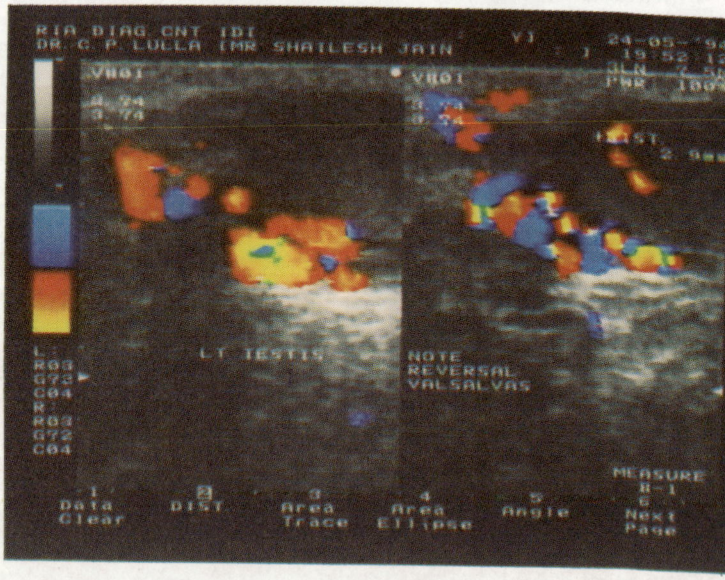

Fig. 9.24. Colour Doppler demonstration of varicocele appearing as multidirectionally flowing venous channels in red and blue colour display

BIOLOGICAL EFFECTS OF ULTRASOUND

In a normal IVF cycle, patients undergo about four exams and oocyte retrieval is inevitably conducted under ultrasound surveillance. In selected circumstances, embryo transfer and GIFT may also be ultrasound-directed. It is possible that in the future, Doppler assessment will play a role in timing ovulation. Considering the degree of ultrasound exposure, it is easy to understand the concern that has existed about its biological effects. No study to date has shown a significant adverse effect. The final conclusion of the 1988 (Hartz) and 1989 (Hartz) US IVF embryo transfer registry report, as well as the collaborative world report on IVF in 1984, emphatically stated that there was no increased risk of fetal anomalies in their total experience (6,500 live births).

REFERENCES

Abramowicz, J.S. et al. (1990). 'Transvaginal Doppler velocimetry of the uterine arteries in *in vitro* fertilization (IVF) patients', Program supplement for 46th annual meeting of the American Fertility Society, Washington, DC (Abstract 0–046).

______(1992). 'Changes in Doppler indices of flow in the ovarian arteries in perimenopausal and menopausal women', NIH Symposium: Exogenous hormones and dysfunctional bleeding, *Bethesda*.

______(1992). 'Transvaginal uterine and ovarian blood flow imaging', in N.J. Alexander, C. d'Alexander (eds.), *Steroid hormones and uterine bleeding.*, AAAS Press, Washington DC, pp. 317–27.

Baber, R. et al. (1988). 'Transvaginal pulsed Doppler Ultrasound assessment of blood flow to the corpus luteum in IVF patients following embryo transfer', *Br. J. Obstet. Gynaecol.*, **95**: 1226–30.

Bazaz-Malik, G. et al. (1983). 'Tuberculous endometritis: a clinicopathological study of 1000 cases', *Br. J Obstet. Gynaecol.*, **90**: 84–6.

Bergh, C. et al. (1992). 'Sonographic evaluation of the endometrium in *in vitro* fertilization (IVF) cycles', *Acta Obstet. Gynecol. Scand.*, **71**: 624–8.

Blankstein, J. et al. (1987). 'Ovarian hyper-stimulation with extogenous pulsatile by number and size of preovulatory ovarian follicles', *Fertil. Steril.*, **47** (4): 597–601.

Bourne, T.H. et al. (1991). 'Intra-follicular blood flow during human ovulation', *Ultrasound Obstet. Gynecol.*, **1**: 53–9.

Butterman, V.C. and R.C. Reiter 'Uterine leiomyomata; etyiology, symptomatology and management', *Fertil. Steril.*, **36**: 433–45.

Charny, C.W. (1965). 'Congenital absences of the vas deferens', *J. Urol.*, **93**: 399–401.

Check, J.H. et al. (1991). 'Influence of endometrial thickness and echo patterns on pregnancy rates during *in vitro* fertilization', *Fertil. Steril.*, **56**: 1173–5.

Coleman, B.G. (1979). 'Endometriosis: Clinical and Ultrasonic correlation', *AJR*, **132**: 747–9.

Coulam, C.B. et al. (1982). 'Ultrasonic evidence for luteinization of unruptured preovulatory follicles', *Fertil. Steril.*, **37**: 460–67.

de Zielger, D. (1990). 'Vascular resistance uterine arterie:dose related effects of endogenous and exogenous estradiol', 46th annual meeting of the American Fertility Society, Washington DC (Abstract 0–068).

Deutinger, J.A. et al. (1989). 'Transvaginal pulsed Doppler measures of blood flow velocity in the ovarian arteries during cycle stimulation and after follicle puncture', *Fertil. Steril.*, **51**: 466–70.

Dicker, D. et al. (1993). 'Severe abdominal complications after transvaginal ultrasonographically guided retrieveal of oocytes for *in vitro* fertilization and embryo transfer', *Fertil. Steril.*, **59**: 1313–5.

Dickey, R.P. et al. (1992). 'Endometrial pattern and thickness associated with pregnancy outcome after assisted reproduction technologies', *Hum. Reprod.*, **7**: 418–21.

______(1993). 'Relationship of endometrial thickness and pattern to fecundity in ovulation induction cycles: Effect of clomiphene citrate alone and in combination with human menopausal gonadotrophins', *Fertil. Steril.*, **59**: 756–60.

Fedele, L. et al. (1988). 'Ultrasonography in the differential diagnosis of '"double" uteri', *Fertil. Steril.*, **48**: 361–4.

Federation CECOS, D. Schwartz and J.M. Mayaux (1982). 'Female fecundity as a function of age results of artificial insemination in 2193 multiparous women with azoopermic husband', *N. Engl. J. Med.*, 306–404.

Feichtinger, W. (1993). 'Transvaginal three-dimensional imaging', *Ultrasound Obstet. Gynecol.*, **59**: 51–53.

Feichtinger, W. and P. Kemefer (1987). 'Conservative treatment for ectopic pregnancy by transvaginal aspiration under sonographic control and methotrexate injection', *Lancet*, **1**: 381–2.

Firedman, H. et al. (1985). 'Endometriosis detection by U/S with the laparoscopic correlation', *Radiology*, **157**: 217–20.

Fleischer, A.C. (1991). 'Ultrasound imaging-2000: Assessment of the utero-ovarian blood flow with the transvaginal color Doppler sonography: Potential clinical applications in infertility', *Fertil. Steril.*, **55**: 684–91.

Fleischer, A.C. et al. (1986). 'Sonography of the endometrium during conception and non-conception cycles of *in vitro* fertilization and embryo transfer', *Fertil. Steril.*, **46**: 442–47.

———(1990). 'Transvaginal sonography: Application in infertility', *Semin. Ultrasound.*, CT M R **11**: 71–81.

Forrest. T.S. et al. (1988). 'Cyclic endometrial changes: US assessment with histologic correlation', *Radiology*, **167**: 233–7.

Friedman, A.J. and R.L. Barbieri 'Leuprolide acetate: Application in gynecology', *Current problems in Obstetric Gynecology and Fertility.*, **9** (6): 209–36.

Genon, Y. and R.F. Casper (1991). 'Prediction of implantation by the sonographic appearances of the endometrium during controlled ovarian hyperstimulation for *in vitro* fertilization (IVF)', *J. In vitro Fert. Embryo Transf.*, **8**: 116–9.

Giotlandio, C. et al. (1987). 'The sonographic picture of the endometrium in spontaneous and induced cycles', *Fertil. Steril.*, **47**: 508–11.

Glissant, A. et al. (1985). 'Ultrasound study of the endometrium during *in vitro* fertilization cycles', *Fertil. Steril.*, **44**: 786–90.

Gonen, Y. et al. (1986). 'Endometrial thickness and growth during ovarian stimulation: A possible predictor of implantation *in vitro* fertilization', *Fertil. Steril.*, **52**: 446–50.

Gongeon A. (1986). 'Dynamics of follicular growth in the human: A model from preliminary results', *Human Reprod.*, **91**: 814–87.

Goswamy, R.K. and P.C. Steptoe (1988) 'Doppler ultrasound studies of the uterine artery in spontaneous ovarian cycles', *Hum. Reprod.*, **3**: 721–6.

Goswamy, R.K. et al. (1988). 'Decreased uterine perfusion a cause of infertility', *Hum. Reprod.*, **3**: 955–9.

Gross, B.H. et al. 'Sonographic features of uterine leimomyomas: Analysis of 41 proven cases', *J. Ultrasound. Med.*, **2**: 401–6.

Grunfeld, L. et al. (1991). 'High resolution endovaginal ultrasonography of endometrium: A noninvasive test for endometrial adequacy', *Obstet. Gynecol.*, **78**: 200–04.

Hackeloer, B.J. et al. (1979). 'Correlation of ultrasonic and endocrinologic parameters of human follicular development', *Am. J. Obstet. Gynecol.*, **135**: 122–8.

Hamilton, S. and J.M. Fitzpatrick (1987). 'Ultrasound diagnosis of a prostatic cysts-causing acute urinary retention', *J. Ultrasound Med.*, **6**: 385–7.

Harger, J.H. et al. (1983). 'Etiology of recurrent pregnancy losses and outcome of subsequent pregnancies', *Obstet. Gynecol.*, **62**: 574.

Hartz, S.C. (1990). '*In vitro* fertilization embryo transfer in the United States: 1988 result from the IVF-ET registry', *Fertil. Steril.*, **53** (1) 13–20.

———(1991). '*In vitro* fertilization embryo transfer (IVF-ET) in the United States: 1989 result from the IVF-ET registry', *Fertil. Steril.*, **55** (1): 14–21.

Heaney, J.A. et al. (1987). 'Giant cyst of the seminal vesicle with renal agenesis', *AJR*, **149**: 139–40.

Husley, V.A. (1991). 'Ultrasound guided embryo transfer: A controlled trial', *Fertil. Steril.*, **55**: 559–62.

Jewelewicz, R. (1975). 'Management of infertility resulting from anovulation', *Am. J. Obstet. Gynecol.*, **122**: 909–20.

Jurkovic, D. et al. (1995). 'Three-dimensional ultrasound for the assessment of uterine anatomy and detection of congenital anomalies: A comparison with hysterosaal-pingography and two-dimensional sonography', *Ultrasound Obstet.Gynecol.*, **5**: 238–40.

Kaneti, J. et al. (1988). 'Aganasis of kidney associated with malformation of the seminal vesicle: Various clinical presentation', *Int. Urol. Nephrol.*, **20**: 29–33.

Kenney, P.J. and M.D. Leeson (1983). 'Congenital anomalies of the seminal vesicles: Spectrum of computed tomographic findings', *Radiology*, **149**: 247–51.

Koos, R.D. (1983). 'Factors that may regulate the growth and regression of blood vessels in the ovary', *Semin. Reprod. Endocrinol.*, **1**: 295–307.

Lenz, S. and J.G. Laurtsen (1982). 'Ultrasonographically guided percutaneous aspiration of human follicles under local anaesthesia: A new method of collection of oocytes for *in vitro* fertilization', *Fertil. Steril.*, **38** (6): 673–7.

Littrup, P.J. et al. (1988). 'Transrectral US of the seminal vesicles and ejaculatory ducts: Clinical correlation', *Radiology*, **168**: 625.

Malatinsky, E. et al. (1987). 'Congenital anomalies of the seminal ducts', *Int. Urol. Nephrol.*, **19**: 189–94.

Malini, S. et al. (1984). 'Sonographic diagnosis and classification of anomalies of the female genetic tract', *J. Ultrasound Med.*, **3**: 397–404.

Matson, P.L. and J.L. Yovich (1986). 'Treatment of infertility associated with endometriosis by *in vitro* fertilization', *Fetil. Steril.*, **46** (3) 432–4.

McClure, R.D. and H. Hricak (1986). 'Scrotal ultrasound in infertile men: Detection of subclinical unilateral and bilateral varicocele', *J. Urol.*, **135**: 711.

McSweeney, M.B. et al. (1988). 'Prediction of IVF and GIFT outcome using transvaginal Doppler assessment of the blood flow', *J. Ultrasound Med.*, 7: 73–9.

Mendelson, E.B. et al. (1985). 'The role of imaging in infertility management', *AJR AMJ Roentgenof*, **44**: 415–20.

O Herlitty, C. et al. (1980). 'Preovulatory follicular size: A comparison of ultrasound and laparascopic measurements', *Fertil. Steril.*, **43** (1): 24–6.

Orsini, L.F. et al. (1985). 'Ultrasonic findings in polycystic ovarian disease', *Fertil. Steril.*, **43**: 709.

Pache, T.D. et al. (1990). 'Growth patterns of non dominant ovarian follicle during the normal menstrual cycle', *Fertil. Steril.*, **54**: 638–42.

Pellerito, J.S. et al. (1992). 'Diagnosis of uterine anomalies: Relative accuracy of mitral regurgitation imaging endovaginal sonography and hysterosalpingography', *Radiology,* **183**: 795–800.

Peters, H. et al. (1975). 'Follicular Growth: The basic-exent in the mouse and the human ovary', *J. Reprod. Fertil.*, **45**: 559.

Picker, R.H. et al. (1983). 'Ultrasonic signs of imminent ovulation', *J. Clin. Ultrasound,* **11** (1): 1–3.

Pierson, R.A. (1992). 'From ovulation to implantation', in R. Jaffe, S.L. Warsof (eds.), *Color Doppler Imaging in Obstetrics and Gynaecology*, McGraw-Hill, New York, pp. 35–59.

Pouly, J.L. et al. (1986). 'Conservative laparoscopy treatment of three hundred and twenty one ectopic pregnancies', *Fertil. Steril.*, **46** (6):1093–7.

Rabinowitz, R. et al. (1986). 'The value of ultrasonographic endometrial measurement in the prediction of pregnancy following *in vitro* fertilization', *Fertil. Steril.*, **45**: 824–8.

Randall, J.M. et al. (1989). 'Transvaginal ultrasonic assessment of endometrial growth in spontaneous and hyperstimulated menstrual cycle', *Br. J. Obstet. Gynaecol.*, **96**: 954–9.

Randolph, J.R. et al. (1996). 'Comparison of real-time ultrasonography, hysterosalpingography and laparoscopy/ hysteroscopy in the evaluation of uterine abnormalities and tubal patency', *Fertil. Steril.*, 828–32.

______(1986). 'Comparison of real-time ultrasonography hysterosalpingography and laparoscopy in the evaluation of uterine abnormalities and tubal patency', *Fertil. Steril.*, **46**: 828–32.

Richman, T.S. et al. (1984). 'Fallopian tubal patency assessed by ultrasound following fluid injection', *Radiology*, **152**: 507–10.

Rock, J.A. and W.D. Schlaff (1985). 'The obstetrics consequences of uterovaginal anomalies', *Fertil Steril.*, **43**: 681.

Rogers, P.A.W. et al. (1991). 'Correlation of endometrial histology, morphometry, and ultrasound appearances after different stimulation protocols for *in vitro* fertilization', *Fertil. Steril.*, **55**: 583–7.

Rossarick, I.K. and W.E. Gibbons (1985). 'Variability of ovarian follicular growth in natural menstrual cycles', *Fertil. Steril.*, **44**: 195–9.

Rubin, S. (1975). 'Congenital absences of the vas deferens', *Scand. J. Urol. Nephrol.*, **9**: 94–9.

Sakamoto, C. et al. (1988). 'Sonographic study of the endometrial response to ovarian hormones in patients receiving ovarian stimulation', *Int. J. Gyneacol. Obstet.*, **27**: 404–14.

Setti, P.E.L. et al. (1993). 'Colour flow imaging and Doppler velocimetry of the uterine arteries in conceptional and nonconceptional ovulatory cycles', *J. Matern. Fetal. Invest.*, **3**: 123–6. (p. 177 Cd inferitliy).

Sher, G. et al. (1991). 'Assessment of the late proliferative phase endometrium by ultrasonography in patients undergoing *in vitro* fertilization and embryo transfer (IVF/ET.)', *Hum. Reprod.*, 7: 232–7.

Sher, G. et al. (1993). 'Management of suboptimal sonographic endometrial patterns in patients undergoing *in vitro* fertilization and embryo transfer', *Human Reprod.*, **8**: 347–9.

Shoham, A. et al. (1991). 'Is it possible to run a successful ovulation induction program based solely on ultrasound monitoring? The importance of endometrial measurements', *Fertil. Steril.*, **56**: 836–41.

Smith. B. et al. (1984). 'Ultrasonic assessment of endometrial changes in stimulated cycles in an *in vitro* fertilization and embryo transfer program', *J. in vitro Fert. Embryo Transf.*, **1**: 233–8.

Steer, C.V. et al. (1992). 'The use of transvaginal color flow imaging in *in vitro* fertilization to identify optimum conditions before embryo transfer', *Fertil. Steril.*, **57**: 372–6.

_____(1990). 'Transvaginal color flow imaging of the uterine arteries during the ovarian and menstrual cycle', *Hum. Reprod.*, **52**: 391–5.

Sterzik, K. et al. (1989). 'Doppler sonographic findings and their correlation with implantation in an *in vitro*-fertilization program', *Fertil. Steril.*, **52**: 825–8.

Tanaka, N. et al. (1989). 'Increase in ovarian blood flow volume during ovulation in the gonadotropin primed immature rat', *Biol. Reprod.*, **40**: 762–8.

Taylor, K.J.W. et al. (1985). 'Ultrasound Doppler flow study of the ovarian and the uterine arteries', *Br. J. Obstet. Gynaecol.*, **92**: 240–46.

Thaler, I. 'Hemodynamic evaluation of the female pelvic vessels using a high frequency transvaginal image-directed Doppler system', *J. Clin. Ultrasound*, **18**: 364–9. (p. 178 Cd infertility).

The American Fertility Society (1988). 'The American Fertility Society classification of adnexal adhesions, distal tubal occlusion, tubal occlusion, secondary to tubal ligation, tubal pregnancies, mullerian anomalies and intrauterine adhesions', *Fertil. Steril.*, **49**: 9944–55.

Timor-Tritsch, I.E. et al. (1989). 'Transvaginal salpingocentisis: A new techniques for treating ectopic pregnancy', *Am. J. Obstet. Gynecol.*, **160**: 459–61.

Toi, A. (1991). 'Asch mitral regurgitation, seminal vesicles: Imaging and intervention using transrectal ultrasound', *J. Ultrasound Med.*, **10**: 19–23.

'Transvaginal sonographic detection of endometrial polyps with fluid contrast augmentation', *Obstet. Gynecol.*, **79**: 1041–43.

Trigauz, J.P. et al. (1991). 'Male genital tract malformations associated with ipsilateral renal agenesis: Sonographic findings', *J. Clin. Ultrasound.*, **19**: 3–10.

Ueno, J. et al. (1991). 'Ultrasonographic appearances of the endometrium in natural and stimulated *in vitro* fertilization cycles and its correlation with outcome', *Hum. Reprod.*, **6**: 901–04.

Valdes, C. et al. (1984). 'Ultrasound evaluation of female genital tract anomalies: A review of 64 cases', *Am. J. Obstet. Gynecol.*, **149**: 285–9.

Walls, W.J. and F. Lin (1975). 'Ultrasound diagnosis of seminal vesicle cyst', *Radiology*, **14**: 693–4.

Welker, B.G. et al. (1989). 'Transvaginal sonography of the endometrium during ovum pickup in stimulated cycles for *in vitro* fertilization', *J. Ultrasound. Med.*, **8**: 549–53.

White-House, G.H. and C.H. Wright (1992). 'Imaging in gynaecology', in R.G. Grainger and D.J. Allison (eds.), *Diagnostic Radiology*, Churchill Livingstone, Edinburgh.

Williams, M.F. (1984). 'The vascular architecture of the rat uterus as influenced by oestrogen and progesterone', *Am. J. Anat.*, **83**: 247–307.

Yaffe, H. et al. (1978). 'Amenorrhea, hypomenorrhea and uterine fibrosis', *Am. J. Obstet. Gynecol.*, **130**: 599–601.

10

Role of Sperm Function Tests

J.C. Calamera, F. Nodar, V. Rawe, Anibal A. Acosta

INTRODUCTION

The main dilemma the andrologist must frequently face when he investigates an infertile couple is the difficulty of carrying out an adequate evaluation of the fertility of the male who wants to conceive. Semen analysis has been gradually developed and now it is accepted that an adequate one, carried out according to the outlines stipulated by WHO (1992), is very important for the basic study of the male. Nevertheless, the results of the sperm analysis do not give a precise diagnosis or prognosis of human male fertility (Aitken et al., 1982; Dunphy et al., 1989). Despite important advances in the last few years, many laboratories and clinics working in human reproduction do not use, or even worse, do not apply correctly the available methods to determine the patient's fertility.

As soon as the techniques of assisted reproduction were accepted for the treatment of the male factor (Acosta, 1992; Testart, 1994), laboratory techniques were considerably improved, not only in order to choose spermatozoa of good quality, but to design new diagnostic methods of sperm function. However, when one looks at the results of a test, it is necessary to consider that different sperm functions may have influenced these results, to avoid reaching false conclusions. Many of these tests have tried to evaluate sperm function, including the fertilizing capacity of the spermatozoa. It is now accepted that the diagnosis of sperm function in human beings cannot be carried out on the basis of a single test, but on a group of determinations, each one directed to test a different organelle. Tests of high specificity must be used to effectively evaluate a special sperm reproductive dysfunction. There are now *in vitro* assays available to check each one of the sperm fertilization steps, from sperm migration to binding to the zona pellucida, and to check also from spermatozoa-oocyte membrane fusion to decondensation of the nuclear chromatin. Researchers continued to develop more precise and objective techniques, in an effort to get a better knowledge of human sperm function and to get a better prediction of the *in vivo* and *in vitro* sperm fertilizing ability.

SPERM PLASMA MEMBRANE

Anatomical and functional integrity of the plasma membrane are essential for sperm viability and its ability to carry out the fertilization process. Considering its configuration and functions, the plasmalemma presents an external glycocalyx composed of charged glycolipids and glycoprotein residues, with oligosaccharide chains extending all over the surface of the cell. Immediately under it, there is a protein matrix embedded in a lipid bilayer, with its hydrophilic terminal directed to the extracellular surface and with its hydrophobic terminal in the intracellular enviromment. It has a submembranous cytofibrillar system composed of microtubules (cytoskeleton) and microfilaments (contractile elements) (Koehler, 1978). The plasma membrane in human beings has been described as an association of phospholipids and sterols in dynamic equilibrium and peripheral and integral membrane proteins (Langlais and Roberts, 1985). Cholesterol is abundant in human spermatozoa, although one part of the sterols is sulfoconjugated (Lalumiere et al., 1976). The cholesterol present in the bilayer of phospholipids reduces the permeability of the membrane (Demel et al., 1972), limits the insertion of proteins in the bilayer as well as the lateral mobility of the functional receptors, and modulates the activity of the membrane proteins. The loss or reduction of cholesterol in the plasma membrane is an important step in the process of capacitation of human spermatozoa. Plasma membrane anatomic integrity and functional activity are also essential for sperm viability: they participate in the physiological changes that take place on the sperm surface during the process of capacitation, acrosome reaction, and binding to the zona pellucida and oolemma.

The traditional methods of determining the integrity of the plasma membrane are based on the supravital stains transit through it (eosin-opal blue, Blom´s eosin-nigrosin or eosin alone) (Dott and Foster, 1972). The discriminant power of these supravital stains depend on the capacity of the membrane, functionally undamaged, to prevent the passage of eosin chromophores into the nuclear compartment of the spermatozoon. The capacity to distinguish viable from nonviable spermatozoa is very important in studies carried out to evaluate the sperm vitality of incubated gametes, or to evaluate different sperm storage methods. There is another problem related to the use of classical supravital stains: they are not adequate for cryopreserved sperm because glycerol may interfere with them (Mixner and Saroff, 1954). It was demonstrated some years ago that up to 4% of glycerol concentration could be compatible with the use of those methods (Almlid and Johnson, 1988). Carboxifluorescein diacetate is a nonfluorescent and plasma membrane-permeating stain. It is hydrolysed by intracellular esterases and the product of this reaction, 6-carboxifluorescein, is highly fluorescent and the membrane is not permeable to it. As a result of this, spermatozoa with an undamaged plasma membrane show a bright green fluorescence and those with membrane problems do not (Garner et al., 1986).

The use of supravital techniques allows for the diagnosis of necrozoospermia because the biochemical changes detected are produced immediately after cellular death. This test is still recommended by WHO as part of the investigation of human semen (WHO, 1992). The clinical significance of these tests in the evaluation of male fertility must be thoroughly considered; they offer diagnostic information of sperm survival, specially in the presence of immotile cells (Wilton et al., 1988). The idea of combining different tests to study the sperm membrane is not new. Ramirez et al. (1992) combined the hypo-osmotic-swelling test (HOST) and the eosin test. One of the combined methods widely used to determine the acrosome status is the triple stain technique, which involves the use of a supravital stain utilized before fixation, Bismark brown and pink of Bengala (Talbot, 1981). Methods of double staining have also been used to evaluate the acrosome status and sperm viability (Didon et al., 1989). Recently, fluorescent tests have been incorporated to get information on sperm viability and the fertilization potential in human beings (see acrosin and acrosome reaction).

Key knowledge of the sperm's physiological mechanisms could be obtained by combining the analysis of the final products of sperm metabolism and sperm kinetics. The main principle involved is the balance between the generation and the consumption of ATP (Kemp et al., 1988).

ATP is an excellent indicator of sperm 'health' because it is the primary generator of energy (Calamera et al., 1982). On the other hand, the number of viable cells correlates with the intracellular levels of ATP; when the cells die, the respiratory activity stops and a quick fall of the nucleotide concentration is detected (Calamera et al., 1989). The ATP content in human spermatozooa has been proposed as a quantitative measure of the sperm fertilizing potential (Comhaire et al., 1983). Although a great deal of effort was made to correlate the nucleotide content with sperm function and fertility, the final conclusion is that it represents only an aspect of the number of living spermatozoa and, probably, its investigation has little clinical relevance (Irvine and Aitken, 1985). The measure of cellular ATP and of the ATP/ADP relation did not show significant differences in oligozoospermic and astenozoospermic populations.

One essential biophysical property of the living cell is its water permeability. It is known that the quality of the cellular membrane reflects on its ability to allow the transit of specific fluids and of certain molecules through it. Water permeability has wide variations among different cells and within a specific cellular type (Stein, 1990). Jeyendran et al. (1984) developed a very simple test called hypo-osmotic swelling test (HOST), commonly used to determine the functional integrity of the plasma membrane. This assay is based on the transit of fluids through an undamaged cellular membrane under hypo-osmotic conditions (150 mOsm/L), until equilibrium between the extra- and intracellular cell compartments is reached. A normal test shows more than 60% of swollen spermatozoa with coiled tails. Due to the fact that the fibres of the tail are under tension, the spaces created make them take a corkscrew shape (Zaneveld and Jeyendran, 1988).When the test values are between 50% and 59%, they are considered to be in a gray area, where it is difficult to make a diagnosis; below 50%, the test is clearly abnormal. The HOST test developers reported that it correlates very well with the hamster oocyte penetration assay, so they proposed it as a simple assay of human sperm function. Other investigators have reported that when the *in vitro* fertilization rate is considered, the method does not have prognostic value (Barratt et al., 1989; Sjoblom and Coccia, 1989).

Lastly, the presence of non saturated lipids in the cellular membrane is a potential danger because of their high lability in the presence of oxygen. Therefore, parameters related to plasma membrane structure and function were converted into good markers of the presence of free radicals that may induce cell injury. (See Other Factors of Prognosis.)

NUCLEAR MATURATION

In early spermatids, chromatin is observed as a group of fibres that appear more densely concentrated near the internal aspect of the nuclear membrane or in other regions around the nucleolus (Bellvé, 1982). Chromatin condensation during spermatogenesis is due to deep physicochemical changes in the nucleus. These changes continue during sperm transit through the epididymis and include the elimination of RNA (Monesi, 1971), the replacement of somatic histones by protamines (Bellvé et al., 1975), and the formation of disulfide bonds that are crucial for chromatin stability (Bedford and Calvin, 1974). This occurs simultaneously with a decrease of free -thiol groups in the nucleus (Saowaros and Panyim, 1979). In human beings, the transit of spermatozoa through the epididymis varies among different people (Rowley et al., 1970) and produces different degrees of nuclear stability (Bedford et al., 1973).

Defects of the sperm nucleus are of great significance in human fertility. In infertile patients, it has been frequently described as intranuclear vacuoles that appear optically empty; they contain pleomorphic inclusions, such as membrane groups, vesicles of different sizes, lipid droplets and cytoplasmic organelles (Zamboni, 1987). These defects are associated with abnormalities in chromatin condensation.

Infertility in patients with sperm nuclear immaturity can be due to its association with other sperm abnormalities, specially hypoplasia of the acrosome (Chemes et al., 1987). According to this, the percentage of ejaculated spermatozoa with an immature nucleus can predict male infertility.

Nowadays, there are several simple tests to detect nuclear maturity. As we have previously reported, somatic histones are rich in lysine, while sperm specific protamines are more basic proteins rich in arginine and cysteine (Auge et al., 1990). In human semen spreads, the presence of morphologically normal spermatozoa whose nuclei are partially or completely stained with aniline blue suggests the presence of proteins rich in lysine, pointing to an alteration in the chromatin condensation and nuclear maturation. Dadoune et al. (1988) reported that the percentage of sperm heads stained with aniline blue was higher in sperm groups that were morphologically abnormal, although 20% of the normal gametes may also show stained heads.

This coincides with ultrastructural observations demonstrating that in some nuclei of normal shape, it is possible to find defects in chromatin condensation (Dadoune et al., 1988; Bartoov et al., 1980).

Although sperm chromatin in mammals is highly condensed and inactive, in human beings, it has the capacity to decondense when it is exposed to a combination of sodium dodecylsulfate (SDS), a detergent-like agent, and EDTA, a chelating agent. SDS breaks the cellular membrane and EDTA removes the Zn ions that stabilize the sulfidryl groups on the protamines involved in the disulfide bonds (Kvist et al., 1980; Huret 1986). Sperm heads with immature nuclei are prone to quick decondensation and they expand or break (Bedford et al., 1973); unfortunately, the rates of decondensation are very different among fertile men (Blazak and Overstreet, 1982). The determination of nuclear stability in the presence of SDS revealed that in a group of 15 fertile donors, 87% had stable nuclei in their ejaculates. (Blazak and Overstreet 1982).

Cervical mucus does not screen for sperm cells with single or multiple abnormalities in the head (Jeulin et al., 1986). Therefore, there is a risk of intrauterine penetration of morphologically normal gametes with noncondensed chromatin. Studies carried out some years ago revealed that the nuclear chromatin decondensation test had good predictive value in a programme of IVF (Liu et al., 1987).

The acridine orange test determines the state and integrity of the sperm nuclear chromatin (Roux and Dadoune, 1989). This technique uses a fluorochrome of acridine orange which, when observed through fluorescence microscopy, gives a green stain if it is bound to native DNA or pink if bound to unnatural DNA (Tejada et al., 1984). There is a good correlation between the results of this test and those obtained with the aniline blue method (Roux and Dadoune, 1989). In general, the percentage of spermatozoa with abnormal DNA, signalled by their red fluorescence, correlates with abnormal morphology (Ibrahim and Pedersen, 1988). A similar but simpler method was proposed by Royere et al. (1988).

The acridine orange test can be carried out using flow cytometry, which has been demonstrated to be an objective method, biologically stable and of high sensitivity for the study of semen quality (Evenson et al., 1991).

CAPACITATION

The fertilizing capacity of spermatozoa depends on functional and structural changes that are produced when the gametes pass through the female reproductive system. This phenomenon, called 'capacitation', was observed for the first time by Austin (1951) and Chang (1951). Although this biological mechanism was described almost 50 years ago, the molecular basis for capacitation is not known in detail. Even though capacitation starts with the separation of spermatozoa from the seminal plasma, it is necessary for its completion that the sperm spend some time in the female reproductive tract. The changes involved in capacitation include important transformations of the plasma membrane, which take place after epididymal maturation.

Within the female reproductive tract, capacitation serves to regulate the acrosome reaction (AR), probably by a mechanism of change in the oocyte-cumulus complex (Bedford, 1983). The biochemical changes that regulate the structure of the cellular membrane during capacitation and AR include alterations of surface charges, modifications in the cholesterol content and changes in the structure of the phospholipids. Among the other changes noticed are the activation of ATPase, the decrease of the free NH2 and SH groups, and the increase in membrane permeability. These changes are associated with the exposure of D-mannose-binding sites, which are probably instrumental in spermatozoa-zona pellucida binding. The loss of cholesterol, indicated by a decrease in the cholesterol-phospholipids ratio, is important in the determination of the AR production capacity (Langlais and Roberts, 1985). During capacitation, there are also intrinsic plasma membrane changes, like the capacity of the intramembranous proteins to move laterally within the plasma membrane. These modifications lead to the formation of patches with rich or poor glycoprotein contents.

The sperm capacitation time varies among species, and is also different if it is produced *in vivo* or *in vitro*. The required time for *in vivo* capacitation in humans seems to be quite variable (Perreault and Rogers, 1982), and it is not yet specified for *in vitro* incubation.

Although different media are able to support capacitation, certain components like serum albumin, Ca++ and CO3H- seem to play an important role (Visconti et al., 1995a). It has been suggested that cAMP as well as protein kinase A (PK A) have an outstanding role in triggering capacitation that increase during the process. Thus, the measurement of the activity of PK A represents a reflection of the intracellular changes in the concentration of cAMP. Besides, inhibitors of PK A block the phosphorylation of tyrosine and capacitation (Visconti et al., 1995 b). In metabolic terms, capacitation is closely related to the activity of adenilcyclase, possibly mediated by adenosine receptors.

There are no direct tests to measure capacitation, even though to assess this process, tests based on plasma membrane surface changes are used. These changes are generally associated with hyperactive sperm movements (Yanagimachi, 1981). The clearest expression of hyperactivation is a change in the sperm movement due to an increase of the proximal flagellar beat (Lindermann and Kanous, 1989), and the result of this is that the transit curve is wider and more winding (Katz et al., 1987a). The functional consequence of hyperactivation is related to gamete transport into the oviduct, and the generation of the necessary forces for sperm penetration through the granulosa cell layer and the zona pellucida of the oocyte (Katz et al., 1987b).

In human semen, the sperm trajectory and shifting modality during capacitation has been studied (Aitken et al., 1985). These observations generally show a tendency to increase the bending and lateral movement of the sperm head (Mortimer et al., 1984). Tests have been designed to quantify these trajectory changes and the descriptions coincide with the hyperactivated motility pattern observed in mammalian spermatozoa (Morales et al., 1988).

In order to understand the mechanisms that regulate sperm movements, we should count on precise methods that quantify the motility of the total population. *In vitro* studies carried out in humans showed different patterns of hyperactivated motility. Three general patterns have been described: (a) Forward progression, characterized by a straight active migration with regular lateral displacement of the head along its progression axis. The flagellar wave is essentially uniform but the magnitude of the proximal wave is larger than that of the sperm in semen. (b) Transition phase: the motility resembles the previous pattern, except that there is a larger and less regular proximal flagellar wave. (c) Hyperactivated motility, characterized by a very wide proximal flagellar wave that seems to expand before its propagation along the tail, which is quicker. This results in a flexion of the head over the axis of the cell (Mortimer and Mortimer, 1990). The heterogeneity of hyperactivated motility observed in humans has made it necessary to develop subclassifications according to the characteristics of the beat pattern. These motility aspects need to be converted into measurable entities if they are to be standardized as a diagnostic test. A simple and quick method of motility analysis is to determine the position of the head at each point of a print left by the spermatozoon at a certain time. The computerized analysis is based on the digitization of video images of cells in movement that are transformed into numbers.

The CASA (computer-assisted semen analysis) measurement systems are part of a technology under continuous development. Many of them were commercialized using methodologies of digital analysis to automate the evaluation of the concentration, motility and other characteristics of spermatozoa (Boyers et al., 1989). Even though they have similar basic principles, they differ in the optic system used, in the technique to capture the image, in the techniques of sperm identification, in the reconstruction of the print and in the algorithms of motility analysis.

The techniques evolve very fast and significant changes are continually made, not only in the software, but also in the hardware. These systems are based on the identification of specific objects by means of the formation of pixels of each video frame (or field) that frequently use the 'edge detection' technique. Each object is made of a continuous group of pixels which have a value opposed to the background. The specific aspects of sperm movement, like speed progression and motility patterns, correlate very well with the cervical mucus penetration test (Eggert-Kruse et al., 1989), with the penetration values in hamster oocytes (Aitken et al., 1984a), and with IVF results (Mortimer et al., 1991).

For the time being, no test has been described that is optimal to judge hyperactivation, but certain basic conditions are important: (a) to carry it out through a CASA method, (b) to use a selection preparation of motile sperm, using a well-known technique that does not hurt spermatozoa, (c) to choose a culture medium able to support sperm capacitation, and (d) to preincubate the samples at 37°C for at least 3 hours in a 5% CO2 incubator.

ACROSOME AND ACROSOME REACTION (AR)

The acrosome covers the anterior portion of the sperm nucleus; it derives from the Golgi system and originates during the first stages of spermatid differentiation. Its final form is the consequence of profound transformation processes involving the nucleus and cytoplasmic components, for instance, the Manchette´s microtubules.

When a fully capacitated spermatozoon is near the fertilization site or it contacts the cumulus oophorus, AR starts. This phenomenon includes the fusion and subsequent vesiculation of the plasma membrane and the external acrosomal membrane, initially creating pores, and the loss of both membranes in the pre-equatorial segment at the end (Nagae et al., 1986). This process produces the release of the acrosomal content and the exposure of the inner acrosomal membrane, with its associated enzymes (Yanagimachi, 1981). Among these changes, there is an activation of the proacrosin-acrosin system (Harrison, 1983).

The roles of ion transport and hydrolytic enzymes in AR is complex, and have been extensively discussed (Meizel, 1984; Yanagimachi, 1988). There is a massive influx of Ca++ due to the activation of the plasma membrane or of the so-called Ca++ bomb. The high intracellular Ca++ concentration inactivates the ATPase of the plasma membrane, resulting in a fast increase of Na+. This results in the release of H+, increasing the intracellular pH that precedes the morphological events of the AR. The role played by Ca++ channels and calmodulin is not yet clear. Ion transport is mediated by cyclic nucleotides which, together with phosphodiesterase inhibitors, stimulate capacitation and AR. The acrosome contains several hydrolytic enzymes, the most important being acrosin; hyaluronidase, esterase, neuraminidase, acid phosphatase, phospholipase, aryl-sulphatase, B-N-acetyl glucosaminidase and collagenase are also present.

A normal acrosome reaction is essential for sperm penetration through the zona pellucida and to prepare the gametes for sperm-oolemma fusion (Sathananthan et al., 1982). Even though the lack of acrosome is rare in male infertility, some infertile patients have been found with a high proportion of acrosomeless sperm (round-headed spermatozoa) (Florke-Gerloff et al., 1984). The AR in humans may be induced by a number of physiological triggers, like follicular fluid (Tesarik, 1985), the oocyte-cumulus complex (Siiteri et al., 1988), the oocytes (De Jonge et al., 1988), the zona pellucida (Cross et al., 1988), and other non-physiological agents like the calcium ionophore, A 23187 (Tesarik, 1985). Some preliminary studies have shown that the proportion of spermatozoa that undergo induced AR by A 23187 or by follicular fluid may predict fertilizing ability either in normal or oligozoospermic men (Aitken et al., 1984 b), although the biological and clinical significance of the absence of AR under these conditions have not been defined as yet.

Among the proteolytic enzymes that the acrosome has, acrosin is the most important and it is believed to play a significant role in the penetration of the zona pellucida (Tesarik, 1989). It has also been suggested that a low activity of acrosin may be associated with male infertility (Schill et al., 1988), and it may also be associated with diminished *in vitro* fertilization rates (Acosta et al., 1986). The conversion of proacrosin into acrosin may occur within the acrosome as an initial feature of AR, before membrane vesiculation. Different tests have been used for the evaluation of this enzyme, taking advantage of its proteolytic, estereolytic and amilolytic properties (Pleban et al., 1990). A RIA (Mohsenian et al., 1982) using competitive binding of an antiacrosin serum in the presence of an iodinated enzyme has been proposed. In spite of the sensitivity of the test, it only measures the total amount of the acrosin-proacrosin complex.

There was also an attempt to use an immunocytochemical method (Francavilla et al., 1992), which is less helpful than the biochemical methods in the diagnosis of infertile patients. The most accurate test determines the estereolytic properties of the enzyme. This technique involves the dispersion of the acrosome at a low pH. The estereolytic activity is determined by varying the pHs of the extraction solutions so that proacrosin changes into acrosin (Goodpasture et al., 1980). To be used clinically, Kennedy et al. (1989) developed a simple amilolytic assay that measures the total amount of acrosin (free, plus proacrosin-convertible). At present, there are commercial kits available and an attempt has been made to correlate the levels of acrosin obtained by these methods to IVF results (Tummon et al., 1991). However, acrosin evaluation is not currently performed in clinical andrology laboratories.

A simple method of acrosomal protease activity determination has been published that can be used in human spermatozoa (Welker et al., 1988). It is based on the digestion halo induced by protease release by the dead spermatozoa, on a slide with a gelatin layer. The enzymes present produce gelatin lysis around the head of the spermatozoon, and the diameter of lysis observed is proportional to the amount of enzyme content in the sperm head (Ficsor et al., 1983). Although it is a simple test, its relevance remains to be demonstrated. Likewise, Hirayama et al. (1989) developed a test to determine the hyaluronidase activity of human spermatozoa, shown by the digestion of a hyaluronic acid substrate present on a slide. These authors state that the activity of hyaluronidase in semen correlates with the proportion of mature oocytes fertilized *in vitro*.

Even though hyaluronidase has traditionally been considered the substance that could facilitate sperm penetration through the cumulus oophorus of fresh oocytes, recent studies have suggested that it is not essential for such penetration. Both tests, acrosin and hyaluronidase determination, are smooth, but uniformity of the thickness of the substrate layers on the slides is difficult to accomplish and this interferes with the measurement of the diameter of the halo.

As we have already stated, AR *in vivo* would take place very near or on the zona pellucida. Tesarik (1989) says that the only physiological AR is the one that is produced by means of the proper biological stimulus, while the spontaneous AR has little biological significance. Then all tests measuring AR should distinguish between the spontaneous and induced ones.

In human spermatozoa, sperm-zona pellucida interaction needs binding by oligosaccharides, which has not been identified yet; a difference in the expression of the binding sites of D-mannose between fertile and infertile human beings (Benoff et al., 1995) has been suggested. These findings trigger research on the relationship between expression of this kind of surface receptors on the sperm after capacitation and the fertilizing potential of the gamete (Tulsiani et al., 1990; Benoff et al., 1993). Progesterone and some zona pellucida-specific glycoproteins of the oocyte (Kamada et al., 1985) are the natural binding sites involved in this process. However, the corresponding sperm receptors have not been identified. Such a complex process cannot be controlled by one type of ligand receptor; it is thought that a multireceptor system may be involved and that those receptors may cooperate positively. They may independently induce a partial AR and altogether a complete one.

The transduction systems, as well as their mechanism of interaction, are not completely known yet. For fertilization to take place, a good binding to the zona pellucida, synchronized with AR, is required. If, for instance, there is a premature AR, the exocytosis of acrosomal vesicles happens before the spermatozoon has interacted with the oocyte. This loss of sites recognition for the zona receptor may risk oocyte-sperm interaction. If, on the other side, the sperm binds to the zona pellucida and the zone is not capable of activating the AR, the spermatozoon will not be able to penetrate the oocyte. In both cases, due to an imperfect synchronization of these processes, fertilization of the oocyte will be seriously affected (Kohn et al., 1997).

The binding events provoke a number of sperm membranes fusion consequences including the increase of Ca++, protein receptors (G binding guanine-nucleotide), and the activation of second messengers, like protein kinase and phospholipase (see New Methods to Measure Spermatic Function).

For a long time, there were no simple techniques for the routine determination of the AR in humans. The methods most commonly used include: (a) Methods that use transmission electron microscopy, which are the most effective for acrosome study; they are hard and expensive to be used in common clinical practice. (b) Methods that use light fluorescense microscopy, including the triple-stain technique (Talbot and Chacon, 1980), Giemsa (Didon et al., 1989) and chlortetracycline (CTC), which provides different distribution patterns on the sperm surface and can be visualized depending on the capacitation and acrosome status of the spermatozoon.The advantage of this method is that it can monitor only capacitation independently of AR. It is believed that the changes in the distribution of the complex Ca++-CTC and the plasmalemma phospholipids are responsible for the different patterns observed.

Methods that use fluorescent lectines have been widely used: Pisum sativum agglutinin (PSA) (Cross and Meizel, 1989), Peanut agglutinin (Mortimer et al., 1987), Concanavalin A (Holden et al., 1990), Ricinus communis agglutinin (Talbot and Chacon 1980), and wheat germ agglutinin (Gabriel et al., 1995). Also, those involving indirect immunofluorescence using antiacrosome antibodies (Wolf et al., 1985), fluorescence-activated cell sorter (Fenichel et al., 1989), or lectines or fluorescent monoclonal antibodies (Henley et al., 1994) have been utilized. A method based on PSA capacity of specific binding to glycoproteins of the acrosome matrix that are released during the AR has been recently designed. The release of the acrosomal content is proportional to the fraction of AR spermatozoa. The glycoproteins present are detected by ELISA (Margalit et al., 1997).

The advantages and disadvantages of these methods have been discussed in detail by Cross and Meizel (1989). The PSA fluorescent method, which is simple and has good reproducibility to be used in the study of the human acrosome (Liu and Baker, 1988), has been the preferred one. The introduction of a supravital dye like Hoechst 33258, or the HOST test coupled with the PSA test, allows for a clear differentiation between live spermatozoa without acrosome from those that have lost it due to degeneration, which is one of the causes of error of the method (Cross et al., 1986). Cummins et al. (1991) described a protocol in which 10 nM of A 23187 is used as a challenger in a modified Hepes-buffer Tyrode medium to induce AR, and introduced the term 'ARIC' (Acrosome Reaction Ionophore Challenge) for this functional test.

ARIC results can demonstrate 2 types of abnormalities: (1) the spermatozoa show low levels of spontaneous AR, with an insufficient increase after ionophore stimulation, and (2) the spermatozoa present an usual high spontaneous AR. Tesarik (1989) has proposed the term 'insufficient spontaneous AR' when it is observed in less than 20% of spermatozoa with less than 15% increase after treatment with the ionophore. It is also possible to have an indirect assessment of AR using the human spermatozoa penetration assay in hamster oocytes (Yanagimachi et al., 1976) (SPA). A simple method of AR determination in spermatozoa bound to the zone pellucida has been recently published that examines the solubilized zona pellucida (Liu and Baker, 1996). There are experiences indicating that the AR in human spermatozoa induced by N-acetylglucosamine-neoglycoprotein can be used to predict *in vitro* fertilization capacity (Brandelli et al., 1995).

When zona pellucida-free oocytes are used, spermatozoa can enter into direct contact with the ooplasm. A test has been developed using female hamsters that are superovulated with pregnant mare serum and human chorionic gonadotrophin. This test was used for a long time as a selective methodology to study the fertilization capacity of human spermatozoa. Only those spermatozoa that have undergone AR are able to bind and penetrate zona-free hamster oocytes (Yanagimachi, 1984). Although the significance of SPA as a predictor of fertilization in humans is still under discussion, there are several papers indicating that low value results have a strong correlation with human infertility (Rogers, 1985). Sperm motility, and particularly morphology, also correlate with the hamster test results (Mortimer, 1989). Yanagimachi (1984) did not find such a correlation between test results and seminal characteristics. It has been proved that immotile spermatozoa from patients with Kartagener syndrome may penetrate the hamster's oocyte (Aitken et al., 1983).

OOCYTE-SPERMATOZOON INTERACTION

A. Binding and zone penetration

Human infertility may be the result of abnormalities in the oocyte-spermatozoon interaction, which includes binding and penetration into the zona pellucida and fusion with the oolemma. Binding of the male gamete to the zona pellucida is species-specific, and it is an important prerequisite for fertilization (Overstreet and Hembree, 1976; Liu et al., 1991). The fertilizing spermatozoon must be capable of binding and penetrating the zona pellucida, and of completing AR before fusion with the oolemma. In the mouse, the spermatozoon binds to the zone pellucida with an intact acrosome, using one of its glycoproteins (ZP3). Then AR is induced by the ZP3 and the acrosome-reacted spermatozoa bind to ZP2. Therefore, evaluation of the oocyte-spermatozoon interaction may be an important method of assessing the fertilizing capacity of the human spermatozoon, since a relatively small number of male gametes are bound to the zona pellucida and only one or very few are able to penetrate into the perivitelline space.

The first sperm penetration test using the human zona pellucida of oocytes from cadavers between 8 and 45 hours post-mortem was described by Overstreet and Hembree in 1976. It was later discovered that the zona pellucida (ZP) of oocytes stored in concentrated saline solution keep their capacity to bind and to be penetrated by human spermatozoa (Yanagimachi et al., 1979). Failure of the sperm to bind to the zona pellucida may be associated with infertility and may indicate a defect in the functional integrity of either the spermatozoa or oocytes (Overstreet et al., 1980). Although Mahadevan et al. (1987) found that oocyte quality influences the number of spermatozoa bound to the ZP, other researchers do not accept the concept (Tesarik et al., 1988). On the contrary, the failure of sperm-zona pellucida binding in IVF is associated more with sperm than oocyte defects (Liu et al., 1988). The hemizona assay (HZA), which is one of the most frequently used at present (Burkman et al., 1988), uses non-viable human oocytes obtained at surgery, at autopsy or through *in vitro* fertilization programmes. These oocytes can be kept for a long time in concentrated saline solution for further utilization.

In the case of the HZA, microdissection of the zona pellucida of individual oocytes is carried out, dividing the zona in two halves using micromanipulators and an inverted microscope, or a simple blade. By means of this technique, the binding capacity of control spermatozoa from normal donors can be compared with the binding of the study male gametes. The clinical value of this test has been evaluated in 106 patients of an IVF programme together with other sperm function tests; it showed a significant correlation with the fertilization rate (Liu et al., 1989). The ability of the spermatozoon to bind to the ZP assesses multiple functions of human gametes (Burkman et al., 1988).

B. Spermatozoon-oocyte fusion

The molecular mechanism of sperm-oocyte fusion is not known in detail and the process is not strictly species-specific. Hamster oocytes previously freed from ZP are easily fused with mammalian spermatozoa. Research on the possible molecular basis and ligands that would act as mediators of the fusion, like the complements Clq and C3b, still continues. The objective of this research is to develop better defined chemical tests for the assessment of sperm function.

Liu et al. (1988) described a sperm-oolemma binding test using oocytes that had failed fertilization in an IVF programme. To carry out this test, the zona pellucida is solubilized with acid pH saline solution (Liu et al., 1989). Then, between 4 to 5 oocytes are incubated with spermatozoa (control and test), marked with different fluorochromes. In the preliminary assays, it was observed that the sperm-oolemma binding relation correlated with the sperm-ZP binding ratio, but less significantly when it was compared with the IVF fertilization rate using logistic regression analysis.

In order to study the sperm-oolemma interaction and the sperm nuclear decondensation that leads to the formation of the male pronucleus, the hamster test has also been used. To obtain a better predictive value, the test has been combined with calcium ionophores sperm treatment. Moreover, it has been described that abnormalities of the postacrosomal sheath may impair the sperm-oolemma fusion test results, as well as the results, of the chromatin decondensation assay.

OTHER TESTS OF PROGNOSTIC SIGNIFICANCE IN INFERTILITY

REACTIVE OXYGEN SPECIES (ROS)

Several studies have been carried out showing that a good number of defects of spermatozoon-oocyte fusion are associated with an abnormal membrane capacity to respond to an intracellular signal of Ca++ release. Human spermatozoa have a great capacity to generate ROS, mainly anion superoxide (O.2) and hydrogen peroxide (H_2O_2). Another source of ROS that may induce sperm peroxidation damage are leucocytes, which may be occasionally found in great amounts in seminal plasma (Aitken and West, 1990).

Even though it is known that the ROS constitute a source of damage in various types of cells, it has been recently suggested that they may be involved in the physiological regulation of capacitation, hyperactivation and AR in humans (de Lamirande and Gagnon, 1993). Neutrophil and macrophage activation involves a cascade of protein phosphorylation reactions; triggering the activation of the oxidase NADPH of the plasma membrane has a similar effect (Aitken et al., 1997). When the natural defence mechanism of the spermatozoa, superoxide dismutase, is overcome, it results in the combination of H_2O_2 with an excess of anion superoxide, triggering the Haber-Weiss reaction which, in the presence of Fe++, generates very powerful cytotoxic free radicals. As has been stated already , human spermatozoa are able to generate ROS or free radicals, and this property is involved in the aetiology of male infertility (Aitken and Clarkson, 1987). Besides the irreversible damage that ROS can cause to the spermatozoa, specially when inappropriate methods of sperm separation are used, the presence of a great number of male gametes with the capacity to produce them will produce an impairment of sperm maturation and/ or morphological abnormalities.

ROS are detected by means of chemiluminescence, using dimetylsulphoxide-solubilized luminol as a test (Aitken et al., 1990). Readings are done in a chamber at 37°C for a total of 30 minutes in an integrated way. To have a more sensitive assay, 3 U of horseradish peroxidase are used, and once a steady state has been reached, the cells are stimulated with 12 myristate 13 acetate phorbol ester (PMA) and monitored for another 15 minutes. Very sensitive chemiluminescent equipment (Berthold LB 9506, LKB Wallac 1221, Hammamatzu, Lumiphotometer T D 4000) has been suggested to ensure good results. Even though the measurement of ROS is technically simple, it requires luminometers of great sensitivity that are the only ones capable of measuring chemiluminescence signals of oxygen-reactive metabolites like H_2O_2 and O.2.

Defects of the sperm middle-piece, associated with the excessive retention of cytoplasmic residues, seem to be associated with excessive generation of ROS and the concomitant peroxidation damage. As a consequence of this, the gametes present high contents of certain enzymes, like lactic dehydrogenase, creatine kinase (CK) and glucose 6-P-dehydrogenase. The determination of these enzymes can be taken as a marker for the presence of cytoplasmic residues. The study of CK has been proposed as an additional test for the determination of sperm function (Huszar et al., 1990). As has been reported, the excessive production of ROS is a perfectly defined pathology responsible for serious sperm disorders (Aitken et al., 1989). In spite of this, its determination is not feasible in routine andrology practice. ROS, as already stated, produces changes in the sperm plasma membrane fluidity, and perhaps on hormone receptors like progesterone (Revelli et al., 1994), cytokines and growth factors. As a result, they may deeply alter sperm function, inducing problems of migration, capacitation, binding and fusion of gametes.

Cytokine determination, like that of interleukin-6, in seminal plasma allows for the detection of the inflammatory process of the accessory glands or excretory ducts of the male reproductive tract (Comhaire et al., 1994). It has also been considered as useful in the determination of other substances that reflect the level of cell division of the seminiferous epithelium, like transferrin as an indicator of Sertoli cell function (Sylvester and Griswold, 1994).

Lipid Peroxidation (LPO)

The mechanism by which ROS damage sperm function involves the peroxidation of nonsaturated fatty acids of the plasma membrane. Plenty of literature has been published to determine the chemical nature of the molecular damage. These studies indicated that lipid peroxidation may be involved in the aetiology of male infertility. Lipid peroxidation induces damage because it reduces sperm membrane fluidity. As a consequence of this damage, membranes are incapable of engaging in fusigenic events. In the studies of Jones et al. (1979), it was demonstrated that the addition of exogens peroxides or the stimulation of endogens peroxides with Fe^{++} results in a loss of cellular viability which, in turn, is followed by a dramatic fall in motility.

The presence of nonsaturated fatty acids in the cells constitutes a potential threat since lipids have a great lability in the presence of oxygen. Peroxidation of fatty acids starts with the catalytic breakdown of pre-existent hydroperoxides to generate alcohoxil radicals (LO.). These start a cascade of reactions in the membrane, subtracting hydrogen atoms of the adjacent lipids. The quick loss of the nonsaturated fatty acids of this structure brings about a concomitant increase in the production rate of malondialdehide (MDA). The chemistry of this reaction has been used to develop a peroxidation assay applicable to human gametes in which the production of MDA is determined after incubating the spermatozoa with catalytic amounts of Fe^{++} and ascorbate (Aitken et al., 1993).

Due to the fact that Fe^{++} ions lead to a quick breakdown of the pre-existent peroxides of the plasmalemma, the measure of peroxidation may be taken as an indicator of the degree of oxidative stress experienced by a sperm population during its life history (Aitken et al., 1993).

Modified Sperm Stress Test (MOST)

The presence of toxic lipid peroxides inevitably induces immobilization, senescence and sperm death. Alvarez et al. (1987), demonstrated that the rate of motility loss *in vitro* in normal spermatozoa, at temperatures between 24°C and 40°C, positively correlates with the endogenous lipid peroxidation potential. These authors later developed a method called Sperm Stress Test, which seems to predict pregnancy rates (Alvarez et al., 1996). To be used in assisted reproductive techniques, we have developed MOST (Modified Sperm Stress Test) to try to predict failures in the fertilization of human oocytes caused by damaged spermatozoa (Calamera et al., 1998). It was demonstrated that motility and strict morphology are the two best predictors of IVF. Nevertheless, neither of them evaluates the changes that spermatozoa may undergo after prolonged incubation, before actual fertilization of the oocytes occurs. Low values of MOST (<0.39) probably indicate an increase in lipid peroxidation, which may interfere with sperm fertilizing capacity. The gametes that have lost motility after incubation (4 hours at 40°C) have a potential of lipid peroxidation incompatible with normal fertilization rates.

Resazurin Test

This is a very simple test. Resazurin is a biochemial indicator which, if reduced, produces colour changes. Reduction of resazurin to risorrufin offers a determination of the reduction capacity of semen. This is demonstrated through a change of colour from purple to violet (Glass et al., 1991).

The test is easy to perform and does not require any equipment. Its results correlate with sperm concentration (Mahmoud et al., 1994), the generation of ROS by the spermatozoa and with prostate functional status (Zalata et al., 1995).

ROLE OF SPERM FUNCTION TEST IN FAILED FERTILIZATION

Fertilization in humans is a process which culminates when the parental genomes unite within the activated oocyte. For this to occur successfully, a series of well-synchronized chronological events must unfold accurately. Failure of these events at any stage is lethal for the zygote and may be the source of some undiagnosed human infertility. While sperm behaviour and the initial encounter of the gametes have been studied in humans, the motility of the sperm and egg nuclei (male and female pronuclei) within the oocyte, which leads to their union, is less well understood.

Today it is possible to analyse the stages at which human fertilization fails with sophistication and precision, using immunofluorescence. The role of the spermatozoon in this process can be studied very closely and its communication with the oocyte, once penetration occurs, can be elucidated.

In the animal species studied so far, the oocytes-activating signal uses calcium as a second messenger. In mammalian oocytes, the source of the calcium participating in these signalling events is predominantly intracellular, although a calcium influx from the extracellular space is also involved. In human oocytes, the sperm-induced calcium oscillations can last for up to 5–6 hours (Sousa et al., 1996); the frequency with which individual calcium spikes appear ranges between one spike every 2 minutes to one every 35 minutes, and is highly variable from oocyte to oocyte, but relatively stable in a single oocyte during the whole calcium oscillation period (Tesarik and Sousa, 1994; Sousa et al., 1996). In human oocytes, the early calcium reaction to the spermatozoon is characterized by an initial group of 3–6 rapidly occurring calcium spikes, which is then followed by lower-frequency spikes for the rest of the calcium period (Tesarik and Sousa, 1994). Any perturbation in the correct pattern of calcium oscillation can cause incomplete Meiotic Promoting Factor (MPF) inactivation, allowing the male nucleus to enter metaphase prematurely and generating premature chromosome condensation (PCC).

Despite the continuous improvement of *in vitro* fertilization techniques, fertilization failure is a recurrent phenomenon. This has been explained mainly in terms of chromosomal alterations. Many years ago, several human studies that showed different types of fertilization failures after conventional *in vitro* fertilization focused on oocytes analysed by cytogenetic techniques (Plachot and Crozet, 1992; Zenzes and Casper, 1992). Although explanations in terms of chromosomal alterations are well documented, the participation of sperm decondensation, meiosis resumption, oocyte activation and pronuclei migration has been less studied. As extensively described by Asch et al. (1995), fertilization failure in mammals may have different causes. Firstly, the injected oocyte can fail to initiate the biochemical processes necessary for oocyte activation (Tesarik, 1998). Alternatively, this process may be initiated but may not occur normally, leading to an incomplete activation. Further, the spermatozoon may remain poorly accessible to oocyte factors required for chromatin decondensation and formation of the female pronucleus (Tesarik and Kopecny, 1989 a, b). Finally, the injection procedure may entail subtle structural changes in oocyte organelles, not detectable by light microscopy.

In brief, in the immunoflourescence analysis, the zona pellucida is removed by a brief incubation in Tyrode's acid, and the oocytes are fixed and permeabilized in a microtubule-stabilizing buffer. As a primary monoclonal antibody, anti α-acetylated tubulin is used to identify the sperm tail, and to analyse the meiotic spindle, the material is incubated with anti β-tubulin-Cy3 monoclonal antibodies. Chromatin is identified by counterstaining with Hoescht 33258. Then, the processed material is mounted between a slide and a coverslip and examined using an epifluorescent microscope.

In order to explore the cellular and molecular aspects of fertilization failure, we studied 248 'non-fertilized' human oocytes after *in vitro* fertilization (IVF) and intracytoplasmic sperm injection (ICSI). No pronuclei were visualized and, in some cases, the extrusion of the second polar body had not occurred after 20–40 hours post-insemination or post-injection.

In this investigation, we observed that the main reason for *in vitro* fertilization failure after IVF is the absence of sperm penetration (54.9%, Table 10.1a). Microtubule and DNA analysis revealed that 45.1% of the oocytes initiate some aspects of the fertilization process, but arrested at specific stages. On the other hand, 13.3% of the 'non-fertilized' oocytes after ICSI did not show any sperm in the ooplasm. These results are in accordance with the previously described findings of Flaherty et al., 1995; Sakkas et al., 1996; and Lopes et al., 1998.

The principal reason of fertilization failure after ICSI, as shown by this study, is oocyte activation failure (36.5%, Table 10.1b). Swann et al. (1990) and Dozortzev et al. (1995) have shown that the sperm contains a temperature-sensitive cytosolic factor called oscilin which, when injected into the oocyte, is able to generate oocyte activation. The absence of this factor or the lack of activity in 'weak' sperm, like the ones used in ICSI procedures, could explain, at least in part, the activation failure observed after ICSI. A higher paternal DNA fragmentation rate, and an even significantly higher rate of DNA fragmentation, in sperm that failed decondensation, compared to sperm that did not, was described by Lopes et al. (1998). The authors suggested that a correlation exists between the rate of DNA fragmentation and a loss of oscilin activity.

When sperm nuclei enter fully mature eggs, they regularly develop into swelling pronuclei, whereas those spermatozoa penetrating oocytes which were arrested at MII undergo conspicuous chromosome condensation. PCC was observed in 6.1% of the oocytes studied after IVF and ICSI. This process was first described by Schmiady et al. (1986), and the essential prerequisite is no activation of the oocyte and the presence of condensing factors (e.g. MPF) in the cytoplasm, preventing the sperm nuclei from transforming into pronuclei.

Defects in pronuclear formation and/or migration has been found in a similar range after IVF and ICSI (23.9% and 21.9%, respectively; Table 10.1). Schatten et al. (1994) have shown that this situation can occur when an inability in the assembly of the microtubules around the paternal centrosome exists. The attraction of γ tubulins towards the centrosome can be generated by specific binding sites, and also by energy-consuming proteins like dynein. Motility and incorporation of maternal components with the paternal centrosome lead to aster enlargement in humans, until parental pronuclei contact occurs. During these processes male pronuclei move towards the centre of the cell to make contact with the maternal pronuclei which have migrated from eccentric position near the oocyte cortex.

The overall fertilization rate gives an indication of the overall effectiveness of IVF and ICSI in overcoming the defects which prevent fertilization, but it does not provide information on the results for individual couples or for variations in the fertilization rate in repeated cycles. Hence, in order to provide a clear diagnosis of failed fertilization in each case, the use of immunofluorescence is needed. Flaherty et al. (1998), have shown that total failed fertilization is a rare event after ICSI (3%), and is most frequent in cycles in which only one or two oocytes are injected. This report is in agreement with those of Liu et al. (1995). Flaherty et al. (1998), reported that the risk of failed fertilization was reduced from 37% when one oocyte was injected to only 0.8% when five or more oocytes were injected. The participation of sperm decondensation, meiosis resumption, oocyte activation and pronuclei migration can be easily studied using techniques like immunofluorescence when failed or poor fertilization occurs. It may concluded that these techniques can be used as a test to identify the causes of failed fertilization and to predict future results in subsequent cycles.

Table 10.1. Immunofluorescence Analysis of Human Oocytes that Failed to Fertilize After IVF and ICSI

Level	IVF (n = 102)	ICSI (n = 137)	Significance
a) No sperm penetration or sperm expulsion	54.9%	13.1%	p<0.01
b) Activation failure	11.4%	36.5%	p<0.01
c) Abortive activation	2.1%	0%	
d) Defects in pronuclear formation/migration	23.9%	21.9%	NS
e) Metaphase arrest	0%	14.6%	
f) Others	19.6%	21.3%	NS

Notes: Total number of studied oocytes: 248

NS: Statistically not significant

REFERENCES

Acosta, A.A. (1992). 'Male factor in assisted reproduction', *Fertil. Steril. Med. Clin. N.Am.*, **3**: 487–503.

Acosta, A.A. et al. (1986). '*In vitro* fertilization and the male factor', *Urology*, **28**: 1–9.

Austin, C.R. (1951). 'The capacitation of the mammalian sperm', *Nature*, **170**: 326–30.

Aitken, R.J. et al. (1982). 'An analysis of sperm function in cases of unexplained infertility: Conventional criteria, movement characteristics and fertilizing capacity', *Fertil. Steril.*, **38**: 212–21.

______(1983). 'Analysis of sperm function in Kartagener´s syndrom', *Fertil. Steril.*, **40**: 696–8.

______(1984 a). 'A prospective study of the relationship between semen quality and fertility in cases of unexplained infertility', *J. Androl.*, **5**: 297–301.

______(1984 b). 'Analysis of human sperm function following exposure to the ionophore A 23187: Comparison of normospermic and oligospermic men', *J. Androl.*, **5**: 321–9.

______(1985). 'Relationship between the movement characteristics of human spermatozoa and their ability to penetrate cervical mucus and zona-free hamster oocyte', *J. Reprod. Fert.*, **73**: 441–5.

______(1989). 'Analysis of the relationship between defective sperm function and the generation of reactive oxygen species in cases of oligospermia', *J. Androl.*, **10**: 214–19.

______(1990). 'Generation of reactive oxygen species, lipid peroxidation and human sperm function', *Biol. Reprod.*, **41**: 183–7.

______(1993). 'Relationship between iron-catalyzed lipid peroxidation and human sperm function', *J. Reprod. Fertil.*, **98**: 257–65

______(1997). 'Reactive oxygen species generation by human spermatozoa is induced by exogenous NADPH and inhibited by the flavoprotein inhibitor diphenylene iodonium and quinacrine', *Mol. Reprod. and Develop.*, **47**: 468–82.

Aitken, R.J. and J.S. Clarkson (1987). 'Cellular basis of defective sperm function and its association with the genesis of reactive oxygen species by human spermatozoa', *J. Reprod. Fertil.*, **81**: 459–69.

Aitken, R.J. and K.M. West (1990). 'Analysis of the relationship between reactive oxygen species production and leucocytes infiltration in fractions of human semen separated on Percoll gradient', *Int. J. Androl.*, **13**: 433–9.

Almlid, T. and L.A. Johnson (1988). 'Effect of glycerol concentration, equilibration time and temperature of glycerol addition on post-thaw viability of board spermatozoa frozen in straws', *J. Anim. Sci.*, **66**: 2899–905.

Alvarez, J.G. et al. (1987). 'Spontaneous lipid peroxidation and production of hydrogen peroxides and superoxide in human spermatozoa: Superoxide dismutase as major enzyme protectant against oxigen toxicity', *J. Androl.*, **8**: 334–48.

Alvarez J.G. et al. (1996). 'The sperm stress test: A novel test that predicts pregnancy in assisted reproductive technology', *Fertil. Steril.*, **2**: 400–05.

Asch R. et al. (1995). 'The stages at which human fertilization arrests: Microtubule and chromosome configurations in inseminated oocytes which failed to complete fertilization and development in humans', *Mol. Hum. Reprod.*, **1**: 1897–906.

Auge, J. et al. (1990). 'Aniline blue staining as a marker of sperm chromatin defects associated with different semen characteristics discriminates between proven fertile and suspected infertile men', *Int. J. Androl.*, **13**: 452–5.

Barratt, C.L.R. et al. (1989). 'The hypo-osmotic swelling test and the sperm mucus penetration test in determining fertilization of human oocyte', *Hum. Reprod.*, **4**: 430–34.

Bartoov, B. et al. (1980). 'Morphological characterization of abnormal human spermatozoa using transmission electron microscopy', *Arch. Androl.*, **5**: 305–22.

Bellvé, A.R. (1982). 'Biogenesis of the mammalian sperm', in R. Amann and G. Seidel (eds.) *Prospects for sexing mammalian sperm*, Colorado Univ. Press., pp. 69.

Bellvé, A.R. et al. (1975). 'Synthesis and amino acid composition of basic proteins in mammalian sperm nuclei', *Dev. Biol.*, **47**: 349–53.

Bedford, J.M. (1983). 'Significance of the need for sperm capacitation before fertilization in eutherian mammals', *Biol. Reprod.*, **28**: 108–113.

Bedford, J.M. and H.I. Calvin (1974). 'The occurrence and possible functional significance of s-s cross links in sperm head with particular reference to eutherian mammals', *J. Exp. Zool.*, **188**: 137–41.

Bedford, J.M. et al. (1973). 'The maturation of spermatozoa in the human epididymis.' *J. Reprod. Fertil.* **18** (suppl.) 199: 213–9.

Benoff, S. et al. (1993). 'Human sperm fertilizing potential *in vitro* is correlated with differential exoression of a head-specific mannose ligand receptor', *Fertil. Steril.*, **59**: 854–62.

Benoff, S. et al. (1995). 'Co-expression of mannose-ligand and non-nuclear progesterone receptors on motile human sperm identifies an acrosome reaction inducible subpopulation', *AJRI*, **34**: 100–115.

Blazak, W.F. and J.W. Overstreet (1982). 'Instability of nuclear chromatin in the ejaculated spermatozoa of fertile men', *J. Reprod. Fertil.*, **65**: 331–9.

Boyers, S.P. et al. (1989). 'Automated semen analysis', *Curr. Probl. Obstet. Gynaecol. Fertil.*, vol. XXII. Year Book Medical Publisher Inc., Chicago.

Brandelli, A. et al. (1995). 'A new predictive test for *in vitro* fertilization based on the induction of sperm acrosome reaction by N-acetylglucose mineneoglycoprotein', *Hum. Reprod.*, **10**: 1751–6.

Burkman, L.J. et al. (1988). 'The hemizona assay (HZA): Development of a diagnostic test for the binding of human spermatozoa to the human hemizona pellucida to predict fertilization potential', *Fertil. Steril.*, **49**: 688–97.

Calamera, J.C. et al. (1982). 'Relation between motility and adenosine triphosphate (ATP) in human spermatozoa', *Andrologia*, **14**: 239–41.

______(1989). 'Effect of lipid peroxidation upon human spermatic adenosine triphosphate (ATP): Relationship with motility, velocity, and linearity of spermatozoa', *Andrologia*, **21**: 48–54.

______(1998). 'Modified sperm stress test (MOST): A simple assay that predicts sperm-related abnormal *in vitro* fertilization', *Hum. Reprod.* (in press).

Comhaire, F. et al. (1983). 'Adenosine triphosphate in human semen: A quantitative estimate of fertilizing potential', *Fertil. Steril.*, **40**: 500–505.

______(1994). 'Cytokines in semen of normal men and of patients with andrological diseases', *Am. J. Reprod. Immunol.*, **31**: 99–103.

Cross, N.L. et al. (1986). 'Two simple methods for detecting acrosome-reacted human sperm', *Gamete Res.*, **15**: 213–26.

______(1988). 'Induction of acrosome reactions by the human zona pellucida', *Biol. Reprod.*, **38**: 235–44.

Cross, N.L. and S. Meizel (1989). 'Methods for evaluating the acrosome status of mammalian sperm', *Biol. Reprod.*, **41**: 635–41.

Cummins, J.M. et al. (1991). 'A test of the human sperm acrosome reaction following ionophore challenger: Relationship to fertility and other seminal parameters', *J. Androl.*, **12**: 98–102.

Chang, M.C. (1951). 'Fertilizing capacity of spermatozoa deposited in fallopian tube', *Nature.*, **168**: 997–1003.

Chemes, H.E. et al. (1987). 'Lack of a head in human spermatozoa from sterile patients: A syndrome associated with impaired fertilization', *Fertil. Steril.*, **47**: 310–16.

Dadoune, J.P. (1988). 'Correlation between defects in chromatin condensation of human spermatozoa stained by aniline blue and semen characteristics', *Andrologia*, **20**: 211–17.

De Jonge, et al. (1988). 'Induction of the human sperm

acrosome reaction by human oocyte', *Fertil. Steril.*, **50**: 949–53.

De Lamirande, E. and C. Gagnon (1993). 'A positive role for the superoxide anion in triggering hyperactivation and capacitation of human spermatozoa', *Int. J. Androl.*, **16**: 21–5.

Demel, R.A. et al. (1972). 'The properties of polyunsaturated lecithins in monolayers and liposomes and the interactions of these lecithins with cholesterol', *Biochem. Biophys. Acta.*, **166**: 24–40.

Didon, B.A. et al. (1989). 'Staining procedure to detect viability and the true acrosome reaction in spermatozoa of various species', *Gamete Res.*, **22**: 51–7.

Dott, H.M. and G.C. Foster (1972). 'A technique for studying the morphology of mammalian spermatozoa which are eosinophilic in a differential live/dead stain', *J. Reprod. Fertil.*, **29**: 443–8.

Dozortsev D. et al. (1995). 'Human oocyte activation following intracytoplasmic sperm injection: The role of the sperm cell', *Hum. Reprod.*, **9**: 2139–44.

Dunphy, B. et al. (1989). 'The clinical value of conventional seemen analysis', *Fertil. Steril.*, **51**: 324–9.

Eggert-Kruse, W. et al. (1989). 'Clinical significance of crossed *in vitro* sperm-cervical mucus penetration test in infertility investigation', *Fertil. Steril.*, **52**: 1032–37.

Evenson, D.P. et al. (1991). 'Individuality of DNA denaturation patterns in human sperm as measured by the sperm chromatin structure assay', *Reprod. Toxicol.*, **5**: 115–19.

Fenichel, P. et al. (1989). 'Evaluation of the human sperm acrosome reaction using a monoclonal antibody, G.B.24 and fluorescence-activated cell sorter', *J. Reprod. Fertil.*, **87**: 699–706.

Ficsor, G. et al. (1983). 'Gelatin-substrate film technique for detection of acrosin in single mammalian sperm', *Fertil. Steril.*, **39**: 548–52.

Flaherty, S.P. et al. (1995). 'Aetiology of failed and abnormal fertilization after intracytoplasmic sperm injection', *Hum. Reprod.*, **10**: 2623–29.

______(1998). 'Assessment of fertilization failure and abnormal fertilization after intracytoplasmic sperm injection', *Hum. Reprod. Supplement.*, **13**: 155–64.

Florke-Gerloff, S. et al. (1984). 'Biochemical and genetic investigation of round-headed spermatozoa in infertile men including two brothers and their father', *Andrologia.*, **16**: 187–202.

Francavilla, S. et al. (1992). 'Sperm acrosin activity and fluorescence microscopic assessment of proacrosin/acrosin in ejaculates of infertile and fertile men', *Fertil. Steril.*, **57**: 1311–15.

Gabriel, L.K. et al. (1995). 'Fluorescein isothiocyanate conjugate: Wheat germ agglutinin staining of human spermatozoa and fertilization *in vitro*', *Fertil. Steril.*, **63**: 894–901.

Garner, D.L. et al. (1986). 'Assessment of spermatozoal function using dual fluorescent staining and flow cytometric analysis', *Biol. Reprod.*, **34**: 127–38.

Glass, R.H. et al. (1991). 'The resazurin reduction test provide an assessment of sperm activity', *Fertil. Steril.*, **56**: 743–6.

Goodpasture, J.D. et al. (1980). 'Acrosin, proacrosin and acrosin inhibitor of human spermatozoa: extraction quantification and stability', *J. Androl.*, **1**: 16–27.

Harrison, R.A.P. (1983). 'The acrosome, its hydrolases and egg penetration', in J. André (ed.) *The sperm cell.*, Martinus Nijhoff, The Hagul.

Henley, N. et al. (1994). 'Flow cytometric evaluation of the acrosome reaction of human spermatozoa: A new method using a photoactivated supravital stain', *Int. J. Androl.*, **17**: 78–84.

Hirayama, T. et al. (1989). 'The measurement of hyaluronidase activity in human spermatozoa by substrate slide assay and its clinical application', *Fertil. Steril.*, **51**: 330–34.

Holden, C.A. et al. (1990). 'Assessment of the human sperm acrosome reaction using concanavalin a lectin', *Reprod. Dev.*, **25**: 247–57.

Huszar, G. et al. (1990). 'Sperm creatine kinase activity in fertile and infertile oligozoospermic men', *J. Androl.*, **11**: 40–45.

Huret, J.L. (1986). 'Nuclear chromatin decondensation of human sperm: A review', *Arch. Androl.*, **16**: 97–101.

Ibrahim, M.E. and H. Pedersen (1988). 'Acridine orange fluorescence as male fertility test', *Arch. Androl.*, **20**: 125–9.

Irvine, D.S. and R.J. Aitken (1985). 'The value of adenosine triphosphate (ATP) measurements in assessing the fertilizing ability of human spermatozoa', *Fertil. Steril.*, **44**: 806–10.

Jeulin, C. et al. (1986). 'Sperm factors to failure of human *in vitro* fertilization', *J. Reprod. Fertil.*, **76**: 735–40.

Jeyendran, R.S. et al. (1984). 'Development of an assay to assess the functional integrity of the human sperm membrane and its relationship to other semen characteristics', *J. Reprod. Fertil.*, **70**: 219-28.

Jones, R. et al. (1979). 'Peroxidative breakdown of phospholipids in human spermatozoa, spermicidal properties of fatty acid peroxidases and protective action of seminal plasma', *Fertil. Steril.*, **31**: 531–7.

Kamada, M. et al. (1985). 'Blocking of human fertilization *in vitro* by sera with sperm immobilizing antibodies', *Am. J. Obstet. Gynecol.*, **62**: 153–328.

Katz, D.F. and R.O. Davis (1987a). 'Automatic analysis of human sperm motion', *J. Androl.*, **8**: 170–75.

Katz, D.F. et al. (1987b). 'The byofisics of sperm penetration of the cumulus and zona pellucida', in H. Mohri (ed.), *New Horizons in sperm cell Research.*, Sci Soc. Press Japan, p. 13.

Kemp, R.B. et al. (1988). 'Comparison of cell death and adenosine triphosphate content as indicator of acute toxicity *in vitro*', *Xenobiotica.*, **18**: 633–9.

Koehler, J.K. (1978). 'The mammalian sperm surface studied with specific labeling techniques', *Int. Rev. Cytol.*, **54**: 75–108.

Kennedy, W.P. et al. (1989). 'A simple clinical assay to evaluate the acrosin activity of human spermatozoa', *J. Androl.*, **10**: 221–9.

Kohn, F.M. et al. (1997). 'Detection of human sperm acrosome reaction: Comparison between methods using double staining, pisum sativum agglutinin, concanavalin A and transmission electron microscopy', *Human Reprod.*, **12**: 714–21.

Kvist, U. et al. (1980). 'The intrinsic mechanism of chromatin decondensation and its activation in human spermatozoa', *Dev. Growth Differ.*, **22**: 543–7.

Lalumiere, G. et al. (1976). 'Cholesteryl sulfate and sterol sulfatasa in the human reproductive tract', *Steroids.*, **27**: 247–56

Langlais, J. and K.D. Roberts (1985). 'A molecular membrane model of sperm capacitation and the acrosome reaction of mammalian spermatozoa', *Gamete Res.*, **12**: 183–224.

Lindermann, C.B. and K.S. Kanous (1989). 'Regulation of sperm motility', *Arch. Androl.*, **23**: 1–22.

Liu, D.Y. et al. (1987). 'Spermatozoal nuclear chromatin decondensation *in vitro*: A test for sperm immaturity composicion with result.

______(1988). 'A human sperm-zona pellucida binding test using oocytes that failed to fertilize *in vitro*', *Fertil. Steril.*, **50**: 782–8.

______(1989). 'A sperm zona pellucida binding test and *in vitro* fertilization', *Fertil. Steril.*, **52**: 281–7

______(1991). 'Horse and marmoset monkey sperm bind to the zona pellucida of salt stored human oocytes', *Fertil. Steril.*, **56**: 764–7.

Liu J. et al. (1995). 'Analysis of 76 total fertilization failure cycles out of 2732 intracytoplasmic sperm injection cycles', *Hum Reprod.*, **10**: 2630–36.

Liu, D.Y. and H.W.G. Baker (1988). 'The preparation of human sperm with poor morphology but normal intact acrosome detected with pisum sativum agglutinin correlates with fertilization *in vitro*', *Fertil. Steril.*, **50**: 288–93.

______(1996). 'A simple method for assessment of the human acrosome reaction of spermatozoa bound to the zona-pellucida lack of relationship with ionophore A 23187 induced acrosome reaction', *Hum. Reprod.*, **11**: 551–7.

Lopes, S. et al. (1998). 'Gamete-specific DNA fragmentation in unfertilized human oocytes after intracytoplasmic sperm injection', *Hum. Reprod.*, **13**: 703–8.

Margalit, I. et al. (1997). 'A novel method for evaluating the acrosomal status of mammalian spermatozoa', *Arch. Androl.*, **39**: 87–99.

Mahadevan, M.M. et al. (1987). 'Effect of oocyte quality and sperm characteristics on the number of spermatozoa bound to the zona pellucida of human oocytes', *J. In Vitro Fert. Embryo Transf.*, **4**: 223–7.

Mahmoud, A.M. et al. (1994). 'Comparison of the resazurin test, adenosine triphosphate in semen and various sperm parameters', *Hum. Reprod.*, **9**: 1688–93.

Meizel, S. (1984). 'The importance of hydrolytic enzymes to an exocytoxic event; the mammalian sperm acrosome reaction', *Biol. Rev.*, **59**: 125–9.

Mixner, J.P. and J. Saroff (1954). 'Interference by glycerol with differential staining of bull spermatozoa', *J. Dairy Sci.*, **37**: 652–8.

Monesi, V. (1971). 'Chromosome activities during meiosis and spermatogenesis', *J. Reprod. Fertil.*, **13**: 1–5.

Morales, P. et al. (1988). 'Changes in human sperm motion during capacitation *in vitro*', *J. Reprod. Fert.*, **83**: 119–23.

Mortimer, D. (1989). 'Objective analysis of sperm motility and kinematics', in B.A. Kell and B.W. Webster (eds.), *Handbook of the Laboratory Diagnosis and Treatment of Infertility.*, Boca Raton, C.R.C. Press, 97–133.

Mortimer, D. et al. (1984). 'Human sperm motility

after migration into and incubation in synthetic media', *Gamete Res.*, **9**: 131–5.

______(1987). 'Specific labelling by peanut agglutinin of the outer acrosomal membrane of the human spermatozoa', *J. Reprod. Fertil.*, **81**: 127–35.

______(1991). 'Hyperactivated motility of human spermatozoa', in B. Baccetti (ed.), *Comparative Spermatology 20 Years After*, Raven Press, N.Y.

Mortimer, S.T. and D. Mortimer (1990). 'Kinematics of human spermatozoa incubated under capacitating conditions', *J. Androl.*, **11**: 195–200.

Mohsenian, M. et al. (1982). 'A study of sperm acrosin in patients with unexplained infertility', *Fertil. Steril.*, **37**: 223–9.

Nagae, T. et al. (1986). 'Acrosome reaction in human spermatozoa', *Fertil. Steril.*, **45**: 701–5.

Overstreet, J.W. and Hembree (1976). 'Penetration of the zona pelucida of non-living human oocytes by human spermatozoa *in vitro*', *Fertil. Steril.*, **27**: 815–31.

Overstreet, J.W. et al. (1980). 'Penetration of human spermatozoa into the human zona pellucida and the zona-free hamster egg: A study of fertile donor and infertile patients', *Fertil. Steril.*, **33**: 534–42.

Perreault, S.D. and B.J. Rogers (1982). 'Capacitation pattern of human spermatozoa', *Fertil. Steril.*, **38**: 258–61.

Plachot, M. and N. Crozet (1992). 'Fertilization abnormalities in human *in-vitro* fertilization', *Hum. Reprod.*, **7**: 89–94.

Pleban, P. et al. (1990). 'Test of sperm function: Acrosin', in A.A. Acosta et al. (eds.), *Human Spermatozoa in Assisted Reproduction.*, Williams and Wilkins, Baltimore, pp. 96–101.

Ramirez, J.P. et al. (1992). 'Sperm plasma membrane integrity in fertile and infertile men', *Andrologia*, **24**: 141–4.

Revelli, A. et al. (1994). 'Steroid receptors in human spermatozoa', *Hum. Reprod.*, **9**: 760–66.

Rogers, B.J. (1985). 'The sperm penetration assay: Its usefulness reevaluated', *Fertil. Steril.*, **43**: 821–40.

Roux, C. and J.P. Dadoune (1989). 'Use of the acridine orange staining on smears of human spermatozoa after heat treatment: Evaluation of the chromatin condensation', *Andrologia*, **21**: 275–81.

Rowley, M.J. et al. (1970). 'Duration of transit of spermatozoa through the human male ductular system', *Fertil. Steril.*, **21**: 390–96.

Royere, D. et al. (1988). 'Freezing and thawing alter chromatin stability of ejaculated human spermatozoa; fluorescens acridine orange staining and Feulgen-DNA cytophotometric studies', *Gamete Res.*, **21**: 51–4.

Sakkas D. et al. (1996). 'Sperm chromatin anomalies can influence decondensation after intracytoplasmic sperm injection', *Hum. Reprod.*, **11**: 837–43.

Saowaros, W. and S. Panyim (1979). 'The formation of disulphide bonds in human protamine during sperm maturation', *Experientia.*, **35**: 191–2.

Sathananthan, A.H. et al. (1982). 'Ultrastructural observations on the penetration of human sperm into the zona pellucida of the human egg *in vitro*', *J. Androl.*, **3**: 356–60.

Schatten G. (1994). 'The centrosome and its mode of inheritance: The reduction of the centrosome during gametogenesis and its restoration during fertilization', *Dev. Biol.*, **165**: 299–335.

Schill W.B. et al. (1988). 'The sperm acrosome; functional and clinical aspects', *Hum. Reprod.*, **3**: 139–45.

Schmiady, H. et al. (1986). 'Prematurely condensed human sperm chromosomes after *in vitro* fertilization (IVF)', *Hum. Genet.*, **74**: 441–3.

Siiteri, J.E. et al. (1988). 'Partial characterisation of a fraction of human follicular fluid that initiated the human sperm acrosome reaction *in vitro*', *Gamete Res.*, **20**: 25–42.

Sjoblom, P. and E. Coccia (1989). 'On the diagnostic value of the hypo-osmotic sperm swelling test in an *in vitro* fertilization IVF program', *In vitro Fertil. Embryo Transf.*, **6**: 41–3.

Sousa M. et al. (1996). 'The role of rianodine-sensitive Ca^{2+} stores in the Ca^{2+} oscillation machine of human oocytes', *Mol. Hum. Reprod.*, **2**: 265–72.

Stein, W.D. (1990). *Channels, carriers and pumps: An introduction to membrane transport.*, Academic Press, N.Y.

Swann K. (1990). 'A cytosolic sperm factor stimulates repetitive calcium increases and mimics fertilization in hamster eggs.' *Development*, **110**: 1295–1302.

Sylvester, S.R. and M.D. Griswold (1994). 'The testicular iron shuttle: A nurse function of the Sertoli cells', *J. Androl.*, **15**: 381–5.

Talbot, P. and Chacon, R.S. (1980). 'A new procedure

for rapidy scoring acrosome reactions of human sperm', *Gamete Res.*, **3**: 211–16.

______(1981). 'A triple-stain technique for evaluating normal acrosome reactions of human sperm', *J. Exp. Zool.*, **215**: 201–8.

Tejada, R.I. et al. (1984). 'A test for the practical evaluation of male fertility by acridine orange (AO) fluorescens', *Fertil. Steril.*, **42**: 87–91.

Tesarik, J. (1985). 'Comparison of acrosome reaction inducing activities of human cumulus oophorus, follicular fluid and ionophore A 23187 in human sperm population of proven fertilizing ability *in vitro*', *J. Reprod. Fertil.*, **74**: 383–8.

______(1989). 'Appropiate time of the acrosome reaction is a major requirement for the fertilizing spermatozoa', *Hum. Reprod.*, **4**: 957–61.

______(1998). 'Oocyte activation after intracytoplasmic injection of mature and immature sperm cells', *Hum. Reprod. Supppl.*, **13**: 117–27.

Tesarik, J. et al. (1988). 'Zona pellucida resistence to sperm penetration before the completion of human oocyte maturation', *J. Reprod. Fertil.*, **83**: 487–95.

Tesarik, J. and V. Kopecny (1989 a). 'Developmental control of the human male pronucleus by ooplasmic factors', *Hum. Reprod.*, **4**: 962–8.

______(1989b). 'Development of the human male pronucleus: Ultrastructure and timing', *Gamet Res.*, **24**: 135–49.

Testart, J. (1994). 'Assisted reproduction and male infertility historical overview', in J. Testant (ed.), *Frontiers in Endocrinology* (vol. 8): *Male Factor in Human Infertility*, Ares Serono Simposia, pp. 208–16.

Tulsiani, D.R.P. et al. (1990). 'Human sperm plasma membranes prossess D-mannosidase activity but not galactosyltransferase activity', *Biol. Reprod.*, **42**: 843–58.

Tummon, I.S. et al. (1991). 'Total acrosinactivity correlaters with fertility potential after fertilization *in vitro*', *Fertil. Steril.*, **56**: 933–8.

Visconti, P.E. et al. (1995 a). 'Capacitation of mouse spermatozoa. I correlation between the capacitation state and tirosine phosphorilation', *Dev.*, **121**: 1129–37.

______(1995 b). 'Tyrosine, phosphorilation and capacitation are regulated by a cAMP- dependent pathway,' *Dev.*, **121**: 1139–50.

WHO. (1992). *Laboratory Manual for Examination of Human Semen and Semen-cervical Mucus Interaction.*, The Press Syndicate of University of Cambridge, U.K.

Wilton, L.J. et al. (1988). 'Human male infertility caused by degeneration and death of sperm in the epididymis', *Fertil. Steril.*, **49**: 1052–58.

Welker, B. et al. (1988). 'Acrosomal proteinase activity of human spermatozoa and relation of results to semen quality', *Hum. Reprod.*, **3** suppl. 75–80.

Wolf, D.P. et al. (1985). 'Acrosomal status evaluation in human ejacultated sperm with monoclonal antibodies', *Biol. Reprod.*, **32**: 1157–62.

Yanagimachi, R. et al. (1976). 'The use of zona-free animal ova as a test system for the assessment of the fertilizing capacity of human spermatozoa', *Biol. Reprod.*, **15**: 471–5.

______(1979). 'Retention of biologic characteristics of zona pellucida in highly concentrated salt solution: The use of salt-stored eggs for assessing the fertilizing capacity of spermatozoa', *Fertil. Steril.*, **31**: 562–7.

Yanagimachi, R. (1981). 'Mechanisms of fertilization in mammalian', in L. Mastroianni and J.D. Biggers (eds.), *Fertilization and Embryonic development in vitro*, Plenum Press, N.Y., pp. 81–9.

______(1984). 'Zona-free hamster eggs: Their use in assessing fertilizing capacity and examining chromosomes of human spermatozoa', *Gamete Res.*, **10**: 187–91.

______(1988). 'Mammalian fertilization', in E. Knobil et al. (eds.), *The Physiology of Reproduction*, vol. 1, Raven Press, N.Y.

Zalata, A. et al. (1995). 'Evaluation of the role of ROS in male infertility', *Hum. Reprod.*, **10**: 1444–51.

Zaneveld, L.S.D. and R.S. Jeyendran (1988). 'Modern assessment of semen for diagnostic purpose', *Semin. Reprod. Endocrinol.*, **6**: 323–7.

Zamboni, L. (1987). 'Sperm ultrastructural pathology and infertility', in B. Gondos and D. Riddick (eds.), *Pathology of Infertility*. Thieure Medical Publishers N.Y., pp. 281–8.

Zenzes, M.T. and R.F. Casper (1992). 'Cytogenetics of human oocytes, zygotes and embryos after *in vitro* fertilization', *Hum. Genet.*, **88**: 367–75.

11

Management of Aspermia and Azoospermia

Rupin Shah

INTRODUCTION

In this chapter, we will focus on the management of two aspects of male infertility that are frequently encountered in assisted reproduction centres—aspermia and azoospermia. Both these problems can be caused by a variety of factors and can be treated in a number of ways. Hence, a proper evaluation protocol is required so that the clinician can select the correct investigations and the appropriate therapy.

ASPERMIA

Aspermia is the absence of an antegrade ejaculate, as opposed to azoospermia in which there is an ejaculate but no sperm.

EVALUATION

Aspermia can result from psychological or organic causes (Table 11.1).

Table 11.1. Causes of Aspermia

- Psychological Anejaculation
  - Situational
  - Complete (anorgasmic anejaculation)
- Organic Anejaculation
  - Failure of emission
    - Neurogenic failure
    - Anatomical block
    - Severe hypogonadism
  - Failure of Antegrade ejaculation
    - Retrograde ejaculation
    - Antegrade obstruction

SITUATIONAL ANEJACULATION

These men can ejaculate in some situations, but are inhibited in others. Usually, this inhibition occurs in the infertility clinic or at the time of ovulation, thus interfering with the therapy. Situational anejaculation can present in a variety of ways (Table 11.2).

Table 11.2. Classification of Situational Anejaculation

Type of Situational Dysfunction	Description
Unexpected ejaculatory failure	Unexpected failure on the day of ovulation
Periovulatory Anejaculation	Inability to ejaculate on day of ovulation, but can ejaculate on other days
Clinic anejaculation	Can collect semen at home, but not in clinic
Masturbatory anejaculation	Ejaculates during intercourse, but cannot collect semen by masturbation
Intercourse anejaculation	Can ejaculate by masturbation, but not during the intercourse

Anorgasmic Anejaculation

This is also termed idiopathic or psychogenic anejaculation. These men have never reached orgasm in the waking state—neither during intercourse nor during masturbation—and hence, have never ejaculated consciously (Shah, 1998).

The diagnosis is based on the history: the man will state that he can have intercourse but does not reach orgasm. However, often the history is not clear, since a man who has never experienced orgasm is uncertain as to how an orgasm feels. We have seen many cases where the man says that he has reached orgasm, and even provides urethral secretions or urine as a semen sample, when in actual fact, he has not reached orgasm! Hence, a high level of suspicion is required to diagnose this problem. A useful pointer is the presence of nocturnal emissions—this rules out organic causes of anejaculation. Unfortunately, this problem has received scant mention in literature. Therefore, many clinicians are unaware of this entity; the diagnosis is often missed, and unnecessary investigations and inappropriate management are common.

Organic Anejaculation

These men reach orgasm but do not ejaculate semen because of failure of emission or failure of ejaculation (Table 11.3).

Failure of emission: The first stage of orgasm involves the emission of sperm from the epididymis, vas and seminal vesicles into the posterior urethra, and is mediated by the lower thoracic and upper lumbar sympathetic fibres (T12 to L2). Damage to these fibres will lead to neurogenic failure of emission. If there is fibrosis of the ejaculatory and prostatic ducts, then emission will not occur due to an anatomical obstruction. In India, this commonly occurs after genital tuberculosis, but may also occur after any infection or inflammation affecting the prostatic fossa.

Failure of ejaculation: The second phase of orgasm involves closure of the bladder neck, again mediated by the thoraco-lumbar sympathetic fibres. If the bladder neck is dysfunctional, semen will follow the path of least resistance and flow retrograde into the bladder. Hence, there will be no antegrade ejaculate.

The third phase of ejaculation results from rhythmic contractions of the bulbocavernosus muscle, which propels the semen forcefully out of the urethra. If there is an obstruction to the outflow, or damage to the bulbocavernosus muscle, then semen will not be ejaculated, and instead, will collect in the anterior urethra and dribble out later or be washed out by urine.

Table 11.3. Organic Causes of Anejaculation

Neurogenic Failure of Emission
– Spinal cord lesions (trauma, myelodysplasia)
– Retroperitoneal lymph node dissection
– Lumbar sympathectomy; anterior lumbar spine surgery
– Abdomino-pelvic surgery (involving aorta, rectum)
– Diabetic autonomic neuropathy
– Sympatholytic drugs
Obstructive Failure of Emission
– Post-infection fibrosis of ejaculatory and prostatic ducts (G.U. tuberculosis)
Retrograde Ejaculation (incompetent bladder neck)
– Congenitally wide bladder neck
– Iatrogenic (bladder neck incision; T.U.R.)
– Bladder neck trauma (rupture bladder)
– Neurogenic paralysis of the bladder neck (diabetes, sympatholytic drugs, spinal cord lesions)
– Idiopathic
Obstruction to Antegrade Ejaculation
– Anterior urethral diverticulum (congenital or acquired)
– Anterior urethral pouch (following urethroplasty)
– Anterior urethral stricture

A diagnostic flow chart incorporating the various possibilities discussed above is presented in Fig. 11.1, A and B.

MANAGEMENT

Treatment of Situational Anejaculation

It can be extremely frustrating when a dozen oocytes are waiting in the incubator and the husband is unable to provide semen at that point. Often, such a situation can be anticipated and prevented, or compensated for, beforehand

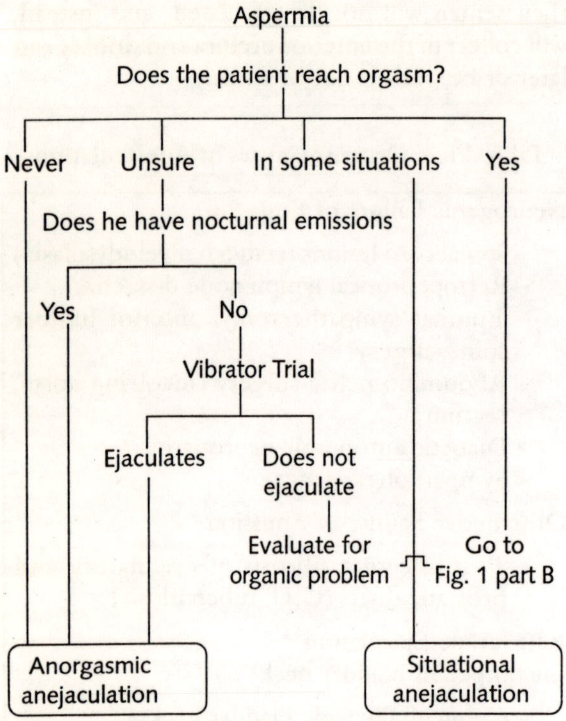

Fig. 11.1A. Flow chart for evaluation of aspermia

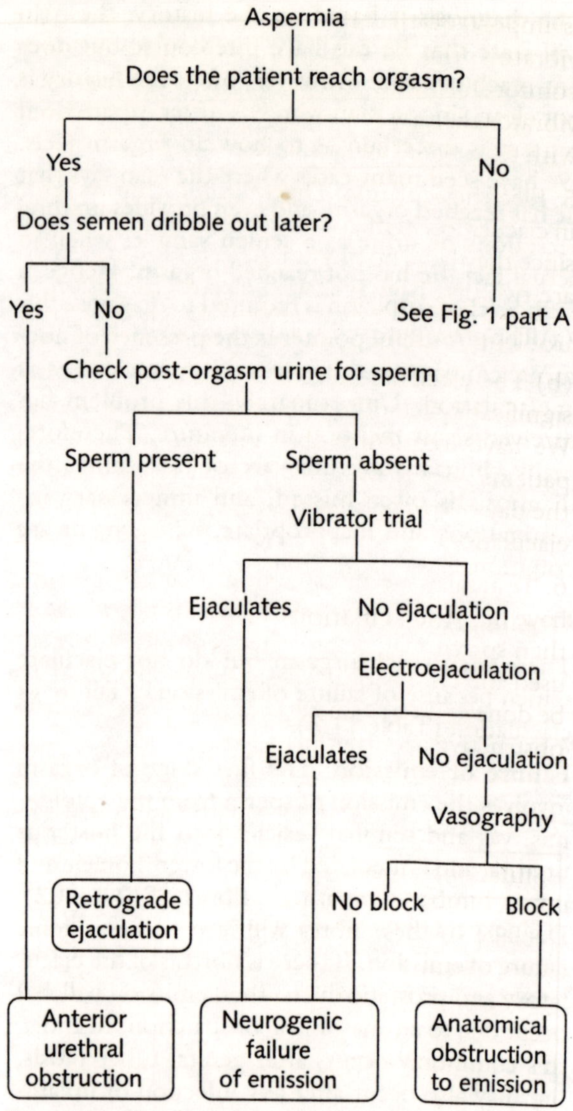

Fig. 11.1B. Flow chart for evaluation of aspermia

(Table 11.4). If this has not been done, special measures for sperm retrieval—vibrator stimulation or electroejaculation—will be required. The following strategies and techniques are used for managing situational anejaculation.

1. Routine cryopreservation of semen: This should be done for all patients scheduled for IVF or ICSI. This allows collection prior to ovulation, at a time when the man is not under pressure. Not only does this ensure that some sperm will always be available, but the fact that a back-up sample is available reduces the patient's stress considerably and facilitates ejaculation when required.

2. Home collection: Most men are far more comfortable collecting semen at home, prior to egg collection, than in the clinic. Therefore, whenever distances permit, it is preferable to ask the man to bring the sample from home.

3. Choice of sperm collection methods: While some men find it easy to ejaculate by masturbation, others need coital stimulation and may need to be instructed about coitus interruptus or provided with non-spermicidal condoms.

4. Erection-facilitating medication: Intrapenile injection of vaso-active drugs (Shah, 1998), or oral medications like sildenafil, can help a nervous man attain an erection and facilitate intercourse and ejaculation in some cases.

5. Vibrator therapy: The strong, prolonged stimulus provided by a vibrator can help a man to reach an orgasm. For men with situational anejaculation, in whom need for a vibrator is anticipated, it

is important that the man practises use of the vibrator prior to ovulation, so that he becomes comfortable with the technique. Properly used, vibrator therapy can succeed in 80 to 90% of men with situational anejaculation.

5. Electroejaculation: This will almost always result in ejaculation in men with situational anejaculation since they have no physical defect. However, there are two disadvantages with electroejaculation.

(a) The procedure needs a short general anaesthesia.

(b) The electroejaculated semen sample is often significantly inferior to naturally-ejaculated semen. We have frequently observed this difference in patients who unexpectedly failed to ejaculate on the day of ovulation and hence, required electro-ejaculation.

6. Testicular sperm extraction: If other measures have failed and electroejaculation is not available, then sperm may be aspirated from the testis and used for ICSI. Epididymal aspiration should *not* be done as it can damage the epididymis and cause obstructive azoospermia.

Treatment of Anorgasmic Anejaculation

Men who have never reached orgasm can be difficult to help. Traditionally, psychosexual therapy aimed at resolving sexual guilt, trauma and misunderstandings, and at improving arousal and sexual stimulation, was used to help these men (Masters and Johnson, 1980). However, progress with such therapy is slow and the outcome is uncertain. When fertility is the main concern, couples do not have the patience to undergo prolonged psychotherapy, and demand more effective and rapid solutions. Hence, the majority of these men are treated with vibratory stimulation or electroejaculation.

Vibrator stimulation induces ejaculation in 60% to 70% of these men. Once ejaculation is achieved, the man continues self-stimulation at home, using a powerful body massager. Subsequent attempts are usually much easier and quicker, and some men learn to ejaculate naturally. Some continue to need vibratory stimulation to approach orgasm, but manage to insert the penis into the vagina as they are approaching ejaculatory inevitability, thus

Table 11.4. Prevention and Management of Situational Anejaculation

Situational Anejaculation	Prevention / Management
Unexpected ejaculatory failure	1. Routine cryopreservation for all patients 2. Collect semen prior to egg collection 3. Intercourse using sildenafil and non-spermicidal condom 4. Vibrator stimulation 5. Electroejaculation 6. Testicular sperm aspiration (ICSI required)
Periovulatory anejaculation	1. Prior cryopreservation 2. Train patient to use vibrator
Clinic anejaculation	1. Home collection 2. Vibrator stimulation in clinic
Masturbatory anejaculation	1. Collection by coitus interruptus (may need medication to support erection if there is also erectile dysfunction) 2. Collection by intercourse using non-spermicidal condom 3. Vibrator stimulation
Intercourse anejaculation	1. Psychosexual therapy to restore natural ejaculation 2. IUI using masturbatory sample

achieving intravaginal ejaculation. Those who are unable to ejaculate intravaginally can achieve pregnancy by insemination of a vibrator-induced ejaculate. Those who fail multiple attempts with the vibrator are treated with electroejaculation. Though electroejaculation is usually successful, it often results in a subnormal ejaculate which necessitates IVF or ICSI (Hovav et al., 1996; Kiekens et al., 1996).

Management of Organic Anejaculation

This will vary with the cause of the problem (Shahban et al., 1997).

Neurogenic failure of emission: If the spinal cord lesion is above thoracic 10 segment, vibratory stimulation is likely to produce ejaculation (Nehra et al., 1996). If the spinal cord is affected at a lower level, or if the lumbar sympathetic ganglia or peripheral sympathetic fibres are affected, then electroejaculation or sperm aspiration is required (Dahlberg et al., 1995). Occasionally, sympathomimetic drugs may restore emission in men whose problem is due to peripheral autonomic neuropathy (Dunsmuir and Holmes, 1996).

Anatomic obstruction causing failure of emission: Unlike men with ejaculatory duct obstruction, who have some ejaculate from the prostatic ducts, men who have complete obstructive failure of emission have extensive fibrosis, which is not amenable to surgical resection. The only therapy possible is ICSI, using sperm aspirated from the epididymis. Occasionally, the fluid aspirated from the vas shows good numbers of actively motile sperm; since these are mature (having traversed the entire epididymis), simple intrauterine insemination may result in pregnancy in such cases.

Retrograde ejaculation: Sympathomimetic drugs (ephedrine 25 mg, four times a day) with anticholinergics (imipramine 50 mg, at night) may restore antegrade ejaculation in some men with sympathetic neuropathy. However, if the bladder neck anatomy is compromised, medical therapy will not work. In such cases, surgical treatment by bladder neck reconstruction can be attempted, but it is a major and complex procedure, and hence, is not preferred unless there is concomitant incontinence. Therefore, if medical therapy fails, the preferred option is to recover sperm from the bladder and use these for insemination.

To facilitate sperm survival in the bladder, the urine must be rendered alkaline and dilute. An alkalinizing substance (sodium bicarbonate or potassium citrate) is administered 6-hourly from the day prior to collection. On the morning of collection, the patient takes the alkalinizer and several glasses of water. He then passes urine every 20 minutes and the pH of the urine is checked. When the pH reaches 7.5 or higher, the patient masturbates to orgasm and then immediately voids urine into a beaker. The sperm-containing urine is centrifuged and the resultant sperm pellet is processed further for IUI.

If this method yields sperm with poor motility, then sperm recovery from medium is tried. The patient takes an alkalinizer, but otherwise remains fasting (to reduce urine output, which would contaminate the medium). He empties his bladder. A small catheter is introduced atraumatically, using mineral oil for lubrication (anaesthetic jelly should not be used as it is spermicidal). Any residual urine is aspirated and 30 mL of sperm-processing medium is introduced into the bladder. The catheter is removed. The patient then masturbates to orgasm and immediately voids the medium into a beaker. Sperm are recovered by centrifugation and processed for IUI. Sperm recovery from medium is often far superior to recovery from urine.

Anterior urethral obstruction: When possible, it is preferable to remove the cause of obstruction. However, often an anterior urethral diverticulum or pouch does not interfere with urination and major surgery does not seem justified. In such cases, milking the urethra after orgasm may result in procurement of an adequate ejaculate. Sometimes, lavaging the urethra with medium can help.

Technique of vibratory stimulation

The vibrator triggers the ejaculatory reflex by providing a strong, prolonged stimulus to the undersurface of the glans. Specially-made, dedicated devices are available. Alternatively, some of the commercially available body massagers, which have strong vibrations, may also be used. The stronger the vibrations, the more likely is the vibrator to succeed (Sonksen, 1994).

Pre-procedure preparatory counselling is very important. The physiology of ejaculation and the procedure are explained. It is emphasized that ejaculation is not under the patient's control: it is a reflex that will take place automatically because of stimulation by the vibrator; all he has to do is apply the vibrator and relax. The patient is shown the vibrator and allowed to handle it and feel the vibratory stimulation so that he is reassured that it is not painful or harmful.

The procedure is carried out in a room with complete privacy. The patient empties his bladder, takes off his clothes and then sits on a bed with his legs apart. He places the vibrator between his legs, with the vibrating surface facing upwards, and allows the penis to rest upon it. After switching on the vibrator, he gently presses the glans on to the vibrating head, such that he feels the maximum sensation without being uncomfortable. Once the vibrator is in place, he is told to divert his attention from the vibrator and fantasize sexually. If he has difficulty fantasizing, visual erotic material is provided—in some men, this is a vital contributor to success. The stimulation is applied for 15 to 20 minutes, followed by a 5-minute break during which he continues to fantasize. Stimulation is continued till ejaculation occurs. If the patient is very tense, an anxiolytic may help.

Some men require as much as two hours of stimulation before they ejaculate the first time. Others succeed only at the second or even third or fourth session. Hence, a confident and experienced physician and perseverance on the part of the patient are vital for success.

Technique of electroejaculation

Electroejaculation induces emission and ejaculation by direct electrical stimulation of the efferent nerves innervating the seminal vesicles and the terminal vas. The procedure is carried out using the Seager electroejaculator, which delivers a sine wave current of up to 1 ampere, at 0 to 50 volts, through 3 electrodes mounted on a rectal probe (Seager and Halstead, 1993).

In neurologically intact men, the procedure is performed under general anaesthesia. After emptying the bladder, the patient is placed in the left lateral or lithotomy position and the rectum is inspected by proctoscopy for any pathology. Then, using adequate lubrication, the probe is introduced transrectally and positioned such that the electrodes face anteriorly and are in close contact with the anterior rectal wall, so that the area above and lateral to the prostate is stimulated. Stimulation is applied by turning the voltage knob up to 5 volts and then back down towards 0. For the second stimulus, the voltage knob is turned up to 6 volts and then down again. The voltage is progressively increased till ejaculation occurs; stimulation is continued at this voltage for as long as ejaculation continues. Then the voltage is further increased till ejaculation occurs again. This is continued till 2 to 3 episodes of ejaculation occur, or 20 to 30 stimulations are completed. If the antegrade ejaculate is scanty, the bladder is catheterized and urine is aspirated and examined for sperm. If the predominant ejaculate is retrograde, for the subsequent attempts, the bladder should be prepared by instilling sperm-washing medium in the bladder; this will minimize contact between the sperm and urine, and thus improve the quality of sperm retrieved from the bladder after electroejaculation. The sperm obtained are used for IUI, IVF or ICSI, depending on the sperm quality.

AZOOSPERMIA

Prior to the advent of ICSI, the evaluation of azoospermia merely entailed identifying obstructive azoospermia that could be surgically treated—all other azoospermic men were advised donor insemination or adoption. Since ICSI offers new therapeutic possibilities for men with obstructive or non-obstructive azoospermia, a new management algorithm has evolved. Further, since cryopreserved epididymal and testicular sperm can be successfully used for ICSI (Fischer et al., 1998), evaluation and treatment have become integrated.

EVALUATION

Azoospermia can have a variety of causes. A functional classification that assists in the clinical management is presented below.

Table 11.5. Clinical classification of Azoospermia

- Hypogonadotropic hypogonadism
  - Idiopathic
  - Intra-cranial tumour
  - Part of syndrome
- Primary testicular failure
  - Congenital
  - Acquired
  - With focal spermatogenesis
  - Without focal spermatogenesis
  - Eugonadotropic (normal FSH)
  - Hypergonadotropic (high FSH)
- Post-testicular obstruction
  - Site of block
  - Possibility of reconstruction
  - Genetic factors

During evaluation the following points should be borne in mind.

In hypogonadotropic hypogonadism:

- Investigate for other hormonal deficiencies
- CT/MRI for intra-cranial SOL

In Primary testicular Failure

- Look for chromosomal abnormalities
  - Numerical—Klinefelter's syndrome
  - Structural—Y chromosome microdeletions
- Look for focal spermatogenesis
  - 20% to 50% of men with testicular failure will have focal areas of sperm production
  - these sperm can be located if multiple testicular biopsies are done
  - hence, even when performing a diagnostic biopsy it is advisable to do a four-quadrant biopsy—this will have greater predictive value
- Reversible causes
  - It may take up to 3 years after chemotherapy or radiotherapy for spermatogenesis to return
  - Occasionally, correction of a large varicocele may result in appearance of sperm in the ejaculate

In post-testicular obstruction:

- Feasibility of reconstructive surgery will depend upon
  - Etiology of block
  - Site of block
  - Nature of block
- Reconstructive surgery v/s ICSI
  Factors to be considered are:
  - Feasibility of surgery
  - Success of surgery
  - Age of couple
  - Cost
  - Couple's preference
- Genetic causes
  - Screening for genetic causes is required to predict the risk to the child born of ICSI

Since a variety of diagnostic tests are available, it is important that the clinician understand the utility and limitations of each test, so that a diagnosis may be reached without unnecessary investigations. Further, the tests required may partly be decided by the therapy being planned. Thus, the evaluation of the azoospermic male must integrate investigation and therapy. Sometimes, a simple biochemical test or hormone assay is all that is required; in other cases, multiple imaging modalities and invasive tests might be needed. The algorithms in Figs. 11.2 A, B and C provide a practical approach to the evaluation of the azoospermic male.

Management

In this section, we will highlight the principles of therapy and important practical points in the management of azoospermia—for specific details the reader may refer to standard texts and to the references cited.

Congenital Bilateral Absence of the Vasa Deferentia

(i) the diagnosis is established clinically (absent fructose, non-palpable vasa);

(ii) exploration is not required to prove absence of vasa;

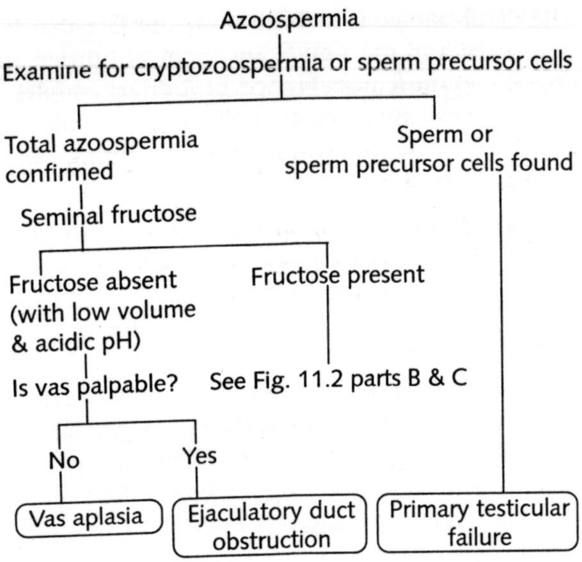

Fig. 11.2A. Flow chart for evaluation of Azoospermia

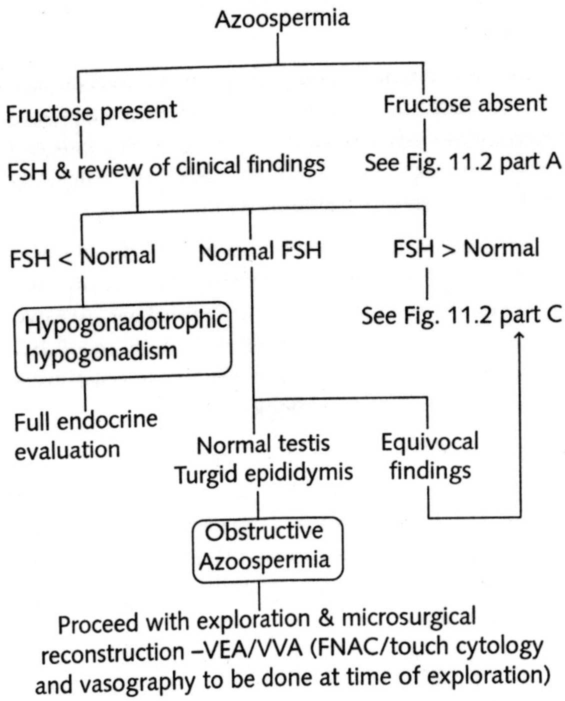

Fig. 11.2B. Flow chart for evaluation of Azoospermia

(iii) testicular biopsy is not routinely indicated since spermatogenesis is normal in these men, unless there is a second pathology which has affected the testes;

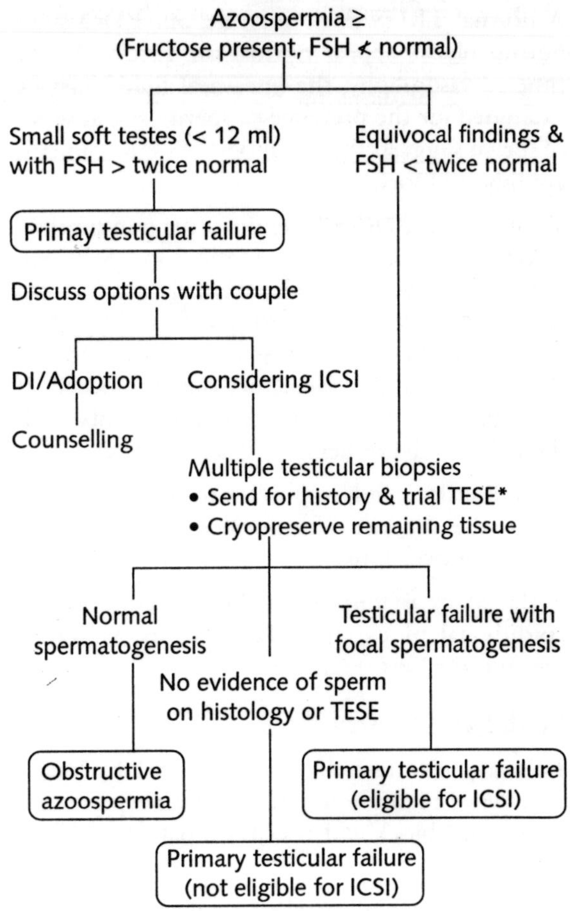

* TESE: Testicular Sperm Extraction

Fig. 11.2C. Flow chart for evaluation of azoospermia

(iv) the only treatment options are epididymal sperm aspiration and ICSI (Tournaye et al., 1994), or donor insemination; spermatoceles have been given up;

(v) if the couple opts for ICSI, they will need to be screened for genetic mutations related to cystic fibrosis (Oates & Amos, 1994).

Ejaculatory Duct Obstruction (EDO)

A transrectal ultrasonography (TRUS) (Jarrow, 1996) and vasography are required to confirm the diagnosis and assess whether the patient has a cystic block that can be opened by transurethral resection.

A normal TRUS does not rule out EDO since fibrous blocks appear normal on TRUS. At the time of vasography, the intravasal fluid must be examined for the presence of sperm; the absence of sperm suggests the likelihood of a concomitant epididymal block.

Treatment of EDO is by endoscopic transurethral resection (TUR) of the prostatic floor (Schlegel, 1997). This deroofs the dilated ejaculatory duct and allows it to drain into the prostatic fossa. However, this is possible only in those cases where just the terminal part of the ejaculatory duct is blocked. If the entire intraprostatic ejaculatory duct is fibrosed, then TUR will not help.

If TUR is done, it is important to simultaneously ensure that the wife is fertile since the obstruction may recur over time.

If the block is fibrous, or there is a secondary epididymal block, then ICSI, using aspirated sperm is the best treatment.

Epididymal Obstruction

This has traditionally been treated by vaso-epididymal anastomosis (VEA), which bypasses the epididymal block and restores a patent pathway for the sperm.

The older macrosurgical procedures have been replaced by microsurgical procedures that allow a direct anastomosis between the epididymal ductule and the vas mucosa. These very delicate and precise surgeries achieve a patency rate of 50% to 60%, and a pregnancy rate of 20% to 30% (Fogdestam et al., 1986).

An alternative to surgery is ICSI, using sperm aspirated from the epididymis or testis (Nagy et al., 1995).

The advantage of VEA over ICSI is that it is less expensive (in India) and enables successful couples to achieve a natural pregnancy. The disadvantage is the need for a specially-trained andrological microsurgeon and the long time taken for sperm to appear after surgery (up to one year).

The advantages of ICSI are a quick result and a high pregnancy rate if multiple attempts are made. The disadvantage is its high cost, the fact that it is artificial and the significant medical burden it imposes on the female. Hence, in younger couples, VEA seems a more reasonable choice, while in couples over 35, for whom time is running out, ICSI is preferable.

If hydrocele surgery has been done previously, the results of microsurgery are very poor and ICSI should be preferred in such cases.

Vasal Obstruction

The commonest cause of vas occlusion is vasectomy. However, the vas can also be damaged iatrogenically during hernia repair or extensive pelvic surgery—in these cases, the extent of damage is variable and may be extensive enough to preclude repair.

Vas occlusion may also occur due to infection; multiple blocks are common and repair is usually not feasible.

If the vasal block is localized, it can be excised and patency restored by vaso-vasal anastomosis (VVA) (Fox, 1994). Microsurgical VVA can have a patency rate of as high as 97% if the duration since vas occlusion is short (Belker, 1991).

Long-standing obstruction leads to back-pressure on the epididymis; this eventually leads to rupture of the epididymal ductule and secondary epididymal obstruction. The longer the duration of obstruction, the more likely it is that there will be a secondary epididymal block.

Hence, it is important to check for sperm in the intravasal fluid that comes out of the testicular end at the time of VVA. If no sperm are found, this fact must be noted, and if the patient remains azoospermic six months after surgery, VEA will be required.

Primary Testicular Failure

Previously, the only options for a man with primary testicular failure were donor insemination or adoption. Now, through ICSI with testicular sperm, many of these men can father a child.

About 50% of men with azoospermia due to

testicular failure will have a few sperm in their testes. These sperm are too few in number to traverse the epididymis and appear in the semen, but can be extracted from the testes and used for ICSI (Friedler et al., 1997).

Even if a single biopsy does not show any sperm, in 20%–50% of such cases, a few sperm may be found if multiple biopsies are taken (since spermatogenesis may be focal) (Tournaye et al., 1997).

Sperm may be found even in men with elevated FSH and small testes.

Multiple testicular biopsies can cause testicular damage and hence, microsurgical techniques must be used to minimize the risk of damage (Schlegel and Su, 1997).

In about 10%–15% of these men, there are numerical chromosomal defects (Skakkebaek et al., 1973), and in another 15%, there are microdeletions on the Y-chromosome (Brandell et al., 1998). If sperm from these men is used for ICSI, there is a risk that the male offspring will be infertile due to an inheritance of the genetic defect—this risk needs to be screened for and explained to the couple (Johnson, 1998).

The use of spermatids or other sperm precursors is still experimental.

Hypogonadotrophic Hypogonadism

If the FSH is lower than normal, the patient should undergo a full endocrine evaluation. If hypogonadotrophic hypogonadism is confirmed, radiological evaluation of the cranium is required to look for a intracranial tumour.

Therapy with gonadotrophins or pulsatile gonadotrophin-releasing hormones is quite successful in initiating spermatogenesis and producing pregnancy (Kliesch et al., 1994).

The main limiting factor is the cost: gonadotrophins are required for one to two years, which means an expense of up to Rs. 200,000. If the patient is unable to afford the full therapy, he should not be made to waste his money on incomplete treatment which will result in no benefit.

CONCLUSION

With the advent of ICSI, the management of severe oligozoospermia and asthenozoospermia has become straightforward. However, aspermia and azoospermia present clinical complexities that require careful diagnosis and choice of therapy. ICSI is just one of many options for these men. Sometimes, a simple measure like vibratory stimulation may produce a dramatic cure, while in others, a drastic solution like multiple testicular biopsies and ICSI may be required. The various options—including their cost, risks and success rates—must be discussed with the couple and the therapy chosen must be individualized to the couple's ages, their personal preferences and financial condition.

REFERENCES

Belker, A. M. et al. (1991). 'Results of 1469 microsurgical vasectomy reversals by the vasovasostomy study group', *J Urol.*, **145**: 505–11.

Brandell, R.A., et al. (1998). 'AZFb deletions predict the absence of spermatozoa with testicular sperm extraction: Preliminary report of a prognostic genetic test', *Hum. Reprod.*, **13**: 2812–5.

Dahlberg, A., et al. (1995). 'Pregnancy results from a vibrator application, electro-ejaculation and vas aspiration programme in spinal cord injured men', *Hum. Reprod.*, **10**: 2305–7.

Dunsmuir, W.D. and S.A. Holmes, (1996). 'The aetiology and management of erectile, ejaculatory, and fertility problems in men with diabetes mellitus', *Diabet. Med.*, **13**: 700–08.

Fischer, R. et al. (1998). 'Use of cryopreserved testicular sperm', in M. Filicori and C. Flamigni (eds.), *Treatment of Infertility: the New Frontiers*, Communications Media for Education, New Jersey, pp. 408–9.

Friedler, S. et al. (1997). 'Intracytoplasmic injection of fresh and cryopreserved testicular spermatozoa in patients with non-obstructive azoospermia—a comparative study', *Fertil. Steril.*, **68**: 892–7.

Fogdestam, I. et al. (1986). 'Microsurgical epididymovasostomy in the treatment of occlusive azoospermia', *Fertil. Steril.*, **46**: 925–9.

Fox, M. (1994). 'Vasectomy reversal—microsurgery for best results', *Br. J. Urol.*, **73**: 449–53.

Hovav, Y., et al. (1996) 'Electroejaculation and assisted fertility in men with psychogenic anejaculation', *Fertil. Steril.*, **66**: 620–23.

Jarrow, J. P. (1996). 'Transrectal ultrasonography in the diagnosis and management of ejaculatory duct obstruction', *J. Androl.*, **17**: 462–74.

Johnson, M.D. (1998). 'Genetic risks of intracytoplasmic sperm injection in the treatment of male infertility: Recommendations for genetic counselling and screening', *Fertil. Steril.*, **70**: 397–411.

Kiekens, C. et al. (1996). 'Pregnancy after electroejaculation in combination with intracytoplasmic sperm injection in a patient with idiopathic anejaculation', *Fertil. Steril.*, **66**: 834–6.

Kliesch, S. et al. (1994). 'High efficacy of gonadotropins or pulsatile gonadotropin-releasing hormone treatment in hypogonadotropic hypogonadal men', *European J. Endocrinol.*, **13**: 347–54.

Masters, W.H. and V.E. Johnson (1980). *Human Sexual Inadequacy,* Bantam Books, New York, pp. 109–29.

Nagy, Z. et al. (1995). 'Using ejaculated, fresh, and frozen-thawed epididymal and testicular spermatozoa gives rise to comparable results after intracytoplasmic sperm injection', *Fertil. Steril.*, **63**: 808–15.

Nehra, A. et al. (1996). 'Vibratory stimulation and rectal probe electroejaculation as therapy for patients with spinal cord injury: Semen parameters and pregnancy rates', *J. Urol.*, **155**: 554–9.

Oates, R.D. and J.A. Amos (1994). 'The genetic basis of congenital bilateral absence of the vas deferens and cystic fibrosis', *J. Androl.*, **15**: 1–8.

Schlegel, P. (1997). 'Management of ejaculatory duct obstruction', in L.I. Lipshulz and S.S. Howards (eds.), *Infertility in the Male*, 3rd ed., Mosby, St. Louis, pp. 385–94.

Schlegel, P.N. and L-M. Su (1997). 'Physiological consequences of testicular sperm extraction', *Hum. Reprod.*, **12**: 1688–92.

Seager, S.W., L.S. Halstead (1993). 'Fertility options and success after spinal cord injury', *Urol. Clin. N. Am.*, **20**: 543–8.

Shah, R.S. (1998). 'Male sexual dysfunction', in S. Dasgupta (ed.), *Recent Advances in Obstetrics and Gynecology*-4, Jaypee Bros, New Delhi, pp. 152–67.

———, (1999) 'Management of anejaculation', in N. Pandiyan (ed.), *Handbook of Andrology*, T.R. Publications, Chennai, pp. 129–139.

Shahban, S.F. et al. (1997). 'Treatment of abnormalities of ejaculation', in L.I. Lipshultz and S.S. Howards (eds.), *Infertility in the Male* , 3rd ed., Mosby, St. Louis, pp. 423–38.

Skakkebaek, N.E. et al. (1973). 'Studies on meiotic chromosomes in infertile men and controls with normal karyotypes', *J. Reprod. Fertil.*, **35**: 23–36.

Sonksen, J., et al. (1994). 'Ejaculation induced by penile vibratory stimulation in men with spinal cord injuries: The importance of the vibratory amplitude', *Paraplegia*, **32**: 651–60.

Tournaye, H. and P. Devroey et al. (1994). 'Microsurgical epididymal sperm aspiration and intracytoplasmic sperm injection: A new effective approach to infertility as a result of congenital bilateral absence of the vas deferens', *Fertil. Steril.*, **61**: 1045–51.

Tournaye, H. and G. Verheyen et al. (1997). 'Are there any predictive factors for testicular sperm recovery in azoospermic patients?' *Hum. Reprod.*, **12**: 80–86.

12

Intracytoplasmic Sperm Injection Assisted Fertilization: Today

Indira Hinduja, Kusum Zaveri and Meheranghiz Minbattiwalla

INTRODUCTION

The advent of assisted reproductive technology (ART) has, to a great extent, deleted the concept of sterility altogether as the application of such technologies corrects most of the causative factors responsible for infertility. The utilization of the ART available bestows the pleasure of gestational, genetic or both parenthood upon the infertile couple.

In vitro fertilization and embryo transfer (IVF-ET) acts as a pivot for ART, as all the other techniques revolve around it. IVF-ET was originally advocated for treating female infertility associated with irreparable tubal damage (Steptoe and Edwards, 1978), and subsequently, to treat male infertility (Lopata et al., 1980; Mahadevan et al., 1983; Ackerman et al., 1984; Lutjen et al., 1984; Hewett et al., 1985). Yovich et al. (1984) have shown that male factor infertility can also be treated with IVF-ET, but the success of this technique remained low (de Kretser et al., 1985; Kruger et al., 1988; Oehninger et al., 1988; Yates et al., 1989). With IVF-ET, fertilization was low, the rate being directly proportional to abnormal semen parameters, resulting in a poor pregnancy rate.

Since a medical or surgical line of treatment did not improve semen quality, efforts were focused on increasing fertilization rates with the existing sperm parameters. As the zona pellucida (ZP) proved to be the major barrier for sperm interaction, attempts were made to overcome this by either weakening or perforating the zona. A revolutionary technique of micromanipulation of human gametes came into vogue in 1988, completely bypassing the ZP and cell membrane (Ng et al., 1988; Palermo et al., 1992).

Direct injection of spermatozoa into the cytoplasm of the oocytes of various animal species has resulted in the birth of live young ones (Markert, 1983). However, this technique did not have much success in humans (Lazendorf et al., 1988). The zonal procedures, such as zona drilling (Gordon et al., 1988), zona cracking (Odawara and Lopata, 1989) and zona dissection (Cohen et al., 1988), followed by macroinsemination methods of assisted fertilization resulted in occasional pregnancies. In 1988, Ng and his associates were the first to report the birth of a baby by injecting spermatozoa into the subzonal space (SUZI); formerly called microinsemination of sperm transfer (MIST). These authors, however, expressed caution as direct ooplasmic sperm injection was an invasive technique with a high incidence of oocyte degeneration (Ng et al., 1991).

Even after four years of experience with zona manipulations, fertilization rates remained low (Cohen et al., 1992). In 1992, Palermo et al. announced the first live human birth by intracytoplasmic sperm injection (ICSI), followed by a series of publications with significantly higher success in fertilization, implantation and live births (Palermo et al., 1993; Van Steirteghem, 1993a). When compared for severe male factor infertility and success rates, ICSI performed better than SUZI (Palermo et al., 1993; Abdalla et al., 1995). Over a period of time, further improvements in the finer aspects of ICSI have facilitated attempts to achieve fertilization and pregnancies with spermatozoa or precursor cells recovered from the ejaculate, epididymes and testes, irrespective of normal or deficient spermatogenesis and regardless of the underlying pathophysiology.

The technique of ICSI has almost replaced the other treatment modalities, such as IVF with modification of insemination (Hall et al., 1995), or improving sperm quality by adding stimulants like pentoxifylline (Wittemer et al., 1996). It, however, still does not solve the underlying andrological problems. Its application and clinical success have progressed far beyond the basic knowledge of the physiological and biochemical events of fertilization. This chapter focuses on the indications in which ICSI could be used to alleviate infertility, and the methodological details and factors that influence the clinical results.

INDICATIONS

The prevalence of ICSI in the treatment of severe male factor infertility is beyond doubt. However, over the years, it has played a predominant role in alleviating other forms of infertility. The indications of ICSI are classified under the following five major categories.

1. Normal Sperm Parameters

1.1 Failed Fertilization in Previous IVF Cycle

Failed fertilization in conventional IVF with normal semen parameters could be related to the inability of the spermatozoa to penetrate the ZP, the primary causes of which may relate to gamete abnormalities, failure of oocyte activation and decondensation of the sperm head nucleus. Currently, ICSI is the most effective form to overcome failure of sperm penetration and subsequent gamete fusion. Rescue ICSI in cases of unfertilized one-day-old oocytes has attained 44% success in the fertilization rate and 14.8% in the pregnancy rate. However, the rate of mosaicism tends to be high in such cases (Morton et al., 1997).

1.2 Lower Number of Oocytes

The pregnancy rate after embryo transfer depends upon the number and quality of the embryos replaced. Patients in a natural cycle, poor responders and oocyte recipients from egg-sharing programmes generally have a low number of oocytes, and consequently, have fewer chances of a successful pregnancy. In such cases, ICSI is the treatment of choice as traditional IVF yields poor results.

1.3 Oocyte Defects

Failure of fertilization is caused by sperm defects and defective sperm-ZP binding (Oehninger et al., 1989; Liu and Baker, 1994). ZP on its own can also impose a major block to fertilization. Liu et al. (1995) have suggested ICSI as an effective treatment for patients with disorders of ZP-induced acrosome reaction, leading to fertilization failure by standard IVF-ET. In a conventional IVF programme, the ZP of fertilized oocytes is significantly thinner than that of unfertilized ones (Bertrand et al., 1995). Oocytes with a thick zona have poor fertilization rates by IVF, but can be fertilized with ICSI, and assisted hatching can further improve the implantation rates.

1.4 Cryopreserved Semen

Cryopreservation has been used to preserve gametes and embryos, and this technique has been particularly useful in patients suffering from cancer. However, on cryopreserving spermatozoa, their survival upon thawing and subsequent fertilizing potential are compromised. Semen samples with normal parameters show decreased motility and viability on thawing after cryopreservation. With ICSI, such impaired spermatozoa can successfully fertilize oocytes (Romero et al., 1996).

2. Abnormal Sperm Parameters

2.1 Oligo Astheno Teratozoospermia

The normal sperm parameters and deviation from these criteria have been reported by the World Health Organization (WHO, 1992), but Tygerberg strict criteria are considered more effective in the assessment of sperm morphology (Kruger et al., 1986, 1988; Menkveld et al., 1990; Yang et al., 1995). Impaired spermatogenesis affects semen properties, including count, motility and morphology (Haidl and Schill, 1993; Grow et al., 1994; Nagy et al., 1995b). It is not rare to find either oligo-, astheno- or teratozoospermia. However, several investigators are of the opinion that a decreased sperm count is also associated with diminished progressive motility and poor morphology (WHO, 1992). ICSI is very useful in the management of male factor infertility caused by Oligo Astheno Teratozoospermia (OAT).

2.2 Azoospermia

Obstructive or nonobstructive azoospermia, except for bilateral obstruction following bilateral vasectomy, was not given any encouragement for treatment by infertility specialists in the past. The causes of obstructive azoospermia could be congenital, surgical or inflammatory. Restoration of fertility in vasectomized patients has been favourable, but extreme damage due to inflammation, failure of recanalization and congenital bilateral absence of the vas deference (CBAVD) has not always been successful in alleviating male factor infertility.

The causes of nonobstructive azoospermia are defective spermatogenesis, including Sertoli cell only syndrome, maturation arrest, orichidectory tubular atrophy, Kleinfelter's syndrome and post-mumps orchitis. In these cases, the chances of recovering spermatozoa are difficult (Tournaye 1996a; Silber et al., 1995, 1996), and it is only through multiple testicular biopsies, performed at different sites in the testes, that occasional spermatozoa can be detected (Hauser et al., 1998).

Various minimally invasive procedures have evolved over a period of time to retrieve spermatozoa from azoospermic men. These include microepididymal sperm aspiration (MESA—Temple-Smith et al., 1985), percutaneous sperm aspiration (PESA—Shrivastav et al., 1994), testicular sperm aspiration (TESA—Craft et al., 1995), testicular sperm extraction (TESE—Silber et al., 1995) and testicular fine needle aspiration (TEFNA—Belker et al., 1996). The application of these techniques in IVF was not very encouraging since the number of spermatozoa recovered for insemination was insufficient. On the other hand, these techniques performed better with ICSI, as it required only one viable spermatozoon per oocyte, irrespective of its morphology. In the absence of mature spermatozoa, the injection of a spermatid or even a sperm nucleus can achieve fertilization and pregnancy (Vanderzwalmen et al., 1995; Tesarik et al., 1995, 1996; Fishel et al., 1995; Yamanaka et al., 1997).

2.3 Immotile Spermatozoa

The motility of spermatozoa plays a vital role in negotiating the ZP. Immotile spermatozoa lack this ability, but can still fertilize the oocyte when mechanically introduced into the ooplasm. Asthenozoospermia may result from either a defect in the protein components of axoneme, including radial spokes, nexin linkage and dynein arms (de Kretser and Kerr, 1994), or from a protein-carboxyl methylase enzyme defect (Tournaye et al., 1998).

The presence of infection due to *E. coli,* chronic prostatitis and male accessory gland infection are also responsible for decreased motility. Treatment with the appropriate antibiotics may improve this condition. Immobilizing antisperm antibodies rendering poor motility has shown a disappointing outcome to the conventional line of treatment. ICSI, on the other hand, has shown significant results in terms of pregnancy rates, irrespective of the causes of impaired motility. But before the commencement of this procedure, it is essential to differentiate immotile viable spermatozoa from necrozoospermia undergoing degeneration by using techniques like the hypo-osmotic test (HOS) and viability staining test. The former indicates both the physical and biochemical integrity of the sperm-plasma membrane, whereas the latter is useful in indicating the physical integrity of the sperm membrane. Casper et al. (1996) revealed that when spermatozoa were selected and ICSI performed after the HOS test, the fertilization rate increased to 41% and the pregnancy rate was 25%.

2.4 Cryptozoospermia

This sperm condition often presents as azoospermia and impaired motility, which is associated primarily with testicular dysfunction and occasionally with partial obstruction of the epididymis or the ejaculatory duct. Chronic infection of the prostate may also be a contributory factor. Spermatozoa recovered by careful centrifugation and sperm wash resulted in occasional pregnancy following ICSI (Ron-El et al., 1997).

2.5 Globozoospermia

Globozoospermia, due to acrosomal defects, is found in 0.1% of all andrological infertility. This condition is characterized by a spherical appearance of the sperm head, and an absence of the acrosome and postacrosomal sheath. They are associated with an abnormality of the mitochondria, midpiece, nuclear packaging and nuclear membrane. Because these spermatozoa are devoid of the acrosome, they lack the ability to penetrate the ZP and the oocyte membrane; but an intracytoplasmic round-headed sperm injection can overcome the inability to negotiate the ZP. There is enough evidence suggestive of a fertilization rate as low as 7% (Battaglia et al., 1997) by globozoospermia. This may be due to the absence of the molecular components that are necessary for oocyte activation (Tournaye et al., 1998).

2.6 Testicular Cancer and Following its Treatment

Testicular cancer is the most common malignancy in men between 20–40 years of age and during the past 50 years, its incidence has increased two- to four-fold. Since the young population, in particular, is at high risk, their reduced fertility due to testicular cancer and the associated side-effects of the treatment are of major concern. The exact aetiology of testicular cancer is not clearly known, but it affects fertility in men in different ways. Testicular cancer may cause obstructive azoospermia, especially in the case of bilateral epididymal tumours, whereas β-hCG-secreting tumours and an increase in scrotal temperature may affect spermatogenesis. Treatment with radiation or chemotherapy may also impair spermatogenesis. Fertility-related problems after surgical treatment include antisperm antibodies, anejaculation and retrograde ejaculation. Cryopreservation of spermatozoa, even of poor quality, should be a part of the treatment schedule.

Until the introduction of ICSI, men with testicular cancer had little or no hope of fathering a child. Since a limited number of spermatozoa of impaired motility are available after cryopreservation, it is important to use these sperm in an optimal way. ICSI has offered promising results in such couples. Nevertheless, no procedure should be performed for 6 months following treatment with chemotherapy, as a high risk of mutogenic effect is expected.

2.7 Genetic Defects in Males

Male infertility is also associated with chromosomal abnormalities. Chandley et al. (1975) have reported a correlation between cytogenetic disorders and semen parameters. Some of the oligospermic (2.1%–6.6%) and azoospermic (14%–16.6%) men exhibit cytogenetic abnormalities.

Bonaccorsi et al. (1997) have reported chromosomal anomalies in 10.6% of oligospermic men and 17.3% of azoospermic patients. The DAZ gene cluster is deleted in 13% of azoospermic men, some of whom harbour fully-formed spermatozoa within their testicular parenchyma; these can be retrieved for use in ICSI (Mulhall et al., 1997). Other abnormalities associated with infertility include 47, XYY Robertsonian translocations and 47, XXY Kleinfelter syndrome (De Brackeleer and Dao, 1991). However, the risk of chromosomal abnormalities being transmitted to a biological offspring remains and hence, counselling of the couple and prenatal cytogenetic analysis are mandatory.

3. Ejaculatory Dysfunction

ICSI has also proved very useful for men with idiopathic anejaculation or retrograde ejaculation. Men with idiopathic anejaculation probably have a psychogenic aetiology, and are unable to achieve orgasm and ejaculation during sexual activity. Men of advanced age, who have failed psychotherapy or sex therapy, can be considered for electroejaculation.

Retrograde ejaculation can be due to spinal cord injury, retroperitoneal lymph node dissection, diabetic neuropathy or multiple sclerosis. These men can initially be treated with sympathomimetic agents. If pharmacological treatment proves unsuccessful, sperm retrieval from the urinary bladder may be considered and the sperm can be processed for IVF or ICSI. The technique of ICSI, however, gives better results than IVF (Gerris et al., 1994).

4. Antisperm Antibodies

The presence of a high level of sperm autoantibodies to spermatozoa is associated with significantly reduced fertilization rates (Witkin et al., 1992; Lahteenmaki, 1993). It is generally believed that antibody-coated spermatozoa are much less likely to bind to the zona (Shibahara et al., 1993). For many years, efforts were made to establish an effective therapy for autoimmune infertility in males. The use of corticosteroids was abandoned after a few years of doubtful results due to its potentially dangerous side-effects (Hendry et al., 1979; Smart et al., 1988). Also, the technique of IVF did not give a satisfactory outcome (Witkin et al., 1992). ICSI was tried for patients in whom the presence of antibodies blocks fertilization (Clarke, 1997). The results of this study have confirmed that fertilization and ongoing pregnancy rates are not dependable on autoantibodies, since the spermatozoa from an antibody positive patient were directly injected into the oocyte cytoplasm. Fertilization, embryonic development and pregnancy rates after ICSI are affected neither by the presence of antisperm antibodies bound to the spermatozoa, nor by the type of immunoglobulin (Nagy et al., 1995c). The quality of embryos and the pregnancy rate improve significantly when ICSI is performed, compared to IVF.

5. Preimplantation Genetic Diagnosis

Preimplantation genetic diagnosis is an important breakthrough in the earliest detection of transmitting genetic disorders. With the use of polymerase chain reaction (PCR) and fluorescent *in situ* hybridization (FISH), the genotype of the embryo can be studied.

IVF leaves a number of spermatozoa attached to the ZP, as well as in the perivitelline space, with the result that blastomere biopsy material may get contaminated and give altered results. This can be overcome by ICSI (Nagy et al., 1995a).

TECHNICAL ASPECTS

Although ICSI was an accidental discovery without much fundamental scientific research, this technique has proved its utility beyond expectation in all forms of male factor infertility. The practice of ICSI has spread, with a good success rate. This part of the chapter describes the technical and methodological details involved in performing ICSI.

1. Skill & Experience Of The Operator

The success of any procedure depends upon the learning curve. The initial few weeks of meticulous training in the injection procedure are of utmost importance. A step-wise observation of the technique performed by experienced staff should be followed by hands-on training in handling manipulators, for immobilization, and aspiration and injection of the spermatozoon. The injection procedure carried out on 2 to 3-day-old oocytes, followed by one-day-old unfertilized oocytes from IVF programmes is the most crucial aspect of the training. The results of one-day-old oocyte injection should be evaluated for fertilization and the incidence of degeneration. After obtaining sufficient experience and gaining confidence, the trainee can be given 2–3 eggs from the ICSI programme for injection. The entire procedure should be carried out under a close-circuit TV and monitored by the senior staff. A critical evaluation of the technique and the results of the procedure performed by the trainee are very important preliminaries before allowing them to perform independently.

2. Microtools & Accessories

The smooth and gentle injection of a spermatozoon into the ooplasm is the key to the success of ICSI. Success also depends upon the use of good quality microtools under optimal magnification, with an appropriate optical system. The type of manipulator, whether hanging or vertical, manual or motorized, is a matter of preference. The glass for the microtools is of special importance, e.g. borosilicate or pyrex. The preparation of microtools is time-consuming and requires extensive experience.

The types of microneedles used are almost universal, with very little variation in the outer diameter of the holding pipette and the bevel, or the angle of the microinjection needles. The outer diameter of the holding pipette varies from 60–100 μm and that of the microinjection needle from 6–8 μm. If the microinjection needle is narrower than 6 μm, it may become difficult to move the spermatozoon in and out of the pipette, and if wider than 8 μm, it may disrupt the oocyte cytoplasm and cause degeneration. The injection needle must be beveled and sharp, with or without a spike. The bevel and the angle of the tip of the needle range from 20°–30° and 35°–50°, respectively.

A number of microscopes, mounted with different optical systems giving depth and differentiation, are available. The operator may decide whether to use the Hoffman modulation with plastic dishes, or the direct interference contrast, or the Normarski system with glass chambers. The essential requirement is the presence of the heating stage on the microscope to prevent fluctuation in temperature, which can cause irreversible damage to the oocyte.

3. Chemicals & Reagents

3.1 Polyvinylpyrrolidone

In order to facilitate the handling of motile and morphologically normal sperm, the use of polyvinylpyrrolidone (PVP) is an important factor in ICSI. The use of 10% PVP solution not only slows down the fast-moving spermatozoa, but also helps to control the flow of fluid in and out of the injection pipette, allowing a very little portion of the vehicle to enter along with the injected sperm into the oocyte. PVP also prevents the sticking of spermatozoa to the injection needle. Sometimes, barely motile spermatozoa may become completely immotile in PVP, making it difficult to distinguish live from dead spermatozoa.

PVP also stabilizes the sperm plasma membrane (Dozortsev et al., 1995b), which delays the calcium oscillation in the oocyte after the injection of the spermatozoa; prevents nuclear decondensation (Clarke and Johnson, 1988); and causes DNA lesion (Ray et al., 1995). Feichtinger et al. (1995) have suggested that chromosomal abnormalities in pregnancy following ICSI could be related to the injection of PVP into the oocyte. Strehler et al. (1998) have proposed that PVP has disintegrating effects on various sperm membranes, and eventually results in a necrotic effect similar to that of infection and inflammation in the seminal fluid. Therefore, it may be worthwhile to wash the spermatozoa in a culture medium after immobilization. However, studies show no detrimental effect on bovine zygotes and developing embryos (Motoishi et al., 1996; Saha et al., 1996).

Long-standing PVP solution gets precipitated, which may interfere with sperm-handling. It is, therefore, essential that freshly-prepared PVP solution is not stored at 4°C for more than a week (Dozortsev, et al., 1995c). Occasionally, precipitates may be mistaken for bacterial contamination. Some investigators have preferred the use of dialyzed and lyophilized PVP (Van Steirteghem et al., 1993b; Palermo et al., 1993), while some advocate the use of PVP of pharmaceutical grade (Lundin et al., 1995; Palermo et al., 1995).

3.2 Enzyme for Denudation of Corona Cumulus Complex

To assess the maturity of the oocyte, i.e. the presence of the germinal vesicle and the presence or absence of the polar body 1 (PB 1), the denudation of the corona cumulus complex is an essential step before ICSI. Hyaluronidase is used to decoronise the human oocyte before the injection of spermatozoa (Mahadeven and Trounson, 1985). However, its use raises the problems of premature activation and degeneration of oocytes. To overcome these problems, different concentrations (760 to 10 IU/mL) of hyaluronidase have been tried. When used at a concentration of 80 IU/mL, the fertilization rate increased and the activation rate decreased drastically (Palermo et al., 1993; Joris et al., 1996). To optimize the concentration of hyaluronidase, Van de Velde et al. (1997) have tried different concentrations of hyaluronidase (78 to 10 IU/mL), along with different sizes of denuding pipettes. These authors demonstrated that a concentration as low as 10 IU/mL, in combination with a pipette size of at least 1000 μm, can be used successfully to denude oocytes for microinjection. Since the source of the hyaluronidase used is either bovine or sheep testes, Trayen et al. (1995) indicated that it was impossible to avoid the risk of exposure to an unknown pathogen, despite the use of the most efficient methods of purification and sterilization of such a product. Therefore, a study was conducted to compare the efficacy of hyaluronidase in denuding oocytes prior to ICSI *vis-à-vis* a plant enzyme preparation containing citric acid, papaine, sodium chloride and phosphate (Coronase; Bio-media, Boussens, France). It was found that the time required for total denudation using coronase was slightly more, but the fertilization rate and the development of embryos were identical and the procedure had no adverse effects on the oocytes. However, careful washing of the oocytes is required after denudation with coronase (Parinaud et al., 1998). The absence of any human or animal compound in coronase avoids contamination by any animal pathogen. In order to have a meaningful comparison, larger studies are required.

3.3 Media

Several media have been evaluated for ICSI, though without significant differences in fertilization and pregnancy rates. The use of simple salt solution compared to that of the highly composite media, both with HEPES buffer, has shown no significant difference in the outcome of ICSI. There is a remote possibility of injecting the HEPES buffer into the oocyte, but there is no evidence of the HEPES buffer having a detrimental effect.

3.4 Oil

Mineral oil or light paraffin oil is used to maintain the pH, osmotic pressure and cleanliness of the culture. It has a tendency to extract lipids from the media and is also a potential toxic substance. It should, therefore, be washed twice and equilibrated before use. However, the use of mineral oil or light paraffin oil should be considered along with the compatibility to the media being used as recommended by the manufacturers.

3.5 Percoll Gradient Centrifugation

Percoll is a colloidal suspension of silica particles coated with PVP. The use of Percoll has been recommended in IVF (Gorus and Pipeleers, 1981) for efficient isolation of motile spermatozoa. It is also considered in order to reduce the generation of reactive oxygen species (ROS) from contaminating cells or abnormal spermatozoa (Aitken and Clarkson, 1988). Subsequent observations have revealed that the Percoll gradient centrifugation is not a prerequisite for a satisfactory ICSI outcome, and many researchers have disregarded the use of Percoll, as the centrifugation process involved damages the sperm cells and decreases the percentage of motile cells (Alvarez et al., 1993). This contention has led to the withdrawal of Percoll for use in IVF programmes. In fact, simple washing of sperm samples is quite adequate for a satisfactory performance of ICSI (de Vos et al., 1997).

4. Procedural Aspects

The activation of the oocyte, by modulation of its internal Ca^{2+} levels, is a major event during fertilization. The spermatozoon carries with it the factors responsible for the modulation of Ca^{2+} in the oocyte during fertilization. Since the activation factor appears to be in the cytosilic fraction of the spermatozoon (Dozortsev et al., 1995d), a calcium response similar to that observed during normal fertilization can also be obtained after ICSI (Tesarik et al., 1994). Therefore, the correct technique of sperm deposition into the ooplasm is an important aspect of ICSI.

4.1 Immobilization of Spermatozoa

A motile spermatozoon injected into the oocyte may get expelled into the perivitelline space. Alternatively, if it remains in the ooplasm, it may damage the cell organelles and cytoskeleton, resulting in the degeneration of the oocyte (Payne et al., 1994; Svalander et al., 1995). Most unfertilized oocytes after ICSI show an intact sperm head in the cytoplasm, along with a single pronucleus, suggesting that the sperm membrane in its capacity may have prevented decondensation of the sperm nucleus, which is aided by the decondensing factors from the oocyte (Dozortsev et al., 1994). Therefore, to ensure sperm decondensation, partial sperm membrane damage prior to the injection is required, which can be achieved by touching the tail with the pipette for immobilizing the spermatozoa (Dozortsev et al., 1995e). Breaking of the sperm membrane evokes physiological and biochemical reactions, releasing oscillin into the cytoplasm of the oocyte, and in turn, the cytoplasmic enzyme in the ooplasm acts on the sperm nucleus decondensation (Tesarik and Kopeeny, 1989; Montag et al., 1992). Chen et al. (1996) cut the spermatozoon tail at 3 different sites: the tip, the midpiece and halfway along the tail. They have suggested that cutting of the tip is easy and it avoids damage to the midpiece, which contains the centriole that plays a major role in cleavage of the embryo.

4.2 Polar Body Position

The positioning of the polar body (PB) is of immense importance for the injection of the spermatozoon. At this stage of oocyte maturity, the microtubule region of the oocyte is situated at the right side of the PB 1 (Dozortsev et al., 1995c). Therefore, the oocyte should be held with the PB kept at either the 12 or 6 o'clock position, so that the needle pierces the oocyte at the 3 o' clock position (Asada et al., 1995). In this manner, the sperm cell will be released in the region away from the point of the spindle occurrence, not disturbing the microspindles (Dozortsev et al., 1995a). However, it is doubtful that the position of the first PB is a reliable reference point for the spindle (Palermo et al., 1995).

4.3 Rupture of Oolemma

There are evidences regarding the best ways to penetrate the vitelline membrane (VM). Svalander et al. (1995) suggest that the needle should breach the oolemma in the same way as it breaches the ZP. Dozortsev et al. (1995d) have proposed penetration of the VM after breaking it by suction aspiration, which has the least risk of damaging the oocyte. Palermo et al. (1996) have described three distinct patterns of membrane breakage: sudden, normal and difficult. They observed a higher incidence of degeneration with sudden breakage than with the other two.

Aspiration of the cytoplasm itself provides a mechanical stimulus to induce the release of intracytoplasmic calcium stores (Tesarik et al., 1994). Gearon et al. (1995) and Tesarik and Sousa (1995) have reported that the mechanical disruption of the ooplasm alone and the degree of cytoplasmic aspiration may increase the activation and fertilization rates. Vanderzwalmen et al. (1996) have reported that when a vigorous aspiration of cytoplasm is performed, the fertilization rate increases from 69% to 83%.

Cytoplasmic aspiration is a delicate part of the ICSI procedure, and a crucial factor appears to be the amount of fluid aspirated and reinjected into the oocyte. It increases the fertilization rate markedly (up to 68%) when an immobilized spermatozoon is injected into the ooplasm after the rupture of the oolemma and the aspiration of the cytoplasm (Vanderzwalmen et al., 1996).

FACTORS INFLUENCING THE RESULTS OF ICSI

The technique of ICSI has overcome a number of events that prohibit fertilization, but as a technique, it still has some limitations regarding successful embryo development and pregnancy. Defect in sperm function is one of the major causes of the failure of fertilization after ICSI (Dozortsev et al., 1995b). The ratio between the seminal plasma and serum carcinoma antigen-125 level may be used as an indirect marker for sperm fertilization potential in IVF and ICSI techniques (Geva et al., 1997). The defects in the spermatozoa could be attributed to oxidative stress arising from ROS (Aitken, 1994). Contaminating leucocytes or spermatozoa themselves might contribute to ROS (Baker et al., 1996). ROS has been linked with chromatin cross-linking (Nackerdien et al., 1991), DNA strand breaks (Martins and Meneghini, 1994; Sakkas et al., 1997), ageing and apoptosis (Yaki, 1993).

ORIGIN OF SPERMATOZOA

Sperm and sperm cells obtained from any segment of the reproductive system have the potential for fertilizing an egg (Ghazzawi et al., 1998), irrespective of the underlying pathology (Nagy et al., 1995a). However, the fertilization rates with epididymal spermatozoa are higher than those with spermatozoa collected from the testes (Silber et al., 1994; Nagy et al., 1995a; Tournaye et al., 1995). However, the resulting embryo quality is inferior when compared with the embryos obtained with spermatozoa from the ejaculates (Palermo et al., 1995).

Recent studies show no significant difference in fertilization rates between spermatozoa from ejaculates in severe OAT, epididymal and testicular spermatozoa in obstructive azoospermia, and testicular spermatozoa in nonobstructive azoospermia (Ghazzawi et al., 1998). The comparison between obstructive and nonobstructive azoospermia indicates that fertilization and pregnancy rates after using testicular spermatozoa in obstructive cases are significantly higher than in nonobstructive cases (Mansour et al., 1997). Patients with an acquired obstruction exhibit a better pregnancy rate than those with a congenital obstruction. Live births per embryo transfer are significantly lower in patients with nonobstructive azoospermia than in those with obstructive azoospermia and OAT. A high abortion rate is reported in cases in which testicular spermatozoa are used (Ghazzawi et al., 1998).

The obstetric outcome in ICSI pregnancies, as a whole, is similar to that of conventional IVF pregnancies. The rate of subclinical pregnancies, abortions and extrauterine pregnancies does not differ in relation to the origin and quality of spermatozoa. The frequency of infants born with low birth weight is higher in the epididymal sperm group than in the ejaculate sperm group, and the rate of intrauterine death is higher in the severe teratozoospermic group than in the normal morphology group (Aytoz et al., 1998).

Sperm Parameters

The application of ICSI has unfolded the fact that there is no difference in the fertilization rates in men with demonstrable or suspected male factor infertility. The specific phenotypic criteria of the semen, such as sperm head characteristics, count and motility, are of lesser importance for fertilization with ICSI (Nagy et al., 1995b).

Count

Males with a low sperm count had no options in the past and, therefore, had to go for either donor sperm samples or adoption. The technique of ICSI has given due respect even to an occasional sperm obtained via ejaculation, epididymal aspiration or testicular biopsy.

Morphology

Abnormal sperm head characteristics are attributed as small or large head size, amorphous head and globozoospermia. Lee et al. (1996) have documented high incidences of structural chromosomal aberrations in spermatozoa with amorphous heads, whereas globozoospermia and small or large spermatozoan heads have not shown significant chromosomal abnormalities (Abramsson et al., 1982; Zambani, 1987). Rybouchkin et al. (1996) have reported fertilization rates to be as low as 7% following an injection of round-headed spermatozoa, because of abnormal sperm head characteristics rather than cytogenetic abnormalities. To improve the low fertilization rate, besides ICSI, parthenogenetic activation with Ca^{2+} ionophore (Battaglia et al., 1997) can be the next best procedure to activate the oocyte and to overcome the lack of oscillin and centrosome that constitute the failure of activation (Levron et al., 1995).

Excellent fertilization and pregnancy rates have been reported in patients with midpiece defects. Likewise, even tail defects are not considered if ICSI is the mode of fertilization.

Motility

The success rate of ICSI drops considerably if immotile spermatozoa are injected into the oocyte. No pregnancy has been reported after injecting totally immotile, non-selected, ejaculated spermatozoa (Nagy et al., 1995a; Kahraman et al., 1996; Nijs et al., 1996). Testicular, totally immature spermatozoa also suffer from a lack of motility as their energetic pathway of motility may not have been switched on (Barros et al., 1997).

Sperm motility may be impaired due to disorders of sperm energy metabolism, such as the availability of ATP (Cummins and Yovich, 1993), wide varieties of ultrastructural abnormalities in the sperm tail (Ryder et al., 1990), defects in the cellular pathways, tail stump syndrome with 100% rudimentary flagella (Stalf et al., 1995), and the immotile cilia syndrome (Barros et al., 1997).

Ageing of the spermatozoa is another factor responsible for controlling motility. An aged spermatozoon can have fragmented DNA. This may result in the process of fertilization and cleavage, but the genome of the spermatozoon will be incapable of completing embryogenesis.

Sperm abnormalities are known to fluctuate from one ejaculate sample to another, randomly providing spermatozoa with normal motility (Barros et al., 1997). However, immotile testicular spermatozoa are still preferred to the ejaculated spermatozoa in men with totally immotile spermatozoa (Kahraman et al., 1996). Nonmotile spermatozoa do not mean cell death; rather, spermatozoa could be viable as identified by the HOS test. In a sample of completely immotile spermatozoa, less than 50% were found to be viable (Barros et al., 1997). Casper et al. (1996) have revealed that when no HOS test is performed, the fertilization rate after ICSI is demonstrated to be 29% with a 0% pregnancy rate. When spermatozoa were selected and ICSI was performed after the HOS test, the fertilization rate increased to 41% and the pregnancy rate to 25%. Thus, ICSI with associated sperm selection techniques can overcome the problem of immotility of spermatozoa to some extent.

Cryopreservation

Spermatozoa or tissue containing spermatozoa become the most valuable material, necessary for preservation especially in patients with incomplete germ-cell aplasia or incomplete maturation arrest, and in male patients undergoing treatment for cancer.

The drawbacks of cryopreservation could be in the form of cryo-injuries, resulting in reduced sperm motility and a decrease in the fertilization rate due to detrimental effects on the acrosomal structure and acrosin activity (Cross and Hanks, 1991). Crypreservation also hampers the integrity of the sperm nucleus and centrosome (Tournaye et al., 1996b). However, the changes have no significant influence on the outcome of ICSI. Friedler et al. (1997) have compared ICSI results with fresh and cryopreserved testicular spermatozoa in patients with nonobstructive azoospermia. They have shown the fertilization rates of fresh and cryopreserved testicular spermatozoa to be 47% and 44%, embryo cleavage rates 94% and 89%, and clinical pregnancy rates 26% and 27%, respectively. These results did not reach any statistical significance.

Female Factors

Female factors cannot be ruled out (Shoukir et al., 1998), as the age of the female and poor oocyte characteristics will not be compatible even with the best-quality sperms.

Age of Female

The physiological decline in female fecundity is related to an advance in maternal age, in natural conception (Schwartz, 1983; Menken et al., 1986), as well as in assisted reproduction (Craft et al., 1988; Padilla and Garcia, 1989; Beral et al., 1990; FIVNAT, 1990; Navot et al., 1991; Stovall et al., 1991; Al-Shawaf et al., 1992). The decline in fertility is associated with a rise in spontaneous abortion in older women (Stein, 1985; Abdalla et al., 1993). Silber et al. (1997) have shown a 46% live birth rate in women in the age-group of 20–30 years, and 4% in women above 40 years. Similar results have been shown by other investigators (Oehninger et al., 1995; Devroey et al., 1996; Spandorfer et al., 1998).

The main reasons for the decrease in the pregnancy rate with advanced maternal age are poor-quality oocytes and embryos, and the low number of embryos available (Navot et al., 1994; Oehninger et al., 1995; Hull et al., 1996; Silber et al., 1997). Age-related oocyte factors have commonly lead to aneuploidy, including mosaicism in cleaving embryos, resulting in the failure of implantation and clinical spontaneous abortion (Angell, 1994; Munne et al., 1995). Fertilization abnormalities, as affected by maternal age, are also due to a high incidence of tripronuclear formation. Such oocytes from older women may be less able to extrude PB 2, leading to an increase in digymy (Sultan et al., 1995; Spandorfer et al., 1998).

The receptivity of the endometrium is also affected by advancing age (Maldrum, 1993; Yarou et al., 1993; Sauer et al., 1994; Hull et al., 1996). The endometrial factors leading to failure of implantation are due to a defective endocrine milieu, poor uterine blood flow and inadequate endometrial proliferation that attributes to reduced endometrial receptivity.

Even though ICSI has changed the prognosis of male infertility, the age of the female partner is vital in ascertaining the outcome. To overcome the low success rate in older women, either an increased number of embryos is transferred (Adonakis et al, 1997; Grimbizis et al., 1998), or egg donation by younger women is considered (Sauer et al., 1990, 1991).

Morphology of Oocyte

The outcome of ICSI depends on the quality of the oocytes retrieved and their maturity, which may account for the variation in the rates of fertilization, embryo cleavage, implantation and continuation of pregnancy (Daya et al., 1995; Alikani et al., 1995). Poor quality oocytes with cytoplasmic inclusions are obtained mostly from women older than 35 years and/or with female factor infertility (Xia, 1997).

To amend failure in fertilization, gross oocyte morphology at metaphase II (M II) is assessed after cumulus corona stripping. Variations in the shape of the oocyte and ZP; the colour, granularity and homogenecity of the cytoplasm; the presence of vacuoles and refractile bodies in the cytoplasm; the size of the perivitalline space (PVS) and the presence of debris in the PVS; and abnormalities of the PB 1 are evaluated. De Sutter et al. (1994, 1996) are of the opinion that oocyte morphology with 1 or 2 abnormal features does not corelate with the fertilization rate and embryo quality after ICSI. However, grading according to PB 1, the size of the PVS and cytoplasmic inclusions has a significant influence not only on the fertilization rate, but also on the embryo quality after ICSI (Xia, 1997). Although normal fertilization and early embryo development were achieved in oocytes with abnormal cytoplasmic morphology, a significantly low implantation rate was recorded by Serhal et al. (1997).

Failed Fertilization

The fertilization failure rate ranges from 30%–40%. This suggests that the direct injection of an apparently normal spematozoon into the ooplasm of a morphologically mature oocyte does not ensure fertilization. The failure may be attributed to either a technical error or gamete deficiencies, which may not result in oocyte activation, sperm decondensation or pronuclear formation. Sakkas et al. (1996) correlated sperm chromatin decondensation failure with chromatin anomalies due to poor chromatin packaging or damaged DNA.

DNA fragmentation was found in 25% of the unfertilized oocytes incapable of reacting to sperm factors, resulting in a lack of activation (Lopes et al., 1998). Fragmented DNA is also associated with a nonfunctional nuclear spindle, which adds to the problem of oocyte activation.

Dubey et al. (1997) have shown that 58% of oocytes lack biochemical modification of the human zona protein, which leads to insufficient cortical granule release, suggestive of incomplete cytoplasmic maturation. Therefore, even an oocyte at the M II stage with cytoplasmic immaturity can be a cause of fertilization failure.

CLINICAL RESULTS

The task force on ICSI was established by the European Society of Human Reproduction and Embryology (ESHRE) in 1994. The world results of 33,903 ICSI cycles from 1993 to 1995, collected from 101 centres, were published by Tarlatzis (1996). Of 33,903 ICSI cycles, 31,276 were performed using ejaculated spermatozoa, 1,611 using epididymal and 1,016 using testicular spermatozoa. The fertilization rate was 61.5% with ejaculated, 57.6% with epididymal and 51.5% with testicular spermatozoa, while the total pregnancy rates per cycle were 28.2%, 31.0%, and 28.2%, respectively. The fertilization rate was significantly low (46.7%) in nonobstructive azoospermia as compared to the other groups.

The survival rate of embryos after thawing was approximately 63% and was affected neither by the origin of the sperm, nor by the aetiology of obstructive or nonobstructive azoospermia. The outcome of the pregnancy was almost the same in the three groups of patients. The major and minor malformations in children were not increased, while the incidence of chromosomal abnormalities in children born following ICSI was slightly elevated (2%).

Our data of 513 ICSI cycles, performed between January 1997 and June 1998, includes 89% using ejaculatory spermatozoa, 7.8% epididymal and 3.2% testicular spermatozoa. The procedure could not be carried out in 4.1% cycles because either there were no M II oocytes, or spermatozoa were not available for microinjection. The mean oocyte retrieval per treatment cycle was 8.8% and mature oocyte in M II was 7%. Successful microinjection was performed in 95% of the oocytes selected for ICSI. The fertilization rate (2 pronuclear stage) of the injected oocytes was 70.2%. Of these, the rate of embryos transferred was 95%. The clinical pregnancy rate was 32%, of which 19.1% ended in first-trimester abortion and 3.2% in ectopic pregnancy. The multiple pregnancy rate was found to be 10.6%. There was one stillbirth due to pregnancy-induced hypertension. Major malformation occurred in three (2.1%) children requiring surgical intervention.

ADVOCATION OF ICSI: HOW FAR AND HOW MUCH?

The successful implementation of ICSI has provided a unique opportunity to allow couples, especially those with severe male factor infertility, to achieve their reproductive goals. But the potential risk factors of genetically transmitted diseases and of conceiving a malformed child still exist. Often the question arises—do the congenital genetic diseases, which could otherwise have been eliminated, get perpetuated in future generations by the use of ICSI?

The complex psychological crisis is an important aspect of infertility and its treatment. It has been hypothesized that men undergoing ICSI would experience more distress during treatment than men undergoing IVF. Nachtigall et al. (1992) found that men with a male factor problem suffered a loss of physical potency and self-esteem.

Knowing the emotional state of couples undergoing ICSI, they need to be warned about the failure of fertilization due to the chromosomal incompatibility of the gametes, or the occurrence of possible genetic abnormalities incorporated in the zygote. But the desire to procreate is so intense in these couples that even when the risks of ICSI are explained to them, their opinion is that the future successes of research and development will help their child either to alleviate infertility or to correct the defect.

Hence, genetic screening is offered to both the partners recruited for ICSI. Prospective PGD should be advocated to the couple for detecting birth defects at the embryo level. Patients should be guided into not allowing 'carrier' embryos to be implanted. Facilities for PGD should be made available at all centres offering ICSI, otherwise the patient should be advised for chorionic villus sampling or amniocentesis. Further, patients should be strongly advised to terminate such pregnancies, in order to nullify the defects in future generations. Long-term monitoring of children from this procedure should be a priority, to decide how far and how much ICSI should be advocated in future as a treatment for infertility.

ACKNOWLEDGEMENTS

We express our gratitude to Drs Sanjay Patil and Prednya Paruleker for expressing their comments in preparing the manuscript and to Mrs Jyotsina Chhabria for her assistance in preparing the manuscript.

REFERENCES

Abdalla, I.H. et al. (1993). 'Pregnancy and miscarriage uterine versus ovarian factor', *Hum. Reprod.*, **8**: 1512–7.

——(1995). 'Comparison of SUZI and ICSI for severe male factor', *Hum. Reprod.*, **10**: 2941–4.

Abramsson, L. et al. (1982). 'Chromosomal aberrations and male infertility', *J. Urol.*, **128**: 552.

Ackerman, S.B. et al. (1984). 'Immunologic infertility and *in vitro* fertilization', *Fertil. and Steril.*, **42**: 474–7.

Adonakis, G. et al. (1997). 'The role of the number of replaced embryos on intracytoplasmic sperm injection outcome in women over the age of 40', *Hum. Reprod.*, **12**: 2542–5.

Aitken, R.J. and J.S. Clarkson (1988). 'Significance of reactive oxygen species and antioxidants in defining the efficacy of sperm preparation techniques', *J. Androl.*, **9**: 367–76.

Aitken, R.J. (1994). 'A free-radical theory of male infertility', *Reprod. Fertil. Devp.*, **6**: 19–24.

Al-Shawaf, T. et al. (1992). 'The influence of ovarian response on gamete intra-fallopian transfer outcome in older women', *Hum. Reprod.*, **7**: 1106–10.

Alikani, M. et al. (1995). 'Intracytoplasmic sperm injection in dysmorphic human oocyte', *Zygote*, **3**: 283–8.

Alvarez, G.T. et al. (1993). 'Centrifugation of human spermatozoa induces sublethal damage: Separation of human spermatozoa from seminal plasma by a dextran swim-up procedure without centrifugation extends their motile lifetime', *Hum. Reprod.*, **8**: 1087–92.

Angell, R.R. (1994). 'Aneuploidy in older women: Higher rates of aneuploidy in oocytes from older women', *Hum. Reprod.*, **9**: 1199–1200.

Asada, Y. et al. (1995). 'Evaluation of the meiotic spindle apparatus in oocytes undergoing intracytoplasmic sperm injection', *Fertil. Steril.*, **64**: 376–81.

Aytoz, A., et al. (1998). 'Outcome of pregnancies after intracytoplasmic sperm injection and the effect of sperm origin and quality on this outcome', *Fertil. Steril.*, **70**: 500–5.

Baker, H.W.G. et al. (1996). 'Protective effect of antioxidants on the impairment of sperm motility by activated polymorphonuclear leukocytes', *Fertil. Steril.*, **65**: 411–19.

Barros, A. et al. (1997). 'Pregnancy and birth after intracytoplasmic sperm injection with immotile sperm recovered from the ejaculate', *Fertil Steril.*, **67**: 1091–94.

Battaglia, D.E. et al. (1997). 'Failure of oocyte activation after intracytoplasmic sperm injection using round-headed sperm', *Fertil. Steril.*, **68**: 118–22.

Belker, A. M. et al. (1996). 'High fertilization and pregnancy rates obtained by non-surgical percutaneous aspiration of testicular sperm', *J. Urol.*, **155**: (Suppl. 1), 364A.

Beral, V. et al. (1990). 'Outcome of pregnancy resulting from assisted conception', *Br. Med. Bull.*, **46**: 753–68.

Bertrand, E., M. Van Den Bergh and Y. Englert (1995). 'Does zona pellucida thickness influence the fertilization rate?' *Hum. Reprod.*, **10**: 1189–93.

Bonaccorsi, A.C. et al. (1997). 'Genetic disorders in normally androgenized infertile men and the use of intracytoplasmic sperm injection as a way of treatment', *Fertil. Steril.*, **67**: 928–31.

Casper, R.F. et al. (1996). 'The hypo-osmotic swelling test for selection of viable sperm for intracytoplasmic sperm injection in men with complete asthenozoospermia', *Fertil. Steril.*, **65**: 972–6.

Chandley, A.C. et al. (1975). 'Cytogenetics and infertility in man: Results of a five-year survey of man attending a subfertility clinic, 1: Karyotype and seminal analysis', *Ann. Hum. Genet.*, **39**: 231–5

Chen, S.U. et al. (1996). 'Intracytoplasmic sperm injection (ICSI) for severe semen abnormalities: Dissecting the tail of spermatozoa at the tip', *Hum. Reprod.*, **11**: 2640–4.

Clarke, G.N. (1997). 'Intracytoplasmic sperm injection for treating infertility associated with sperm autoimmunity', *Fertil. Steril.*, **68**: 112–7.

Clarke, R.N. and L.A. Johnson (1988). 'Factors related to successful sperm microinjection of hamster eggs: The effect of sperm species, technical experience, needles dimensions, and incubation medium on egg viability and sperm decondensation', *Theriogenology*, **30**: 447–60.

Cohen J. et al. (1988). 'Implantation of embryo after partial opening of oocyte zona pellucida to facilitate sperm penetration', *Lancet*, **2**: 162.

Cohen, J. et al. (1992). 'Microsurgical fertilization procedures: The absence of stringent criteria for patients selection', *J. Ass. Reprod. Genet.*, **9**: 197–206.

Craft, I. et al. (1988). 'Analysis of 1071 GIFT procedure the case for a flexible approach to treatment', *Lancet*, **2**: 1094–7.

Craft, I. et al. (1995). 'Percutaneous epididymal sperm aspiraion and intracytoplasmic sperm injection in the management of infertility due to obstructive azoospermia', *Fertil. Steril.*, **5**: 1038–42.

Cross, N.L. and S.E. Hanks (1991). 'Effects of cryopreservation on human sperm acrosomes', *Hum. Reprod.*, **6**: 1279–83.

Cummins, J. and J. Yovich (1993). 'Sperm motility enhancement *in vitro*', *Semin. Reprod. Endocrinol.*, **11**: 56–71.

Daya, S. et al. (1995). 'Oocyte morphology as a predictor

of pregnancy for intracytoplasmic sperm injection (ICSI)', The 51st Annual Clinical Meeting of The Society of Obstetricians and Gynaecologists of Canada. Calgary, Canada, *Abstract.,* 013-REL. p. 47.

De Brackeleer, M. and T.M. Dao (1991). 'Cytogenetic studies in male infertility: A review', *Hum.Reprod.*, **9**: 245–50.

de Kretser, D.M. et al. (1985). 'The use of *in vitro* fertilization in the management of male infertility', in R. Rolland, et al. (eds.), *Gamete Quality and Fertility Regulation, Excerpta medica,* Amsterdam, pp. 213–23.

de Kretser, D.M. and J.B. Kerr (1994). 'The cytology of the testis', in E. Knobil and J.D. Neill (eds.), *Physiology and Reproduction*, Raven Press, New York, pp. 1177–290.

De Sutter, P. et al. (1994). 'Influence of oocyte morphology on the outcome of intracytoplasmic sperm injection', Xth Meeting of IVF Contact Group, Brussels, Belguim, 29 January, *Abstract*, p. 8.

De Sutter, P. et al. (1996). 'Oocyte morphology does not correlate with fertilization rate and embryo quality after intracytoplasmic sperm injection', *Hum. Reprod.*, **11**: 595–7.

De Vos, A. et al. (1997). 'Percoll gradient centrifugation can be omitted in sperm preparation for intracytoplasmic sperm injection', *Hum. Reprod.*, **12**: 1980–84.

Devroey, P. et al. (1996). 'Female age predicts embryonic implantation after ICSI: A case-controlled study', *Hum. Reprod.*, **11**: 1324–7.

Dozortsev, D. et al. (1994). 'Behaviour of spermatozoa in human oocytes displaying no or one pronucleus after intracytoplasmic sperm injection', *Hum. Reprod.*, **9**: 2139–44.

Dozortsev, D. et al. (1995a). 'Timing of sperm and oocyte nuclear progression after intracytoplasmic sperm injection', *Hum. Reprod.*, **10**: 3012–7.

______(1995b). 'Oocyte activation and ICSI', *J. Assist. Reprod. Rev.*, **5**: 32–9.

______(1995c). 'Methodology of intracytoplasmic sperm injection in the human', *J. Assist. Reprod. Rev.*, **6**: 38–44.

______(1995d). 'Human oocyte activation following intracytoplasmic sperm injection: Role of the sperm cell', *Hum. Reprod.*, **10**: 403–7.

______(1995e). 'Sperm plasma membrane damage prior to intracytoplasmic sperm injection: A necessary condition for sperm nucleus docondensation', *Hum. Reprod.*, **10**: 2960–64.

______(1997). 'Sperm-associated oocyte-activating factor is released from the spermatozoon within 30 min after injection as a result of the sperm-oocyte interaction', *Hum. Reprod.*, **12**: 2792–6.

Dubey, A.K. et al. (1997). 'Failed fertilization after intracytoplasmic serm injection: The extent of paternal and maternal chromatin decondensation', *Fertil. Steril.*, **68**: 714–7.

Feichtinger, W. et al. (1995). 'Sex chromosomal abnormalities and intracytoplasmic injection', *Lancet*, **346**: 1566.

Fishel, S. et al. (1995). 'Pregnancy after intracytoplasmic injection of spermatid', *Lancet*, 245: 1641–2.

FIVNAT—Piette, C. et al. (1990). '*In vitro* fertilization: Influence of women's age on pregnancy', *Hum. Reprod.*, **5**: 56–9.

Friedler, S. et al. (1997). 'Intracytoplasmic injection of fresh and cryopreserved testicular spermatozoa in patients with non-obstructive azoospermia—a comparative study', *Fertil. Steril.*, **68**: 892–7.

Gearon, C.M. et al. (1995). 'Factors affecting activation and fertilization of human oocytes following intracytoplasmic injection', *Hum Reprod.*, **10**: 896–902.

Gerris, J. et al. (1994). 'Pregnancy after intracytoplasmic injection of metaphase II oocytes with spermatozoa from a man with complete retrograde ejaculation', *Hum. Reprod.*, **9**:1293–6.

Geva, E. et al. (1997). 'The ratio between carcinoma antigen-125 levels in the seminal plasma and serum may be a marker for fertilization in intracytoplasmic sperm injection', *Fertil. Steril.*, **68**: 1120–24.

Ghazzawi, I.M. et al. (1998). 'Comparison of the fertilizing capability of spermatozoa from ejaculates, epididymal aspirates and testicular biopsis using intracytoplasmic sperm injection', *Hum. Reprod.*, **13**: 348–52.

Gordon, J.M. et al. (1988). 'Fertilization of human oocytes by sperm from infertile males after zona pellucida drilling', *Fertil. Steril.*, **50**: 68–73.

Gorus, F.K. and D.G. Pipeleers (1981). 'A rapid method for the fractionation of human spermatozoa according to their progressive motility', *Fertil. Steril.*, **35**: 662–5.

Grimbizis, G. et al. (1998). 'Intracytoplasmic sperm

injection results in women older than 39: According to the age and the number of embryos replaced in selective or non-selective transfer', *Hum. Reprod.*, **13**: 884–9.

Grow, D.R. et al. (1994). 'Sperm morphology as diagnosed by strict criteria probing the impact of teratozoospermia on fertilization rate and pregnancy outcome in a large *in vitro* fertilization population', *Fertil. Steril.*, **62**: 559–67.

Haidl, G. and W.B. Schill (1993). 'Sperm morphology in fertile men', *Arch. Androl.*, **31**: 153–7.

Hauser, R. et al. (1998). 'Multiple testicular sampling in non-obstructive azoospermia—is it necessary?' *Hum. Reprod.*, **13**: 3081–5.

Hendry, W.F. et al., (1979). 'Steroid treatment of male subfertility caused by antisperm antibodies', *Lancet*, **ii**: 498–501.

Hewett, J. et al. (1985). 'Treatment of idiopathic infertility, cervical mucus hostility and male infertility: Artificial insemination with husband's semen or *in vitro* fertilization?' *Fertil. Steril.*, **44**: 350–55.

Hull, M.G.R. et al. (1996). 'The age-related decline in female fecundity: A quantitative controlled study of implantation capacity and survival of individual embryo after *in vitro* fertilization', *Fertil. Steril.*, **65**: 783–90.

Joris, H. et al. (1996). 'Comparison of different concentration of hyaluronidase used to remove surrounding cells from oocytes for ICSI', Abstract Book, 12th Annual Meeting of the European Society for Human Reproduction and Embryology.

Kahraman, S. et al. (1996). 'Pregnancies achieved with testicular and ejaculated spermatozoa in combination with intracytoplasmic sperm injection in men with totally or initially immotile spermatozoa in the ejaculate', *Hum. Reprod.*, **11**: 1343–6.

Kruger, T.F. et al. (1986). 'Sperm morphologic features as a prognostic factor in *in vitro* fertilization', *Fertil. Steril.*, **46**: 1118–23.

Kruger, T.F. et al. (1988). 'Predicting value of abnormal sperm morphology factor in *in vitro* fertilization', *Fertil. Steril.*, **49**: 112–7.

Lahteenmaki, A. (1993). '*In vitro* fertilization in the presence of antisperm antibodies detected by the mixed antiglobulin reaction (MAR) and the tray agglutination test (TAT)', *Hum. Reprod.*, **8**: 84–8.

Lazendorf, S.E. et al. (1988). 'A preclinical evaluation of pronuclear formation by microinjection of human spermatozoa into human oocytes', *Fertil. Steril.*, **49**: 835–42.

Lee, J.D. et al. (1996). 'Analysis of chromosome constitution of human spermatozoa with normal and aberrant head morphology after injection into mouse oocytes', *Hum. Reprod.*, **11**: 1942–6.

Levron, J. et al. (1995). 'Highly effective method of human oocyte activation', *Zygote*, **3**: 157–61.

Liu, D.Y. and H.W.G. Baker (1994). 'A new test for the assessment of sperm zona pellucida penetration: Relationship with results of other sperm tests and fertilization *in vitro*', *Hum.Reprod.*, **9**: 489–96.

Liu, D.Y. et al. (1995). 'Fertilization and pregnancy with acrosome intact sperm by intracytoplasmic sperm injection in patients with disordered zona pellucida-induced acrosome reaction', *Fertil. Steril.*, **64**: 116–21.

Lopata, A. et al. (1980). 'Use of *in vitro* fertilization in the infertile couple', in R.J. Pepperell et al. (eds.), *The Infertile Couple*, Churchill Livingstone, Edinburgh, pp. 209–28.

Lopes, S. et al. (1998). 'Gamete-specific DNA fragmentation in unfertilized human oocytes after intracytoplasmic sperm injection', *Hum. Reprod.*, **13**: 703–8.

Lundin, K. et al. (1994). 'Fertilization and pregnancy after intracytoplasmic micro injection of acrosomeless spermatozoa', *Fertil. Steril.*, **62**: 1266–7.

______(1995). 'The significance of the PVP used for ICSI', *J. Assist. Reprod. Genet.*, **12** (suppl.), 755.

Lutjen, P. et al. (1984). 'The establishment and maintenance of pregnancy using *in vitro* fertilization and embryo donation in a patient with primary ovarian failure', *Nature (London)*, **307**: 174–5.

Mahadevan, M.M. et al. (1983). 'The relationship of tubal blockage, infertility of unknown cause, suspected male infertility and endometriosis to success of *in vitro* fertilization and embryo transfer', *Fertil. Steril.*, **40**: 755–62.

Mahadevan, M.M., and A.O. Trounson (1985). 'Removal of the cumulus oophorus from the human oocyte for *in vitro* fertilization', *Fertil. Steril.*, **43**: 263–7.

Maldrum, D.R. (1993). 'Female reproductive aging-ovarian and uterine factors', *Fertil. Steril.*, **59**: 1–5.

Mansour, R.T. et al. (1997). 'Intracytoplasmic sperm

injection in obstructive and non-obstructive azoospermia', *Hum. Reprod.*, **12**: 1974–9.

Markert, C.L. (1983). 'Fertilization of mammalian eggs by sperm injection', *J. Exp. Zool.*, **228**: 195–201.

Martins, E.A.L. and R. Meneghini (1994). 'Cellular DNA damage by hydrogen peroxide is attenuated by hypotonicity', *Biochem. J.*, **299**: 137–40.

Menken, J. et al. (1986). 'Age and infertility', *Science*, **233**: 1389–94.

Menkveld, R. et al. (1990). 'The evaluation of the morphologic characteristics of human spermatozoa according to stricter criteria', *Hum. Reprod.*, **5**: 586–92.

Montag, M. et al. (1992). '*In vitro* decondensation of mammalian sperm and subsequent formation of pronuclei-like structures for micromanipulation', *Mol. Reprod. Dev.*, **33**: 338–46.

Morton, P.C. et al. (1997). 'Reinsemination by intracytoplasmic sperm injection of 1-day-old oocyte after complete conventional fertilization failure', *Fertil. Steril.*, **68**: 488–91.

Motoishi, M. et al. (1996). 'Examination of the safety of intracytoplasmic injection procedures by using bovine zygotes', *Hum. Reprod.*, **11**: 618–20.

Mulhall, J.P. et al. (1997). 'Azoospermic men with deletion of the DAZ gene cluster are capable of completing spermatogenesis: Fertilization, normal embryonic development and pregnancy occur when retrieved testicular spermatozoa are used for intracytoplasmic sperm injection', *Hum. Reprod.*, **12**: 503–8.

Munne, S. et al. (1995). 'Embryo morphology development rates, and maternal age are correlated with chromosomal abnormalities', *Fertil. Steril.*, **64**: 382–91.

Nachtigall, R.P. et al. (1992). 'The effect of gender-specific diagnosis on men's-women's response to fertility', *Fertil. Steril.*, **57**: 113–21.

Nackerdien, Z. et al. (1991). 'Chemical nature of DNA—protein cross-links produced in mammalian chromatin by hydrogen peroxide in the presence of iron or copper ions', *Biochemistry (USA)*, **30**: 4873–9.

Nagy, Z. et al. (1995a). 'Comparison of fertilization, embryo development and pregnancy rates after intracytoplasmic sperm injection using ejaculated, fresh and frozen-thawed epididymal and testicular spermatozoa', *Fertil. Steril.*, **63**: 808–15.

Nagy, Z.P. et al. (1995b). 'The result of intracytoplasmic sperm injection is not related to any of the three basic sperm parameters', *Hum Reprod.*, **10**: 1123–9.

———(1995c). 'Results of 55 intracytoplasmic sperm injection cycles in the treatment of male-immunological infertility', *Hum. Reprod.*, **10**: 1775–80.

Navot, D. et al. (1991). 'Poor oocyte quality rather than implantation failure as a cause of age related decline in female fertility', *Lancet*, **337**: 1375–7.

———(1994). 'Age-related decline in female fertility is not due to diminished capacity of the uterus to sustain embryo implantation', *Fertil. Steril.*, **61**: 97–101.

Ng, S-C. et al. (1988). 'Pregnancy after transfer of multiple sperm under the zona', *Lancet*, **ii**: 790.

Ng, S-C. et al. (1991). 'Microinjection of human oocytes: A technique for severe oligoasthenoteratozoospermia', *Fertil. Steril.*, **56**: 1117–23.

Nijs, M. et al. (1996). 'Fertilizing ability of immotile spermatozoa after intracytoplasmic sperm injection', *Hum. Reprod.*, **11**: 2180–85.

Odawara, Y. and A. Lopata (1989). 'A zona opening procedure for improving *in vitro* fertilization at low sperm concentration: A mouse model', *Fertil. Steril.*, **51**: 699–704.

Oehninger, S. et al. (1988). 'Failure of fertilization in *in-vitro* fertilization: The "occult" male factor', *J. IVF. ET.*, **5**: 181–7.

———(1989). 'Hemizona assay: Assessment of sperm dysfunction and prediction of *in vitro* fertilization outcome', *Fertil. Steril.*, **51**: 665–70.

———(1995). 'Intracytoplasmic sperm injection achievement of high pregnancy rates in couples with severe male factor infertility is dependent primarily upon female and not male factor', *Fertil. Steril.*, **64**: 977–81

Padilla, S.I. and J. Garcia (1989). 'Effects of maternal age and number of *in vitro* fertilization procedure on pregnancy outcome', *Fertil. Steril.*, **52**: 270–73.

Palermo, G. et al. (1992). 'Pregnancies after intracytoplasmic injection of a single spermatozoon into an oocyte', *Lancet*, **340**: 17–18.

———(1993). 'Sperm characteristics and outcome of human-assisted fertilization by subzonal insemination and intracytoplasmic sperm injection', *Fertil. Steril.*, **59**: 826–35.

Palermo, G. D. et al. (1995). 'Intracytoplasmic sperm injection: A novel treatment for all forms of male factor infertility', *Fertil. Steril.*, **63**: 1231–40.

______(1996). 'Aggressive sperm immobilization prior to intracytoplasmic sperm injection with immature spermatozoa improves fertilization and pregnancy rates', *Hum. Reprod.*, **11**: 1023–29.

Parinaud, J. et al. (1998). 'Use of a plant enzyme preparation (Coronase) instead of hyaluronidase for cumulus cell removal before intracytoplasmic sperm injection', *Hum. Reprod.*, **13**: 1933–5.

Payne, D. et al. (1994). 'Successful treatment of severe male factor infertility in 100 consecutive cycles using intracytoplasmic sperm injection', *Hum. Reprod.*, **9**: 2051–7.

Ray, B.D. et al. (1995). 'Testing the mutagenic potential of polyvinylpyrrolidone and methyl cellulose by sister chromatid exchange analysis prior to use in intracytoplasmic sperm injection procedures', *Hum. Reprod.*, **10**: 436–8.

Romero, J. et al. (1996). 'Fertilization after intracytoplasmic sperm injection with cryopreserved testicular spermatozoa', *Fertil. Steril.*, **65**: 877–9.

Ron-El, R. et al. (1997). 'Extended sperm preparation: An alternative to testicular sperm extraction in non-obstructive azoospermia', *Hum. Reprod.*, **12**: 1222–6.

Rybouchkin, A. et al. (1996). 'Analysis of the oocyte activating capacity and chromosomol complement of round-headed human spermatozoa by injection into mouse oocyte', *Hum.Reprod.*, **11**: 2170–75.

Ryder, T. et al. (1990). 'A survey of the ultrastructural defects associated with absence of impaired human sperm motility', *Fertil. Steril.*, **53**: 556–60.

Saha, S. et al. (1996). 'Normal calves obtained after direct transfer of verified bovine embryos using ethelene glycol trehalose, and polyvinylpyrrolidone', *Cryobiology*, **33**: 291–9.

Sakkas, D. et al. (1996). 'Sperm chromatin anomalies can influence decondensation after intracytoplasmic sperm injection', *Hum. Reprod.*, **11**: 837–43.

Sakkas, D. et al. (1997). 'Chromatin packaging anomalies and DNA damage in human sperm: Their possible implications in the treatment of male factor infertility', in C. Barratt et al. (eds.), *Genetics of Human Male Fertility*, EDK Press, Paris, pp. 205–21.

Sauer, M.V. et al. (1990). 'A preliminary report on oocyte donation extending reproductive potential to women over 40', *N. Engl.J.Med.*, **323**: 1157–60.

______(1991). 'Oocyte and pre- embryo donation to women with failure and extended clinical trail', *Fertil.Steril.*, **55**: 39–43.

______(1994). 'Three hundred cycles of oocyte donation at the university of Southern California assessing the effect of age and infertility diagnosis in pregnancy and implantation rates', *J. Assist. Reprod. Genet.*, **11**: 92–6.

Schwartz, D. (1983). 'The measurement of fecundity of couple's contribution by age of partners', *Contracept. Fertil. Sex.*, **11**: 897–900.

Serhal, P.F. et al. (1997). 'Oocyte morphology predicts outcome of intracytoplasmic sperm injection', *Hum. Reprod.*, **12**: 1267–70.

Shibahara, H. et al. (1993). 'Effects of sperm immobilizing antibodies on sperm-zona pellucida tight binding', *Fertil. Steril.*, **60**: 533–9.

Shoukir, Y. et al. (1998). 'Blastocyst development from supernumerary embryos after intracytoplasmic sperm injection: A paternal influence', *Hum. Reprod.*, **13**: 1632–7.

Shrivastav, P. et al. (1994). 'Percutaneous epididymal sperm aspiration for obstructive azoospermia', *Hum. Reprod.*, **9**: 2058–61.

Silber, S.J. et al. (1994). 'Conventional IVF versus ICSI for patients requiring microsurgical sperm aspiration', *Hum. Reprod.*, **9**: 1705–9.

______(1995). 'High fertilization and pregnancy rates after intracytoplasmic sperm injection with spermatozoa obtained from testicular biopsy', *Hum. Reprod.*, **10**: 148–52.

______(1996). 'Normal pregnancies resulting from testicular sperm extraction and intracytoplasmic sperm injection for azoospermia due to maturation arrest', *Fertil. Steril.*, **66**: 110–17.

______(1997). 'The effect of female age and ovarian reserve on pregnancy rate in male infertility: Treatment of azoospermia with sperm retrieved and intracytoplasmic sperm injection', *Hum. Reprod.*, **12**: 2693–700.

Smart, S.C. et al. (1988). 'Effect of therapy on infertile couple with antisperm antibodies', *Am. J. Obstet. Gynecol.*, **158**: 969–73.

Spandorfer, S.D. et al. (1998). 'Effect of parental age on fertilization and pregnancy characteristics in couples treated by intracytoplasmic sperm injection', *Hum. Reprod.*, **13**: 334–8.

Stalf, T. et al. (1995). 'Pregnancy and birth after intracytoplasmic sperm injection with spermatozoa from a patient with tail stump syndrome', *Hum. Reprod.*, **10**: 2112–4.

Stein, Z.A. (1985). 'Women's age: Child bearing and child rearing', *Am. J. Epidemiol.*, **121**: 327–42.

Steptoe, P.C. and R.G. Edwards (1978). 'Birth after the re-implantation of a human embryo (letter)', *Lancet.*, **2**: 366.

Stovall, D.W. et al. (1991). 'The effect of age on female fecundity', *Obstet. Gynaecol.*, 77: 33–6.

Strehler, E. et al. (1998). 'Detrimental effects of polyvinylpyrrolidone on the ultrastructure of spermatozoa', *Hum. Reprod.*, **13**: 120–23.

Sultan, K.M. et al. (1995). 'Chromosomal status in unipronuclear human zygotes following *in vitro* fertilization and intracytoplasmic sperm injection', *Hum. Reprod.*, **10**: 132–6.

Svalander, P. et al. (1995). 'Factors of importance for the establishment of a successful programme of intracytoplasmic sperm injection treatment for male infertility', *Fertil. Steril.*, **4**: 828–37.

Tarlatzis, B. (1996). 'Report on the activities of the ESHRE task force on intracytoplasmic sperm injection', in A. Van Steirteghem et al. (eds.), *Genetics and Assisted Human Conception*, Oxford University Press, Oxford, pp. 160–167.

Temple-Smith, P.D. et al. (1985). 'Human pregnancy by *in vitro* fertilization (IVF) using sperm aspirated from the epididymis', *J. In Vitro Fertil. Embryo Transf.*, **2**: 119–22.

Tesarik, J. and V. Kopeeny (1989). 'Developmental control of the human male pronucleus by ooplasmic factors', *Hum. Reprod.*, **4**: 962–8.

Tesarik, J. et al. (1994). 'Human oocyte activation alter intracytoplasmic sperm injection', *Hum. Reprod.*, **9**: 511–8.

______(1996). 'Spermatid injection into human oocyte. II. Clinical application in the treatment of infertility due to non-obstructive azoospermia', *Hum. Reprod.*, **11**: 780–83.

Tesarik, J. and M. Sousa (1995). 'More than 90% fertilization rates after intracytoplasmic sperm injection and artificial induction of oocyte activation with calcium ionophore', *Fertil. Steril.*, **63**: 343–9.

Tesarik, J. et al. (1995). 'Viable embryos from injection of round spermatids into oocytes', *N. Engl. J. Med.*, **333**: 525.

Tournaye, H. et al. (1995). 'Recent concepts in the management of infertility because of non-obstructive azoospermia', *Hum. Reprod.*, **10** (Suppl. 1): 115–9.

______(1996a). 'The use of testicular sperm for intracytoplasmic sperm injection in patients with necrozoospermia', *Fertil Steril.*, **66**: 331–4.

______(1998). 'Sperm parameters, globozoospermia, necrozoospermia and ICSI outcome', in Marco Filicori and Carlo Flamigini (eds.), *Treatment of Infertility: The New Frontiers*, Communications Media for Education, U.S.A.

Tournaye, H. et al. (1996b). 'Correlation between testicular histology and outcome after introcytoplasmic sperm injection using testicular spermatozoa', *Hum. Reprod.*, **11**: 127–32.

Trayen, U. et al. (1995). 'There is nothing permanent except change: The emergence of new virus diseases', *Vet. Microbiol.*, **43**: 103–22.

Van de Velde, H. et al. (1997). 'Effect of different hyaluronidase concentrations and mechanical procedures for cumulus cell removal on the outcome of intracytoplasmic sperm injection', *Hum. Reprod.*, **12**: 2246–50.

Vanderzwalmen, P. et al. (1995). 'Fertilization of an oocyte micro-inseminated with a spermatid in an *in vitro* fertilization programme', *Hum. Reprod.*, **16**: 502–3.

______(1996). 'Two essential steps for a successful intracytoplasmic sperm injection of immobilized spermatozoa after rupture of the oolema', *Hum. Reprod.*, **11**: 540–47.

Van Steirteghem, A.C. et al. (1993a). 'Higher success rate by intracytoplasmic sperm injection than by subzonal insemination: Report of a second series of 300 consecutive treatment cycles', *Hum Reprod.*, **8**: 1055–60.

______(1993b). 'High fertilization and implantation rates after intracytoplasmic sperm injection', *Hum Reprod.*, **8**: 1061–66.

Witkin, S.S. et al. (1992). 'Relation between antisperm antibodies and the rate of fertilization of human oocyte *in vitro*', *G. Ass. Repro. Genet.*, **9**: 9-13.

World Health Organization (1992). *Laboratory manual for Examination of human semen and sperm-cervical mucus interaction*, 3rd ed., Cambridge University Press, New York.

Xia, P. (1997). 'Intracytoplasmic sperm injection:

Correlation of oocyte grade based on polar body, perivitelline space and cytoplasmic inclusions with fertilization rate and embryo quality', *Hum. Reprod.*, **12**: 1750–55.

Yaki, K., (1993). 'Lipid peroxidase, free radicals and disease', in K. Yaki (ed.) *Active Oxygens, Lipids Peroxidase and Antioxidants,* CRC Press, Boca Raton, pp. 1–38.

Yamanaka, K. et al. (1997). 'Ooplasmic round spermatid nuclear injection procedure as an experimental treatment for non-obstructive azoospermia', *J. Assist. Reprod. Genet.*, **14**: 55–62.

Yang, Y.S. et al. (1995). 'The correlation between sperm morphology using strict criteria in original semen and swim-up inseminate and human *in vitro* fertilization', *Arch. Androl.*, **34**: 105–13.

Yarou, Y. et al. (1993). 'Endometrial receptivity: The age-related decline in pregnancy rates and the effect of ovarian function', *Fertil.Steril.*, **60**: 314–8.

Yates, C.A. et al. (1989). 'Male factor infertility and *in vitro* fertilization', 4th. International Congress in Andrology, Florence, Italy 14–18 May 1989, *Abstract*, p. 263.

Yovich, J.L. et al. (1984). 'Treatment of male infertility by *in vitro* fertilization', *Lancet*, **2**: 169–70.

Zambani, L. (1987). 'The ultrastructural pathology of the spermatozoon as a cause of infertility: The role of electron microscopy in the evaluation of semen quality', *Fertil. Steril.*, **48**: 711.

13

Role of Testicular Spermatozoa and Spermatids

Nijs Martine and Vanderzwalmen Pierre

INTRODUCTION

A new era in the treatment of human infertility began with the report of pregnancies after the injection of a single spermatozoon into the ooplasm by Palermo et al. in 1992. The procedure was called intracytoplasmic sperm injection (ICSI). Patients suffering from severe oligo astheno teratozoospermia, who had little chance of having offspring, were given a realistic hope by this technique.

The management of all male factor indications was even more revolutionized when it was demonstrated that spermatozoa retrieved from the testis (and thought to be immature and incapable of fertilizing) could activate an oocyte and lead to viable embryos and healthy pregnancies (Schoysman et al., 1993; Silber et al., 1995). Patients suffering from obstructive and nonobstructive azoospermia enrolled for application of this technique. The results became comparable to those of ejaculated spermatozoa, especially for obstructive azoospermic men (Vandervorst et al., 1996; Mulhall et al., 1997). Cryopreservation of testicular sperm, which has shown good survival and fertilization rates, is the latest development in this domain: if a small number of viable sperm is retrieved surgically, the excess of testicular tissue and/or spermatozoa can now be frozen for another attempt.

When no spermatozoa could be found in patients with partial or complete failure of spermiogenesis, the injection of immature germ cells (spermatids) was shown to be successful, especially for elongating or elongated spermatids (Vanderzwalmen et al., 1996; Fishel et al., 1996). It is clear that the application of all these techniques in the treatment of infertile patients has to be safe since genetic factors can be involved.

This chapter summarizes the evolution of the use of testicular spermatozoa and spermatids in infertility treatment, and tries to evaluate the power and safety of all the techniques applied.

THE PROCESS OF SPERMATOGENESIS AND SPERMIOGENESIS

Arising from the albuginae, the septa divide the testis into about 250 lobules with vascular supply. Each lobule contains 1–4 very convoluted seminiferous tubulus (Van de Casseye, 1994). Each tubule has a diameter of 150–250 microns and a maximum length of 30–70 cm. The total amount of seminiferous tubules form over 90% of the volume of the testis. The remaining connective tissues contain, in addition to blood vessels, a few lymphocytes, plasma cells and clumps of Leydig cells, the secretors of testosterone. The tubules themselves are lined by spermatogenetic epithelium, which is made of gametogenic cells at different stages of maturation: a cross-section of any normal seminiferous tubule will show 4 or 5 distinct generations of germ cells (Fig. 10.1 a, b and c). The Sertoli cells are big and tentacular cells, clinging to the basal membrane. Their cytoplasm is poorly defined and extends from the basal membrane to the lumen of the tubule. The germinal cells bulge into the cytoplasm of the Sertoli cells, receiving nutritional and hormonal supply. The mature spermatozoa can be seen attached to and surrounding the Sertoli cells prior to release. Normal spermatogenesis covers a period of approximately 70

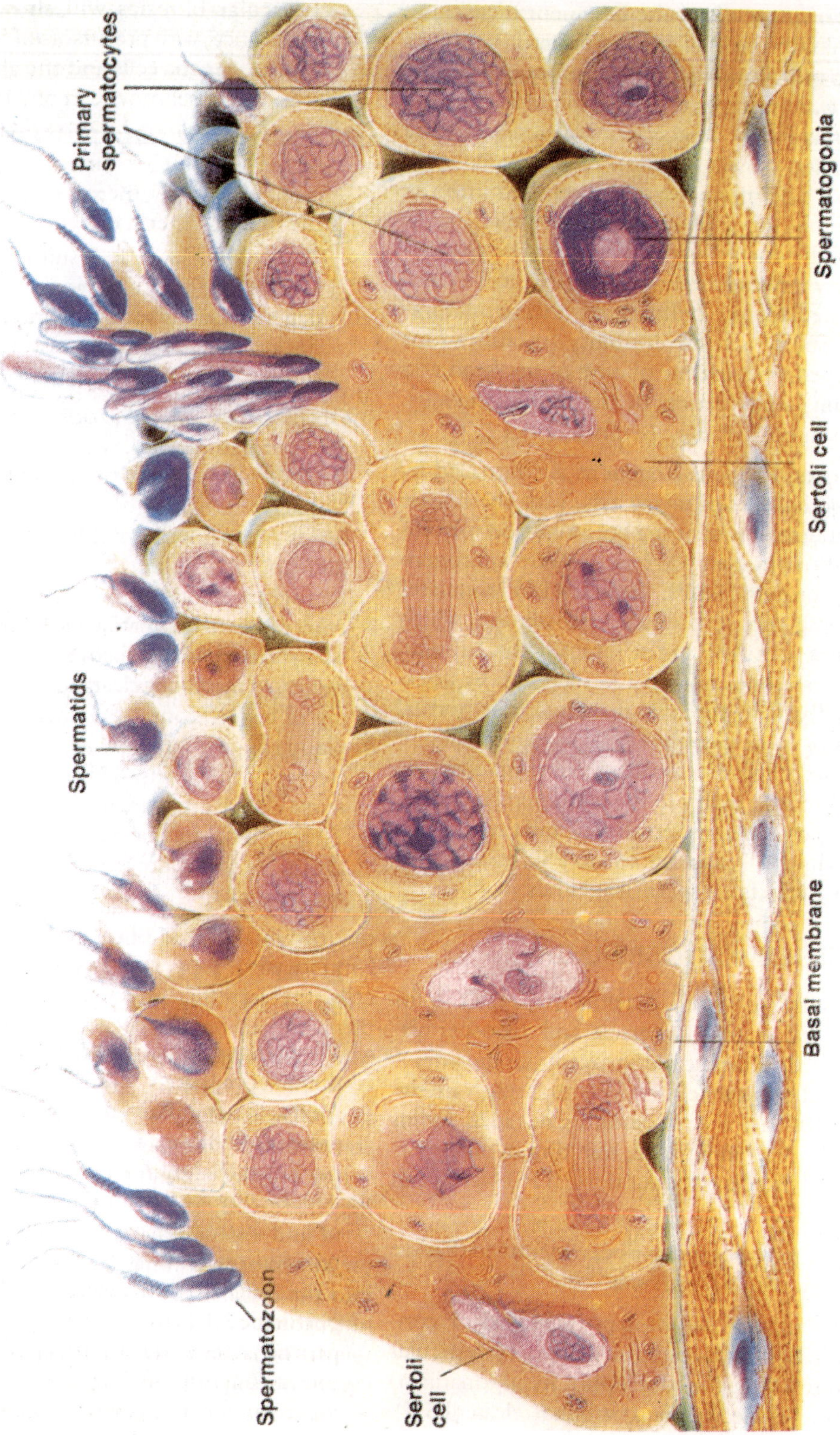

Fig. 13.1. Section of the germinal epithelium of a seminiferous tubule. Clearly recognizable are the groups of germ cells at different stages of maturation: spermatogonia, primary spermatocytes, spermatids and spermatozoa

days. *Spermatogonia* at the basement membrane and lamina propria of the seminiferous tubules undergo meiosis through the *primary and secondary spermatocyt stages*, to form haploid *spermatids*. Spermatids then undergo spermiogenesis, elongate and develop flagella to form recognizable spermatozoa. The spermatozoa are released into the seminiferous tubular lumen, and via the rete testis through the ducti efferentia, arrive in the epididymis. They traverse the epididymis in 2 to 14 days. Here, they acquire cellular and nuclear maturation, mobility and fertilizability (modifications in the sperm plasma membrane of the head and flagellum, stabilization of the sperm nucleus, changes in c-AMP, etc.; Bedford, 1994).

The process of spermatogenesis is controlled by the hypothalamic-pituitary axis, with the release of gonadotrophin-releasing hormones. Sertoli cells respond to pituitary FSH and secrete androgen-binding protein (ABP). Pituitary LH stimulates the Leydig cells to produce testosterone, which combines with ABP in the seminiferous tubules, and testosterone controls LH secretion by negative feedback to the hypothalamus. For normal spermatogenesis, Sertoli cells also produce inhibin, which has a negative feedback effect on pituitary FSH secretion. Injury to the seminiferous epithelium, which damages Sertoli cells and thus inhibin production, will cause the serum FSH to rise, with resulting effects on spermatogenesis.

CAUSES OF AZOOSPERMIA

Damage by toxins or ischaemia may result in focal or total maturation arrest and azoospermia. When a whole tubule is destroyed, this disorder is associated with a much-reduced testis size, with the absence of Sertoli cells, resulting in raised serum FSH. Lesions can be focal, resulting in oligospermia of varying severity, but normal FSH levels can be measured.

Different pathologies have been identified that are associated with *azoospermia*.

a) Pre-testicular pathologies (acquired or congenital), which result in secondary testicular failure (hypogonadotrophic hypogonadism) due to a decreased gonadotrophin release (FSH). Testicular biopsies will show a prepubertal appearance, with precursors of Sertoli cells, prespermatogenetic cells and the absence of Leydig cells (Hadziselimovoc et al., 1986).
b) Androgen resistance: partial or complete defect in the amount or function of the androgen receptor. Usually, there is no maturation beyond the primary spermatocyte.
c) Testicular failure can result in different appearances in the testicular biopsy: sclerosing tubular degeneration is seen in Klinefelter's syndrome, disorganization with extensive hyalinization and tubular atrophy is seen after orchitis.

Obstructive causes of azoospermia will show normal spermatogenesis, with some sloughing off of the superficial layers of the seminiferous epithelium. Congenital absence of the vas deferens, cystic fibrosis or acquired epididymal blocks by TB, or gonococcal or chlamydial infection are described. Retrograde ejaculates also result in azoospermia. The other causes of spermatogenic failure or disorder may be associated with defective testosterone synthesis, decreased metabolic clearance rates, increased binding of testosterone to plasma proteins, increased plasma oestradiol, and low, normal or moderately elevated FSH levels. This can be induced by systemic illness, exposure to drugs or industrial toxins. The germinal aplasia (Sertoli cell only—SCO) syndrome, or the failure of Leydig cells also shows total azoospermia.

HELPING THE AZOOSPERMIC PATIENT

The fertilizing ability of testicular spermatozoa and the first pregnancy following the use of testicular spermatozoa obtained by testicular biopsy in a patient in whose case epididymal sperm retrieval has failed (Schoysman et al., 1993) offers a new opportunity for patients suffering from obstructive or nonobstructive azoospermia. Different surgical retrieval methods for testicular tissue are used. TESE refers to testicular sperm extraction, usually performed by an open biopsy under local or general anaesthesia: a small incision is made in the tunica albuginae, and the small portion of extruding testicular tissue is removed for sperm extraction and identification (Schoysman et al., 1993). When no spermatozoa are found, the surgeon repeats the biopsy in another area of the testis until a minimum amount of spermatozoa for ICSI are found. This technique is usually applied in the case of patients suffering from nonobstructive azoospermia with a poor prognosis, or for spermatid recovery. For men with an active spermatogenesis, with or without obstruction, or in situations where no spermatozoa are retrieved after epididymal sperm aspiration, one can apply a blind testicular fine needle aspiration (TEFNA, TESA) (Craft and Tsirigotis, 1995). The needle is introduced in the testis and by suction, tubular material is removed and flushed back into the culture medium. A 23-gauge needle or biopsy gun needle are usually used for this technique. Different areas, if necessary, can be 'hit' by the needle. This method yields clearly a much lower amount of spermatozoa for ICSI or for freezing as compared to an open biopsy method for the same type of pathology.

The laboratory preparation of surgically retrieved spermatozoa has also developed in the last ten years. Preparation of testicular samples is more complex then preparing epididymal spermatozoa. The standard method for exposing seminiferous tubule contents in order to expose spermatozoa is to shred the biopsy sample (whether a large open biopsy piece or a small needle biopsy sample), by repeatedly pulling the sample apart with tuberculine needles or glass slides. The sample is then crushed by glass slides, vortexed and examined under high power to look for spermatozoa (Kahraman et al., 1996). Modifications to the technique are maceration with micro-grinders or enzymic treatment of the sample with erythrocyte lysing buffer (Nagy et al., 1997). Stewart (1998) unravels individual tubules with a forceps and squeezes them from the middle to the end, so the content is deposited in the petridish, ready for inspection.

Fresh testicular sperm samples can be further processed either by washing in medium or by centrifugation over a discontinuous Percoll gradient to remove blood cells, Sertoli cell nuclei and other debris. Fifty per cent of testicular sperm samples show no motility at the time of preparation, but can still be used for injection: totally immotile spermatozoa that are freshly collected have the same fertilizing potential as motile spermatozoa after 4 h of culture (Nijs et al., 1996). However, when the sample is placed in culture, the proportion of motile sperm is usually the highest (91%) after 24 h of incubation (Nijs et al., 1997), and it is easier to identify the living spermatozoa. Therefore, flexibility is possible in the timing of the testis biopsy, and biopsies the day before oocyte retrieval are scheduled in our routine.

ICSI with testicular spermatozoa is similar to ICSI with ejaculated spermatozoa. After the selection of a morphologically normal, preferably motile spermatozoa from the sperm droplet, the sperm is immobilized in PVP and injected in the oocyte. The outcome of testicular spermatozoa after ICSI is similar to that of ICSI with ejaculated spermatozon (Silber et al., 1995; Mulhall et al., 1997). Due to the small number of viable sperm needed to carry out an ICSI cycle, a single surgical procedure can provide enough sperm for several ICSI attempts. There is good reason to minimize the number of surgical procedures on the testicle, as it has been suggested that the TESE procedure and even the TEFNA or TESA can devascularize regions of the testis and may adversely affect sperm production up to six months post-operatively (Schlegel and Su, 1997). Since freezing techniques for testicular spermatozoa have improved even the freezing of a single spermatozon (Walmsley et al., 1998) and similar results are being obtained as with fresh samples, excess sperm should, therefore, be frozen at the time of the biopsy (even at the time of a diagnostic procedure) (Romero et al., 1996; Oates et al., 1997). Such an approach obviates the need to have donor semen back-up at the time of the ICSI.

CONSIDERATIONS FOR ICSI WITH TESTICULAR SPERMATOZOA

While the combination of surgically retrieved spermatozoa and ICSI has allowed us to help all but a small proportion of azoospermic men to have a chance to become genetic fathers, the technology is not without consequence for the offspring. Consideration should be given to the link between cystic fibrosis and congenital bilateral absence of the vas deferens (CBAVD), and preferably all patients with CBAVD should be screened for potential CF mutations. Consideration should also be given to cytogenetic abnormalities in azoospermic men presenting for treatment. In a review, 13.7% of azoospermic males had an abnormal karyotype (Van Assche et al., 1996), with sex chromosome abnormalities (mainly 47XXY) predominating. Karyotyping should perhaps be a mandatory part of the pretreatment screening process for all men referred for TESE treatment.

A small number of men were found to have detectable lesions on the long arm of the Y chromosome. It was proposed that this was a site of a spermatogenesis gene or azoospermia factor (AZF), with three or more discrete spermatogenesis loci in theYq11 (Voght et al., 1996). Care must be taken since some men with deletions in this area show to be oligospermic and not azoospermic. It appears also that these deletions can appear *de novo* or can be inherited by the son.

As for the future fertility potential of male offspring after testicular sperm injection, it is not known whether this will leave the offspring fertile or infertile. There is as yet no evidence that these assisted reproductive techniques may compromise the reproductive health of the progeny by transmission of the genetic deletions associated with azoospermia. Patients undergoing these procedures should be properly counselled.

THE USE OF SPERMATIDS

In some men showing severe testicular dysfunction, no spermatozoa could be found, either in the ejaculate or in the testicular tissue. After encouraging investigations with rodent spermatids (Ogura et al., 1993, 1994; Ogura and Yanagimachi, 1995; Sofikitis et al., 1996; Kimura and Yanagimachi, 1995a; Ogura et al., 1996), an attractive challenge was to apply the injection of the spermatids collected from the ejaculate, or from testicular material, to the treatment of men with nonobstructive azoospermia. This new approach gives hope in cases of azoospermia which, until recently, were considered untreatable. At the start of the human application, the use of testicular haploid germ cells was considered in two groups of men according to the severity of the testicular dysfunction: the first group included patients with occasional failure of spermiogenesis (*partial spermiogenesis failure*). The second group (*complete spermiogenesis failure*) included men suffering from azoospermia due to primary testicular disorder, caused by different aetiological factors. In the latter, previous histological examination(s) of the testis showed a total absence of complete spermatogenesis in the history of the patient.

Viable embryos were obtained after injection of different types of immature sperm cells: elongated spermatids (Vanderzwalmen et al., 1995, 1997; Fishel et al., 1995, 1997; Tesarik et al., 1996; Chen et al., 1996; Mansour et al., 1996; Antiniori et al., 1997; Araki et al., 1997; Kahraman et al., 1998; Sofikitis et al., 1998a), or round spermatids retrieved from semen (Tesarik et al., 1995, 1996; Barak et al., 1998) or from testis tissue (Hannay, 1995; Fishel et al., 1997; Antiniori et al., 1997; Amer et al., 1997; Vanderzwalmen et al., 1997; Yamanaka et al., 1997; Kahraman et al., 1998).

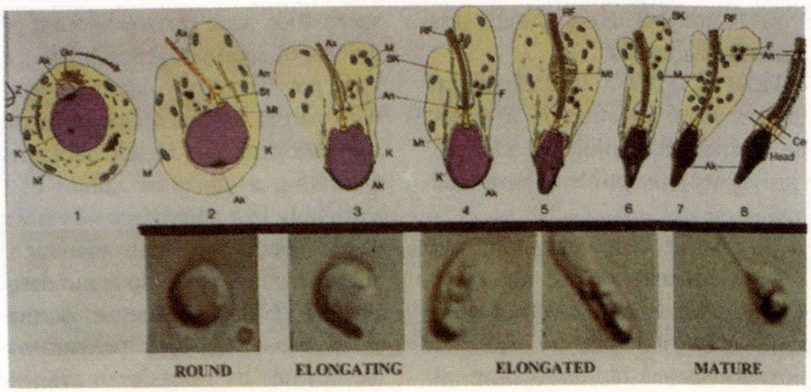

Fig. 13.2: Spermiogenesis: differentiation of a spermatid into a spermatozoon:
–classification after staining and light and electron microscopy
–classification of spermatids in a wet preparation under Hoffman Modulation Contrast

Classification and Identification of Sperm Cell Precursor

One of the problems of spermatid injection is the need for an accurate morphological approach and selective tools for the identification of haploid living cells (Tesarik, 1997; Vanderzwalmen et al., 1998). The studies of Clermont (1963), de Krester and Kerr (1969), and Holstein and Roosen-Runge (1981), using staining techniques under light or electronic microscopy, established a classification making an accurate distinction between the different developmental stages.

In situ, without cytological techniques and under the conventional light microscopic technique, it is more difficult to make a strict distinction between the different developmental stages. Four categories of spermatids can be observed in the wet preparation under the Hoffman Modulation Contrast system, according to the shape, the amount of cytoplasm and the size of the tail: the round, the elongating, the elongated and the mature spermatids just before their release from the Sertoli cells (Fig. 13.2).

It is clear that the methodology for ROS isolation and purification (Yamanaka et al., 1997; Aslam et al., 1998) is a major factor affecting the outcome of spermatid injection, and that such morphological criteria are highly susceptible to intra- and extra-observer variations. Therefore, in order to feel more confident and ascertain that the identification of ROS on the basis of morphological characteristics in the wet preparation are valid, we need tools to confirm our ability to select ROS. Different techniques for the isolation of spermatids with minimum loss of viability were reported by using the fluorescent-activated cell sorter (FACS) method (Aslam et al., 1998), after using computer-assisted image analysis and confocal scanning laser microscopy (Yamanaka et al., 1997), with the use of correct phase-contrast optics on an inverted microscope in order to identify the acrosomal vesicle (Verheyen et al., 1998).

Clinical Results

The injection technique of spermatids into the ooplasm was similar to the conventional ICSI method with mature spermatozoa, using an injection pipette with an inner diameter of 6–7 μm (Vanderzwalmen et al., 1996; Tesarik and Mendoza, 1996). Fertilization, embryo quality and pregnancy rates are affected by the type of male germ cells (round, elongating, elongated spermatids) found in the testicular biopsies (Fig. 13.3) and injected into oocytes (Vanderzwalmen et al., 1997). This was confirmed by Fishel et al. (1997), who observed, using sibling oocytes, that the overall fertilization rate with ROS was significantly lower than that with elongated cells isolated from testicular tissue. Considering the normality of the centrosome (Simerly et al., 1995), the nuclear protein maturation (Souza et al., 1998) and an easy identification, the elongated spermatids (ELS) stage should be more suitable for injection.

The presence of these different cell types depends on the severity of testicular pathology (Vanderzwalmen et al., 1997). We observed only cells in the

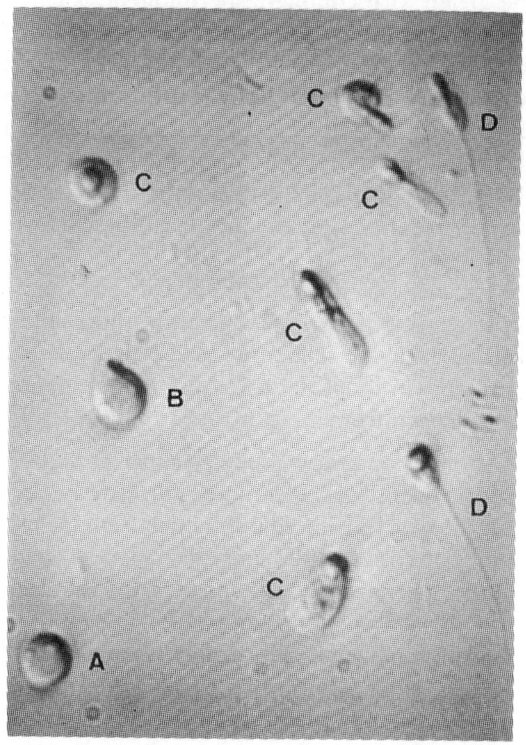

Fig. 13.3. Identification of different types of spermatids
A. round spermatid with acrosome protrusion
B. elongating spermatid
C. elongated spermatid at different stages of development
D. mature spermatids removed from the germinal epithelium cells—immature spermatozoa

elongation stage (elongating, elongated and mature) in the group, with occasional failure of complete spermatogenesis. Histopathological examination clearly showed a correlation between the probability of finding spermatids in the elongation phase and the percentage of seminiferous tubules showing some spermatozoa. Histopathological examination of testes exhibiting a complete failure of spermiogenesis showed an extremely low percentage of tubules (<10%) containing few ROS, presenting a picnotic nucleus, in degenerated or atrophic phase, and also some desquamated spermatids (van de Casseye, 1994).

For patients with complete spermatogenesis arrest, fertilization rates are extremely poor (8%). In the group with previous active spermatogenesis in few tubules, acceptable fertilization rates after spermatid injection were obtained (54% with ELS and 27% with ROS) (Vanderzwalmen et al., 1997). In the group with complete spermiogenesis failure, specific alterations induce an absolute inability to produce mature spermatozoa in few seminiferous tubules. The morphological identification and isolation does not, however, reveal anything about the viability or the genomical normality of the ROS. Aslam et al. (1998) evaluate the viability of the germ cells using the Trypan blue exclusion test. It was shown that 97% of ROS are viable at the moment of collection. But without staining or destroying the cell, it is currently impossible to distinguish living cells from dead cells, to identify spermatids in apoptose and to differentiate genomically normal from abnormal spermatids.

We showed previously (Vanderzwalmen et al., 1997) that the quality of the embryos correlated directly with the type of haploid cells which were injected. In fact, the number of embryos of good quality selected for transfer was low when ROS were used, and especially when the embryos originated from a man with complete spermiogenesis failure. Janny and Menezo (1994) identified a strong paternal effect on embryo development and blastocyst formation.

Acceptable pregancy rates have already been reported after the injection of elongated spermatids (Fishel et al., 1996; Mansour et al., 1996; Araki et al., 1997; Vanderzwalmen et al., 1997). But the results obtained after the injection of round spermatids remain dramatically lower. Until today, the birth of only seven babies has been achieved after ROS, 3 using spermatids from the ejaculates (Tesarik et al., 1995, 1996; Barak et al., 1998), and 5 using ROS extracted from testicular tissue (Antiniori et al., 1997; Vanderzwalmen et al., 1997). In all these cases, the male patient did present in his past history the presence of spermatozoa or ELS in the ejaculate or in the testicular tissue. On the contrary, in all cases where the male patient showed a complete absence of ELS or spermatozoa in previous ejaculate or testicular biopsy, no pregnancy has been obtained so far with the use of ROS (Hannay, 1995; Amer et al., 1997; Vanderzwalmen et al., 1997; Barros et al., 1998; Bernabeu et al., 1998; Kahraman et al., 1998; Sofikitis et al., 1998 a,b). Can we still consider spermatid injection in cases of patients showing a complete block of spermiogenesis in preliminary explorative biopsy? Can we still consider, in such a situation, ROS injection as a useful therapy?

It is reported that an explorative testicle biopsy showing SCO syndrome or maturation arrest at the level of the spermatocyte I does not preclude the possibility of finding ELS or spermatozoa for injection (Amer et al., 1997; Vanderzwalmen et al., 1997; Barros et al., 1998; Bernabeu et al., 1998; Kahraman et al., 1998; Sofikitis et al., 1998b). Therefore, the diagnostic testicles biopsy should be taken only as a prognostic factor and the result should not be an exclusion criterion for the patients. Thus, a trial should always be offered to azoospermic patients.

Couples who want to enter this treatment should be advised about the hazards, risk and the extremely low efficacy of the procedure of ROS. The risk of genetic transmission of Y chromosome deletions and of genomic imprinting anomalies should not be overlooked, and care should be taken to avoid the serious consequences of such pathologies. In fact, some paternally expressed genes must be imprinted during spermatogenesis for later function in the offspring. The excellent health of all of the offspring observed in the animal model after ROS (Ogura et al., 1994; Sofikitis et al., 1996; Kimura and Yanagimachi, 1995a), or secondary spermatocyte injection (Kimura and Yanagimachi, 1995b), and their fertility potential suggest that such cells can provide the paternally imprinted genes needed for embryonic development, and that the nucleus of ROS is genetically ready to participate in a normal fertilization process (Ogura and Yanagimachi, 1995). A better knowledge of the different imprinted genes, of their consolidation and the mechanism of reactivation of normally silent allele could reduce epigenetic risk factors which might turn out to be involved.

CONSIDERATIONS CONCERNING SPERMATID INJECTIONS

In conclusion, it now seems that there should be a reconsideration of the earlier enthusiasm to help men suffering from extremely severe testicular disorder with the use of the spermatid injection procedure. At the present state of this approach, the spermatid indication seems more favourable for azoospermic men who have previously proved their capacity to produce spermatozoa, albeit only a few. However, in severe pathological cases, the usefulness of ROS remains to be proved on a large scale. Therefore, these data suggest that spermatid injection should be considered only as an option in case of an unexpected absence of spermatozoa. In the case of patients with a complete block of spermiogenesis, ROS should not be proposed to couples as a therapy.

If spermatid therapy with ROS can be considered as a treatment in view of the actual results, further research is needed first to evaluate the required *in vitro* culture conditions to induce progression of spermatocyte I or spermatocyte II (extremely rare in humans) into the ROS stage, and finally, into a more elongated stage. Secondly, an alternative to improve the feasibility of the method should consist of finding a viability selection test in the case of ROS injection.

A possible avenue is offered by the results of culture attempts of round spermatids until the appearance of the flagellum (Aslam and Fishel, 1998; Tesarik et al., 1998). Because this kind of approach seems very promising, there is a need that several groups start research programmes in an attempt to find the appropriate protocols (maturation with FSH alone, maturation with the whole spermatogenic population or by using isolated cells, presence of testicular tissue, optimization of the temperature condition) that could successfully mature, *in vitro*, the ROS and spermatocyte I up to the elongated stage or even mature spermatozoa at an acceptable rate. Both in the mice species (Kimura and Yanagimachi, 1995b) and in the human (Sofikitis et al., 1998c), pregnancies have been obtained after injection of secondary spermatocytes.

Still, it remains mandatory that we should make careful investigations concerning the gene expression and genomic imprinting when using prespermatozoal cells in clinical application. Since genomic imprinting is an epigenetic process, a disruption of normal imprinting can cause human genetic diseases and promote the development of malignant childhood tumours. Therefore, when using immature cells for conception, the screening of the patients is recommended. Clearly, this goes well beyond a simple karyotype and demands further work on the genes of the Y chromosome.

CONCLUSION

It now appears that most types of male infertility, even the extreme cases like maturation arrest, Sertoli cell only, post-chemotherapy azoospermia and Klinefelter syndrome, can be succesfully treated. Ironically, female age and ovarian reserve, rather than the source, quantity or quality of the spermatozoa, are the major determinants of the success of assisted reproductive treatment in these patients.

REFERENCES

Amer, M. et al. (1997). 'Is complete spermiogenesis failure a good indication for spermatid conception?' *Lancet*, **350**: 116.

Antiniori, S. et al. (1997). 'Fertilization with human testicular spermatids: four successful pregnancies.' *Hum. Reprod.*, **12**: 286–91.

Araki, Y. et al. (1997). 'Intracytoplasmic injection with late spermatids: A successful procedure in achieving childbirth for couples in which the male partner suffers from azoospermia due to deficient spermatogenesis', *Fertil. Steril.*, **67**: 559–61.

Aslam, I. and S. Fishel (1998). 'Short-term *in vitro* culture and cryopreservation of spermatogenic cells used for human *in vitro* conception', *Hum. Reprod.*, **13**: 634–8

Aslam, I., A. Robin, K. Dowell et al. (1998). 'Isolation, purification and assessment of viability of spermatogenic cells from testicular biopsies of azoospermic men', *Hum. Reprod.*, **13**: 639–45.

Barak, Y. et al. (1998). 'Pregnancy and birth after transfer of embryos that developed from single-nucleated zygotes obtained by injection of round spermatids', *Fert. Steril.*, **70**: 67–70.

Barros, A. et al. (1998). 'Intracytoplasmic injection of ejaculate and testicle spermatids: Report on 35 cycles', *Hum. Reprod.*, **13**: 154–6.

Bernabeu, R. et al. (1998). 'Successful pregnancy after spermatid injection', *Hum. Reprod.*, 1899–1900.

Bedford, J. (1994). 'Epididymal physiology: It's implications for epididymal microsurgery', in R. Schoysman (ed.), *Microsurgery of Male Infertility*, Fondatione per gli studi sulla riproduzione umana, pp. 71–100.

Craft, I. and M. Tsirigotis (1995). 'Simplified recovery, preparation and cryopreservation of testicular spermatozoa', *Hum. Reprod.*, **10**: 1623–7.

Chen, S.U. et al. (1996). 'Fertilization and embryo cleavage after intracytoplasmic spermatid injection in an obstructive azoospermic patient with defective spermiogenesis', *Fertil. Steril.*, **66**: 157–60.

Clermont, Y. (1963). 'The cycle of the seminiferous epithelium in man', *Amer. J. Anat.*, **112**: 35–51.

de Krester, M. and J.B. Kerr (1969). 'The cytology of the testis', in E. Knobil and J.D. Neill (eds.), *The Physiology of Reproduction*, Raven, New York.

Elder, K. and Elliot (eds.) (1995). *The Use of Testicular and Epididymal Sperm in I.V.F.*, Ladybrod Publishing.

Fishel, S. et al. (1995). 'Pregnancy after intracytoplasmic injection of spermatid', *Lancet*, **245**: 1641–2.

______(1997). 'Human fertilisation with round and elongated spermatids', *Hum. Reprod.*, **12**: 336–40.

Fishel, S. et al. (1996). 'Spermatid conception: A stage too early, or a time too soon?' *Hum. Reprod.*, **11**: 1371–5

Hannay, T. (1995). 'New Japanese IVF method finally made available in Japan', *Nature Med.*, **1**: 289–90.

Hadziselimovoc, F. et al. (1986). 'The significance of postnatal gonadotropin surge for testicular development in normal and cryptochidic testes', *J. Urol.*, **136**: 274–6.

Holstein, A. and E. Roosen-Runge (1981). *Atlas of Human Spermatogenesis*, Grosse Verlag, Berlin.

Janny, L. and Y. Menezo (1994). 'Evidence for a strong paternal effect on human preimplantation embryo development and blastocyst formation', *Mol. Reprod., Dev.*, **38**: 36–42.

Kahraman, S. et al. (1996). 'High implantation and pregnancy rates with testicular sperm extraction and ICSI in obstructive and non-obstructive azoospermia', *Hum. Reprod.*, **11**: 673–6.

Kahraman, S. et al. (1998). 'Multiple pregnancies obtained by testicular spermatid injection in combination with intracytoplasmic sperm injection', *Hum. Reprod.*, **13**: 104–10.

Kimura, Y. and R. Yanagimachi (1995 a). 'Mouse oocytes injected with testicular spermatozoa or round spermatids can develop into normal offspring', *Dev.*, **121**: 2397–405.

______(1995 b). 'Development of normal mice from oocytes injected with secondary spermatocyte nuclei', *Biol. Reprod.*, **53**: 855–62.

Mansour, R. et al. (1996). 'Pregnancy and delivery after intracytoplasmic injection of spermatids into human oocytes', *Middle East Fertil. Soc. J.*, **1**: 223–5.

Mulhall, J. et al. (1997). 'Presence of mature sperm in testicular parenchyma of men with non-obstructive azoospermia: Prevalence and predictive factors', *Urology*, **49**: 91–5, (discussions) 95–6.

Nagy, Z. et al. (1997). 'An improved treatment procedure for testicular biopsy specimens offers more efficient sperm recovery: Case series', *Fertil. Steril.*, **68**: 376–9.

Nijs, M. et al. (1996). 'Fertilizing ability of immotile spermatozoa after ICSI', *Hum. Reprod.*, **11**: 10, 2180–5.

______(1997). '*In vitro* culture of testicular spermatozoa: An improvement for the ICSI outcome?' Abstr. 10th World Congress on IVF, Vancouver.

Ogura, A. et al. (1993). 'Behaviour of hamster and mouse round spermatid nuclei incorporated into mature oocytes by elecrofusion', *Zygote*, **1**: 1–8.

______(1994). 'Birth of normal young after elecrofusion of mouse oocytes with round spermatids', *Proc. Natl. Acad. Sci.* USA, **91**: 7460–2.

Oates, R. et al. (1997). 'Fertilization and pregnancy using intentionally cryopreserved testicular tissue as the sperm source for ICSI in 10 men with nonobstructive azoospermia', *Hum. Reprod*, **12**: 734–9.

Ogura, A. and R. Yanagimachi (1995). 'Spermatids as male gametes', *Reprod. Fertil. Dev.*, 7: 165–9.

Ogura, A. et al. (1996). 'Mouse oocytes injected with cryopreserved round spermatids can develop into normal offspring', *J. Ass. Reprod. Genetics.*, **13**: 431–4.

Palermo, G. et al. (1992). 'Pregnancies after intracytoplasmic injection of single spermatozoon into an oocyte', *Lancet.*, **340**: 17–8.

Romero, J. et al. (1996). 'Fertilization after ICSI with cryopreserved testicular spermatozoa', *Fertil. Steril.*, **65**: 877–9.

Silber, S. et al. (1995). 'High fertilization and pregnancy rate after intracytoplasmic sperm injection with spermatozoa obtained from the testicle biopsy', *Hum. Reprod.*, **10**: 148–52.

Schlegel, P. and L. Su (1997). 'Physiological consequences of testicular sperm extraction', *Hum. Reprod.*, **12**: 1688–92.

Schoysman, R. et al. (1993). 'Pregnancy after fertilization with human testicular sperm', *Lancet*, **342**: 1237.

Simerly, C. et al. (1995). 'The paternal inheritance of the centrosome, the cell's microtubule-organizing center, in humans, and the implications for infertility', *Nature Med.*, **1**: 47–52.

Sofikitis, N. et al. (1996). 'Beneficial effects of electrical stimulation before round spermatid nuclei injections into rabbit oocytes on fertilization and subsequent embryonic development', *Fertil. Steril.*, **65**: 176–85.

______(1998). 'Ooplasmic injection of elongating spermatids for the treatment of non-obstructive azoospermia', *Hum. Reprod.*, **13**: 709–14.

Sofikitis, N. et al. (1998b). 'Micro- and macro-consequences of ooplasmic injections of early haploid male gametes', *Hum. Reprod. Update*, **4**: 197–212.

______(1998c). 'Delivery of a healthy male after ooplasmic injection of secondary spermatocytes', *J. Androl.* (suppl), **57**.

Souza, M. et al. (1998). 'Current problems with spermatid conception', *Hum. Reprod.*, **13**: 255–8.

Stewart, B. (1998). '*The use of testicular and epididymal sperm in I.V.F.*', in Elder, K. Elliot (ed.), Ladybrod Publishing.

Tesarik, J. et al. (1995). 'Viable embryos from injection of round spermatids into oocytes', *N. Engl. J. Med.*, **333**: 525.

______(1996). 'Spermatid injection into human oocytes II: Clinical application in the treatment of infertility due to non-obstructive azoospermia', *Hum. Reprod.*, **11**: 780–83.

Tesarik, J. et al. (1998). 'Differentiation of spermatogenic cells during *in vitro* culture of testicular biopsy samples from patients with obstructive azoospermia: Effect of recombinant follicle stimulating hormone', *Hum. Reprod.*, **13**: 2772–81.

Tesarik, J. and C. Mendoza (1996). 'Spermatid injection into human oocytes, I: Laboratory techniques and special features of zygote development', *Hum. Reprod.*, **11**: 772–9.

Tesarik, J. (1997). 'Sperm or spermatid conception', *Ferti. Steril.*, **68**: 214–6.

Vanassche, E. et al. (1996). 'Cytogenetics in infertile men', *Hum. Reprod.*, **11**: Suppl. 4, 1–24, (discussion) 25–6.

Van de Casseye M. (1994). 'The pathology of the testis and epididymis', in *Microsurgery of male infertility*, Fondazione per gli studi sulla riproduzione umana. 51–70.

Vandevorst, M. et al. (1996). 'Surgical recovery of sperm for ICSI', J. Studd (ed.), *The yearbook of the RCOG*, RCOG Press, 167–77.

Vanderzwalmen, P. et al. (1995). 'Fertilization of an oocyte microinseminated with a spermatid in an *in vitro* fertilization programme', *Hum. Reprod.*, **10**: 502–3.

______(1996). 'Two essential steps for a successful intracytoplasmic sperm injection: Injection of immobilized spermatozoa after rupture of the oolemma', *Hum. Reprod.*, **11**: 540–7.

______(1997). 'Intracytoplasmic injection of spermatids retrieved from testicular tissue: Influence of testicular pathology, type of selected spermatids and oocyte activation', *Hum. Reprod.*, **12**: 1203–13.

Vanderzwalmen, P. et al. (1998). 'The problems of spermatid microinjection in the human: The need for an accurate morphological approach and selective methods for viable and normal cells', *Hum. Reprod.*, **13**: 515–9.

Verheyen, G. et al. (1998). 'Simple and reliable identification of the human round spermatid by inverted phase-contrast microscopy', *Hum. Reprod.*, **13**: 101–8

Voght, P. et al. (1996). 'Human Y chromosome azoospermia factors (AZF) mapped to different subregions in Yq11', *Hum. Mol. Genet*, **5**: 933–43.

Yamanaka, K. et al. (1997). 'Ooplasmic round spermatid nuclear injection procedures as an experimental treatment for nonobstructive azoospermia', *J. Assist. Reprod. Genet.*, **14**: 55–62.

Walmsley, R. et al. (1998). 'The first birth and ongoing pregnancies associated with sperm cryopreservation within evacuated egg zonae', *Hum. Reprod. Suppl.*, **4**: 61–70.

14

Route of Embryo Transfer and Implantation: A Dilemma

Michelle Hutchison, Jesse J. Hade, and Alan H.DeCherney

INTRODUCTION

In vitro fertilization-embryo transfer (IVF-ET) is a relatively recent addition to the field of reproductive gynaecology. It has been in use since the 1970s and offers significant hope to couples suffering from infertility. The use of assisted reproductive technologies (ART) is offered to patients with tubal factor infertility and to couples in whom alternative treatments have failed. Since the success rate of IVF-ET is only 20%–30% improvements in both practice and techniques are needed.

OVUM CAPTURE, TRANSPORT, AND IMPLANTATION

Oocyte fertilization and embryo development is a complex process, with many obstacles. Upon the release of the dominant follicle, the ovum is captured by the lush folds of the fimbria and begins its descent into the uterus. Although the human fallopian tube measures only 8 to 13 cm, the transport time through the fallopian tube is approximately 80 hours (Croxatto et al., 1978). The majority of this time (72 hours) is spent in the ampullary portion of the tube. The cilia located on the mucosal ridges of the ampulla create a turbulent stream within the tube when a functioning tubal muscularis and secretory glandular activity are present. This turbulent stream is responsible for the transport of the embryo from the ampulla to the endometrial cavity.

The embryo enters the endometrial cavity as a morula approximately three days after fertilization, and continues to develop into a blastocyst. The hatching of the blastocyst from the zone pellucida occurs by day six to seven and initiates the process of implantation. Once hatched, the blastocyst continues to grow and attaches itself to the epithelium of the endometrium on days 6 to 8. It then moves through the basement membrane of the uterine epithelium into the stroma.

The attachment of the blastocyst to the endometrial surface epithelium is dependent upon the expression of adhesion molecules. The adhesion molecules believed to be involved in this process include immunoglobulins (ICAM, VCAM, PECAM and Modcan-1), fibronectin, vitronectin, integrin $\alpha_v\beta_3$, as well as other potential factors (Lessey et al., 1992).

Next, the penetration of the stroma by the invading trophoblast occurs. The developing embryo secretes a collagenase enzyme which digests the basement membrane of the extracellular matrix (Puistola et al., 1989). The other enzymes involved in this process include metalloproteins, proteinases, gelatinases, stromelysins, metallolastases and urokinase (Queenan et al., 1987).

Local oedema occurs as a result of prostaglandin release during the degradation process and permits the trophoblast to completely invade through to the stroma. As the trophoblast invades, it sends long protrusions between the tight junctions of the epithelial cells and ruptures these adhesive bands. This enables direct contact between the trophoblast and subepithelial zone. The trophoblast then attaches itself preferentially to the basement membrane components, laminin and fibronectin which surround the decidual cells (Loke, 1989).

The depth of penetration by the trophoblast cells is regulated, in part, by decidual protease inhibitors (Marshall, 1987). Upon reaching the stroma, the trophoblast synthesizes and secretes an extracellular matrix protein, which facilitates attachment to the surrounding tissue.

The developing embryo is a semiallograft since it contains both paternal and maternal gene products. The antigens contained on the surface of the embryo are unique and considered immunologically foreign to the maternal host. It is believed that the conceptus is able to continue growing and implants by escaping detection by the maternal immune system. One likely explanation proposes that the invading trophoblast at the maternal-fetal interface does not express the classic major histocompatibility complex (MHC) class I or II molecules (Gudice, 1994). However, a distinct form of MHC class I, termed HLA-G, is expressed (Wegmann, 1989). It is believed that the function of the HLA-G is to regulate the natural killer cells (NK cell) activity within the uterus. Through this and other unknown mechanisms, the implanting blastocyst is capable of regulating immune and complement factors which may otherwise have had deleterious effects on its development, implantation and growth.

Embryo Transfer

An integral yet critical component of the IVF process is the embryo transfer procedure. The most common method of embryo transfer is through a transcervical route. The other methods include laparoscopic-guided tubal transfers and sonographic-guided transmyometrial transfers. The transcervical technique involves the use of a special catheter, which traverses the cervical canal to the endometrium and allows for the injection of the embryo directly into the uterine cavity (Tan, 1990). However, this method is not always simple since cervical factors may cause technical difficulty with this procedure. Multiple attempts at embryo transfer can cause cervical trauma and ultimately, a reduced pregnancy rate (Visser et al., 1993).

One method of embryo transfer that avoids cervical manipulation and trauma is the transmyometrial approach. This technique involves the transvaginal ultrasound-guided transmyometrial placement of the embryo. It was initially believed that this method would benefit those patients with cervical stenosis, as well as those with failed prior attempted transfers. However, no benefit was achieved by performing a transmyometrial transfer compared to the transcervical approach (Groutz et al., 1997).

Laparoscopic-guided tubal transfer allows the embryo to develop in the fallopian tube rather than in culture media. This method of embryo transfer closely mimics a natural conception cycle. Embryos that are transferred by this method spend an average of only 26 hours in culture media, compared to 72 hours with current transcervical methods. This is advantageous since the transfer occurs at the pronuclear stage of development and more embryos can be salvaged for transfer and freezing. Tubal transfer enables the embryo to arrive at the uterine cavity at the appropriate stage of development and reduces the deleterious effects of uterine trauma that are associated with a transcervical approach.

Studies which compare tubal versus transcervical methods of embryo transfer have not revealed any advantage when 'fresh' embryos are used (Tanbo, 1990). However, when cryopreserved embryos are used, a statistically higher pregnancy rate is achieved during the tubal transfer cycles compared to intrauterine-placed embryos (68% versus 24%, respectively) (Van Voorhis, 1995). Factors which influence pregnancy rates during the frozen embryo transfer cycles include patient age, and the number and quality of embryos transferred (Toner, 1993).

Zygote Intrafallopian Transfer Improves The Pregnancy Rate In Select Patients

There are several different types of *in vitro* fertilization (IVF), such as the standard transcervical embryo transfer (ET), zygote intrafallopian transfer (ZIFT), gamete intrafallopian transfer (GIFT), tubal embryo transfer (TET), and peritoneal oocyte and sperm transfer (POST). Despite the myriad advances in assisted reproduction, the clinical pregnancy rate remains at 20–25% (SART, 1992; 1996). For unclear reasons, the majority of embryos obtained by IVF fail to implant. Modifications of the standard IVF-ET, including modifying the ET catheter, changing patient position during ET, using general anaesthesia for ET (Diedrich, 1989), using six or more embryos for ET (Azem, 1995), and using fibrin sealant (Ben-Rafail-Z, 1995), have also failed to improve implantation and pregnancy rates.

In a study by Levran et al. (1995), the authors investigated the value of ZIFT in a case-control study of patients with repeated failure of implantation with IVF-ET. They included patients with at least three previous failures of implantation in IVF-ET cycles, in which a minimum of three embryos were transferred. This criteria for infertility consisted of male factor or unexplained infertility, with same criteria control patients who also underwent an additional cycle of the standard IVF-ET in that same period. They examined 70 patients undergoing 92 ZIFT cycles. A summary of the results showed that the pregnancy rates and implantation rates were significantly higher in the ZIFT group, measuring 34.2% and 8.7%, respectively, compared to the controls with 17.1% and 4.4%, respectively. The authors concluded that repeated failure of implantation in standard IVF-ET is a criterion for IVF-ZIFT, with a need for further randomized studies to support their observations.

ZIFT successfully supports embryonal growth in the natural tubal environment and the subsequent transfer of the embryos into the uterus via more physiological regulations (Yovitch, 1988). ZIFT is also thought to prevent spillage of embryos out of the uterus following transcervical ET (Schulman, 1986). Several prospective randomized studies in the early 1990s showed no difference in implantation rates and pregnancy rates in IVF-ZIFT compared to standard IVF-ET (Fluker et al., 1993; Toth et al., 1992). Patient selection plays a role in the success of different treatment methods. In the study by Levran et al., their patients had a history of repeated failure of implantation in standard IVF-ET prior to undergoing ZIFT. In addition to the higher implantation and pregnancy rates per cycle with ZIFT compared to standard IVF-ET, their study also demonstrated that those patients with poor-quality embryos had relatively higher pregnancy rates with ZIFT than with the standard IVF-ET. Indices such as regularity of blastomeres, degree of fragmentation and rate of cleavage determine embryo quality (Goryeth et al., 1995; Staessen et al., 1992). Perhaps the benefits of ZIFT, such as the more physiological culture conditions in the tube, help explain the improved pregnancy rate with the use of this procedure. Thus, low-quality embryos in IVF cycles may be a proposed criterion for ZIFT, as well as the criterion of a history of repeated IVF-ET failures. More research with prospective randomized studies could further support these findings.

Delay Of Embryo Transfer Improves The Outcome Of IVF

Despite advances in the field of ARTs, there remains much room for improvement, with the pregnancy rate for IVF being only 21% for the year 1994, according to the Society for Assisted Reproductive Technology (SART, 1996). The aetiology of this low success rate is unclear, whether it may be secondary to a suboptimal *in vitro* environment or an inability to select good quality embryos, or both. Some studies have turned to examining the clinical outcomes of using different culture media for IVF and ET and different time frames. Traditionally, IVF includes ET on day number two (48 hours after retrieval), with two- to four-cell embryos. This is different from the *in vivo* embryo that reaches the uterus for implantation on day four or five (Harper, 1994). With the advent of an improved embryo culture media (Bavister, 1995; Post et al., 1998), and assisted hatching on day three after retrieval (Cohen et al., 1990; Schooleroff et al., 1994), ET with IVF was delayed to day number three after oocytes retrieval. Previously, the standard culture media was human tubal fluid medium. A change was then made in 1994 at the University of Louisville/Alliant Health System programme from human tubal fluid to a glucose- and phosphate-free medium compatible with human embryo development and pregnancy (Conaghan, et al., 1993; Quinn et al., 1995). It is also shown that glucose and phosphate are inhibitory to various animal species embryo development (Sehsagiri and Bavister, 1991).

Given the favourable outcomes obtained with this media, a delay of ET from day two to day three was instituted in 1995. With such a delay, it was thought that the differences in cell number would facilitate selecting those embryos that were rapidly dividing for ET. A review of these patients for the year 1995 was performed, comparing day-two and day-three ET. The results showed an improvement in the pregnancy rate outcomes in the day-three ET which, in 1996, propagated a delay of ET to day three. Carrillo et al. then published a retrospective review that demonstrated these improved clinical outcomes of day-two versus day-three ET, using a culture media with no glucose or phosphate in 176 IVF-ET patients (Carillo et al., 1998). In their study, Carrillo et al. noted a significantly greater number of blastomeres in embryos transferred on day three. Their results also showed a significantly higher clinical pregnancy rate in day-three ET than that with day-two transfer, measuring 51% versus 29%, respectively ($p < 0.01$). In addition, the implantation rate was again higher in the day-three group than in to the day-two group, at 24% versus 13%, respectively ($p<0.01$). No significant difference in the rate of multiple pregnancies was discerned. The day-three transfer group had in overall greater number of blastomeres, with 85% of the embryos beyond the four-cell stage and 49% with eight or more cells. In comparison, the day-two group had a majority of embryos in the two and four cell stages, measuring 86% and 43%, respectively. The study also calculated the pregnancy rates in comparison to the cell number per embryo and found that higher pregnancy rates were associated with greater cell number per embryo. Thus, this study supported the observations that good-quality embryos are more successful in developing beyond the 4-cell stage than poor-quality embryos, as noted by the increased pregnancy rates in this study by Carrillo and in previous studies (Bolton et al., 1989; Braude et al., 1988). Waiting the additional 24 hours allows one to select such developing embryos and these higher-cell-number embryos will increase the pregnancy rate of the IVF-ET cycle (Claman et al., 1987; Staessen et al., 1992). After the four-cell stage, the embryos undergo a transition from the maternal to the embryonic genome; only a successful transition leads to viable embryos (Telford et al., 1990).

Several other studies have examined the differences in the outcomes of day-two versus day-three ET and the results vary. Both Edwards et al. (1984) and van Os et al. (1989) found no change in the pregnancy rate between day-two and day-three transfers. A large retrospective study by Dawson et al. (1995), reported a significantly higher implantation rate and lower embryo loss rate in the day-three ET group. However, no change in the pregnancy rate or clinical abortion rate was noted (ibid., 1995).

Varying results have also been obtained with the delay of ET to days four and five. One study showed no effect on the pregnancy rate by waiting till day five, while other studies found higher implantation rates but no change in the pregnancy rate when the transfer was delayed to day four (Scholtes 1996; Hunsman et al., 1994). However, all studies that were performed prior to the study by Carrillo et al. (Carillo et al., 1998) used traditional media, and not glucose and phosphate-free media. This may explain the discrepancy in the results observed by different authors.

As mentioned earlier, both glucose and phosphate have proven to be inhibitory to embryo growth in other species, and to inhibit human embryo development. Glucose levels are relatively lower in the fallopian tube during the time of fertilization than the level of sugar in the uterus (Gardner et al., 1996). Keeping the embryo in a glucose-free environment may have a subtle effect that influences the development of a select group of embryos, thus accounting for the varying results for the timing of ET. However, a plentitude of successful pregnancies have been achieved with both glucose- and phosphate-rich media and with early return of ET, which shows that more research is needed to further understand the nutritional and metabolic needs of the human embryo.

The Blastocyst And Assisted Hatching

A delay of ET to the blastocyst stage improves the implantation rate. By waiting till day five or six, ET is thought to be more physiological, and only the most viable embryos will bypass the four- to eight-cell block and survive the blastocyst and hatching stages. Assisted hatching of the zona pellucida has been associated with increased implantation rates. In this procedure, an opening is made in the zona pellucida in order to facilitate the embryo's emergence. In addition, it has been postulated that if the zona pellucida is enzymatically softened so that zona-free blastocysts can be transferred, improved cell-cell interactions and anchoring of the embryo to the endometrium will occur.

In a recent prospective study by Fong et al. (Fong et al., 1998), the pregnancy rate was reviewed in a group of patients after the transfer of day-five blastocysts with enzymatic treatment of the zona pellucida. The clinical PRs per cycle and implantation rates were improved over the standard, measuring 53% and 33%, respectively. Thus, zona-manipulated blastocysts implant relatively well, possibly due to better anchorage and dialogue of the embryo with the endometrium.

FACTORS THAT INFLUENCE ET OUTCOME

A major limiting factor of ET is failure of implantation. Factors which may interfere with the success of ET include endometriosis, hydrosalpinx, and cervical infections. These factors may play a critical role in the outcome of an IVF-ET cycle, and should be addressed and managed prior to starting a fertility cycle.

Effect Of Cervical Infections On IVF

Infections caused by Chlamydia, gonorrhoea and other pathogenic organisms have recently been linked to decreased implantation and pregnancy rates in IVF cycles (Witkin et al., 1994). It is speculated that direct contamination of the embryos with microorganisms colonized in the cervix can also cause a reduction in implantation. Microbial organisms, such as *E. coli* and Streptococcus species, have been detected as possible organisms responsible for reduced implantation rates during IVF-ET cycles (Renato et al., 1998). However, further investigation is needed to determine if the treatment of cervical colonization by microorganisms prior to ET improves the implantation and pregnancy rates.

Endometriosis And IVF

Endometriosis is defined as the presence of ectopic glands and stroma outside of the uterus. It is a progressive disease that can lead to both pelvic pain and infertility. Approximately 3–10% of women in the reproductive age-group and 25–35% of women with infertility have the disease (Olive and Schwartz, 1993; Cramer, 1993). It is thought that endometrial cells can spread by mechanical methods or can arise via means of metaplasia, whereas disease progression may be determined by immune mechanisms.

Endometriosis was first described by John Sampson in 1927. He postulated that a retrograde flow of endometrial tissue from the uterus, through the tubes, into the peritoneal cavity is the aetiology of this disease (Sampson, 1927). Investigations performed by others have validated his theory (Liu and Hitchchock, 1986; Ishimaru and Masuzaki, 1991; Jenkins et al., 1986). He also believed that vascular and lymphatic transport is responsible for the dissemination of endometriosis to distant sites (Ueki, 1991).

Another theory involves the transformation of the coelomic epithelium into endometrial-type glands (Suginami, 1991). This theory has its limitations since it does not explain how endometriosis arises in distant sites (Ueki, 1991). Likewise, Sampson's theory does not account for the women with menstrual reflux who do not develop endometriosis. Genetic and immunological factors have also been implicated as possible causes, of this disease. It is known that women with endometriosis have an increased prevalence of humoral antibodies to endometrial and ovarian tissue (Mathur et al., 1982). However, this theory has its limitations as well.

In situations of dysmenorrhoea, dyspareunia, and/or infertility, endometriosis should be suspected. The symptoms of endometriosis may include diffuse pelvic pain, or sometimes localized pain, often in the rectum. Low back pain and premenstrual spotting have also been reported. CA-125, a cell surface antigen found on derivatives of the coelomic epithelium, is often elevated with endometriosis and may correspond with the severity of the disease (Barbieri et al., 1986; Pittaway, 1990). Note that increased CA-125 levels are also seen with early pregnancy, fibroids, menses and acute pelvic inflammatory disease (PID). On examination, the uterus is often fixed and retrofitted, and the ovaries may palpate as enlarged. Uterosacral ligament and cul-de-sac nodularity is detected in one-third of patients. Confirmation of the disease prior to the initiation of treatment is made with laparoscopy, in which lesions ranging in colour from red, black, blue to white may be seen. In addition, adhesions, peritoneal defects, and the classic 'chocolate cyst' of the ovary filled with blood, also called the endometrioma, may be observed (Jansen, 1986). Both ultrasound and magnetic resonance imaging can diagnose the endometrioma, but neither is able to visualize small peritoneal implants or adhesions (Friedman et al., 1985; Arrive et al., 1989).

Endometriosis has been identified as a cause of infertility, with decreased rates of fecundity in women with the disease as compared to those without it (Candiani et al., 1991). An obvious effect is when adhesions caused by endometriosis block tubal motility and pick-up of the oocyte. This results in a mechanical interference with fertility. However, when no adhesions are present and a minimal amount of endometriosis exists, fertility rates are still lower than expected. Despite having lower pregnancy rates, women diagnosed with minimal amounts of endometriosis have a long-term cumulative pregnancy rate that is high even without treatment (Badaway et al., 1988).

Other theoretical causes of infertility secondary to endometriosis include the production of prostaglandins by the implants, which may have a detrimental impact on tubal motility, folliculogenesis and corpus luteum function (Drake et al., 1980; Drake et al., 1981). This cause remains controversial as many studies dispute whether prostaglandins are elevated in the peritoneal fluid in patients suffering from infertility and endometriosis (Rock et al., 1982; Rezai et al., 1987). Another cause may be the peritoneal macrophage with increased activation associated with endometriosis (Halme, 1984; Chacho et al., 1986). These macrophages secrete interleukin-1, which has been found to be toxic to mouse embryos (Mori et al., 1992). Ultrasound studies have shown a correlation between growth retardation in follicles and endometriosis, which suggests that the disease may cause disordered follicle growth and ovulatory dysfunction (Doody et al., 1988).

The question remains as to whether patients with minimal or mild endometriosis should be treated to improve their infertility. Several studies conclude that treatment improves endometriosis associated infertility, but these studies are limited by the lack of control groups (Olive and Haney, 1986). Further, the literature cites comparative pregnancy rates in women with expectantly managed minimal endometriosis and those with treatment (Fedele et al., 1992). Specifically, Badway et al. (Badaway et al., 1988) reported a 90% cumulative pregnancy rate after 5 years in women with expectantly managed minimal endometriosis. Treatment for endometriosis encompasses both a hormonal and surgical approach. Using conservative surgery by laparotomy, Buttram and Betts reported a 73.2% pregnancy rate within 15 months of therapy in their study of 56 patients with mild endometriosis, and an average duration of infertility of 37 months (Buttram and Betts, 1979). Fayez et al. (Fayez et al., 1988) compared different modalities of treatment of women with mild endometriosis and found higher pregnancy rates with laparoscopic excision of the disease, as compared to a hormonal approach treatment with danazol. Still, Olive and Lee concluded in their study that conservative surgery has no advantage over expectant management based on monthly fecundity rates and life table analyses (Olive and Lee, 1986).

Significance Of Hydrosalpinx In IVF

A classic indication for IVF-ET is tubal factor infertility. In essence, IVF-ET may be performed in an attempt to bypass abnormally functioning fallopian tubes. In this situation, one would expect high pregnancy rates. However, the success of IVF-ET remains, on an average, only 20%–25% (SART, 1996). Tubal hydrosalpinges are an example of extreme tubal disease that is linked to decreased pregnancy rates with assisted reproduction.

Several theories attempt to explain why a lower-than-expected pregnancy rate exists. It is speculated that adhesion tissue products, which are released from a hydrosalpinx, have deleterious effects on both gametes and embryos. Abnormal tubal epithelium may secrete toxic hormones or growth factors. An altered uterotubal flow may also affect implantation (Hill et al., 1986). The presence of a hydrosalpinx reduces the expression of the endometrial integrin $\alpha_2\beta_3$ which is speculated to cause a decrease in embryo implantation.

Hydrosalpinx is essentially fluid collection in the fallopian tube. It has been cited as a complication of ovarian stimulation, and results in an emptying of fluid into the uterine cavity. To date, no specific inhibitory component of such fluid has been successfully identified. Mukherjee et al., in 1996, showed that human hydrosalpinx fluid has an embryotoxic effect on murine embryogenesis *in vitro* (Mukherjee et al., 1996). Several other studies in the literature have looked at the effect of hydrosalpinges on assisted reproduction, and Zeyneloglu et al. examined these studies in their meta-analysis on the subject (Zeyneloglu et al., 1988). Their analysis concurred with the contention that hydrosalpinx is, indeed, associated with decreased implantation rates, along with an increased risk of pregnancy loss. From their search, they analysed 13 studies and 10 abstracts, all of which had a cohort design. They found that the pregnancy rate of those patients with tubal factor infertility and hydrosalpinx was only half the PR of those without hydrosalpinx. In patients with tubal infertility who received IVF-ET, the presence of hydrosalpings ranged from 10% to 13% by ultrasound, and 25%–30% when diagnosed by hysterosalpingogram (HSG) or operative findings. Only 34% of patients with hydrosalpinx detected by HSG are successfully diagnosed with transvaginal ultrasound (Atri et al., 1994).

Given this correlation of decreased implantation and pregnancy rates and increased pregnancy losses in the face of hydrosalpinges, several theories exist to explain this. For instance, David and Czernobilsky (David et al., 1969) described the fibrotic wall of a hydrosalpinx with an impaired epithelial lining. As mentioned earlier, Mukherjee et al. showed that hydrosalpinx fluid was embryotoxic, and that correcting the often high pH of the fluid (with normal pH levels fluctuating between 7.2 and 7.7, and low levels of protein and bicarbonate) did not significantly alter the outcome. Mansour et al. (1991) reported an inability of IVF-ET treated patients with hydrosalpinges to conceive. In his patients, he described the drainage of brownish fluid from the cervix. When the proximal end of a tube with hydrosalpinx communicates with the uterine cavity, a direct flow of a myriad substances exists. This flow may include microorganisms, toxic debris, lymphocytes, cytokines, and prostaglandins, which may prove detrimental to the transferring embryo. The highest rates of pregnancy obtained with IVF-ET occurred with pure mechanical factor infertility, such as having a history of previous bilateral tubal ligation, as reported by Oehniger et al. (1989). In this study, they reported poorer results associated with more severe tubal disease, but no change in follicle development or the pregnancy rate in patients with tubal factor secondary to bilateral salpingectomy or other tubal surgery. These studies included in the meta-analysis by Hulusi et al., although limited by the fact that none is prospective in design, do all seem to depict the strong effect that hydrosalpinx has on the pregnancy rate in IVF cycles.

Effect Of Bedrest On Outcome On IVF

Assisted reproduction with embryo transfer has been available for infertile couples for almost 20 years. The exact mechanism of implantation, which occurs approximately four to seven days following fertilization, is not yet fully understood. It is recognized that the failure of implantation with ET is the most likely cause of IVF failure. With the many changes surrounding ART, bed rest following ET has remained a steady factor. Bedrest varies in length from several minutes to 24 hours (Leeton, 1984; Bonnicksen, 1989; Damewood and Meng, 1990). One line of thought is that mechanical reasons, such as the embryo dropping out, may be the cause of the failure of implantation (Schulman, 1984). However, there is no scientific data to support this. On the contrary, a recent large cohort-control study looked at over 1,000 IVF cycles without bedrest following ET that showed no difference in the clinical pregnancy rate per cycle of IVF (Khaldoun et al., 1998). This study by Sharif et al., although limited as it is not the golden-standard randomized prospective study, does follow a large patient population of 1,091 IVF cycles without bedrest, performed from June 1994 to August 1996 at the Birmingham Women's Hospital in the UK. In their study, they reported a clinical pregnancy rate of 23.5% per cycle of IVF, which they then compared to a historical control of 19,697 IVF cycles in the UK national data-base, which reported a rate of 18.6% for the year 1994 (Human Fertilization and Embroylogy Authority, 1996). Indeed, the patients in the group studied by Sharif in Birmingham had a statistically higher clinical pregnancy rate per cycle (P=0.0001), which shows that bedrest following ET is not beneficial.

COMPLICATIONS OF IVF

Risk Of Ectopic Pregnancy With IVF

The developing embryo is capable of communicating with maternal tissue, and modifies the metabolism of the uterus and other organs during the implantation process. Ectopic implantation indicates that the uterus is not essential for embryonic survival; the embryo has an intrinsic ability to implant in any tissue.

Ectopic pregnancy is a well-known complication of IVF-ET, the incidence being approximately 4%–5% (twice that of normal). Among patients participating in an ART procedure, the incidence of combined pregnancy is about 1% (incidence in the general population is 1/5,000 to 1.30,000) (Molloy et al., 1990; Dor et al., 1991). In a case-control study, Fernandez et al. (Fernandez et al., 1991) identified the causes of ectopic pregnancy with ART as high hormone levels secondary to the stimulation protocols and multiple ovulations. Further analysis of the risk factors for ectopic pregnancy with IVF has been done by Marcus et al. (Marcus and Brinsden, 1995) and Ribic-Pucelj et al. (Ribic Pucelj et al., 1995). Close monitoring of ART patients with ultrasound and hCG titres is important for early detection to prevent a hazardous delay in the treatment of ectopic pregnancy.

An uncommon but important subset of ectopic pregnancy is the cornual or interstitial pregnancy. Although rare, the cornual pregnancy warrants careful attention because of the risk of early rupture with severe haemorrhage. The rate of cornual pregnancy after natural conception is about 2% of all ectopic implantations (Crvendovic et al., 1995). All cases are published, but given the low numbers, not much is known about the incidence and risk factors for cornual pregnancy in patients undergoing IVF. In the literature, the published number of patients with reported cornual pregnancies after IVF remains small. Six studies have reviewed the incidence of cornual pregnancy as a complication of IVF. In a total of 4,323 pregnancies achieved by IVF-ET, 183 total ectopic pregnancies were noted, of which 25 (13.7%) were cornual pregnancies (Chen et al., 1998). Specifically, Chen et al. reviewed 1,014 IVF cycles from October 1990 to October 1996 that resulted in 245 pregnancies; of these, 11 (4.5%) were ectopic, and 3 (27.3%) were cornual. Thus, it may be deducted that the risk of cornual pregnancy after IVF-ET may be significantly higher than that after natural conception. This increased risk may be due to pre-existing tubal disease or other risk factors for ectopic pregnancy in general.

A possible cause of cornual pregnancy with IVF-ET may be related to catheter misplacement or reflux of the culture medium into the cornu, with placement of embryos in the cornu. Agarwal et al. (1996) noted that causes of tubal dysfunction, a history of prior salpingectomy, or even uterine contractions may lead to cornual pregnancy. In 1986, Pavic et al. (1986) described the first case report of a cornual pregnancy after IVF-ET in a patient whose history was significant for a prior bilateral salpingectomy. In the study by Chen et al., 2 of the 3 cornual pregnancies had a history of bilateral salpingectomy before the IVF cycles. Thus, history of bilateral salpingectomy does not exempt a patient from the risk of ectopic or cornual pregnancy.

Ultrasound has been imperative in detecting cornual pregnancies. Crvenkovic et al. described the typical sonographic findings of the cornual pregnancy, including eccentrically located versus lateral gestational sac, thin or incomplete myometrial mantle that covers the gestational sac, and the presence of myometrium between the uterine cavity and sac. One must also pay close attention to the multiple gestation pregnancy, in which there may be concomitant intrauterine and ectopic pregnancies. Beck et al. (1990) first reported a heterotopic gestation following IVF, in which a ruptured cornual pregnancy was detected.

For the prevention of ectopic pregnancy, some experts have proposed the benefit of the prophylactic removal or cornual occlusion of nonfunctioning tubes prior to the onset of IVF (Hewit et al., 1985). However, while salpingectomy may reduce the risk of ectopic pregnancy, it cannot eliminate the risk of cornual pregnancy. Cornual resection cannot eliminate the risk of interstitial implantation. Thus, close monitoring for ectopic pregnancy, and not prophylactic salpingectomy, is warranted in patients with prior tuboplasty or salpingectomy with cornual patency who are receiving IVF.

THE RISK OF MULTIPLE PREGNANCY WITH IVF

With the increasing use of IVF and its successful development, a new dilemma emerges in medicine: the multiple gestation. In order to maximize the success of IVF, multiple embryos are usually transferred per cycle, which leads to a higher risk of multiple pregnancies. In fact, there exists an approximately twentyfold (20X) increase in the risk of having twins and a four hundredfold (400X) increase in the risk of having triplets (Kauma, 1997). This is important since multiple gestations correlate with a higher incidence of fetal/infant morbidity and mortality (a sixfold increase for twins and a twentyfold increase for triplets) as compared to singleton gestations, as well as a higher cost of medical care (Luke and Keith, 1992; Callahan et al., 1994). Procedures such as selective fetal reduction can decrease the incidence of multiple gestations and births. This procedure can decrease the incidence of fetal morbidity and mortality by lowering the risk of preterm labour and delivery, and ultimately, the demise of all fetuses involved (Berkowitz et al., 1996).

Martin et al. performed a statistical analysis to calculate the probabilities of specific pregnancy outcomes after a single completed IVF cycle (Martin and Welch, 1998). They looked at two variables: the implantation rate and the number of embryos transferred. A computation of exact binomial probabilities for singleton and multiple pregnancies was done. They incorporated implantation rates varying from 5% to 50%, and a number of embryos varying from one to eight. The study revealed a direct relationship between the number of embryos transferred and the incidence of pregnancy. When more embryos were transferred, the chance of pregnancy increased. However, the chance of multiple gestations increased and the probability of having a singleton pregnancy decreased.

The regulation of the number of embryos transferred during an IVF cycle is controversial (Jones, 1995; Bronson, 1997). Currently, some restrictions addressing this issue exist in western Europe, as well as in other regions of the world (Elsner et al., 1997). Nonetheless, the low implantation rates caused by poor embryo quality mandate the transfer of a higher number of embryos to maintain the adequate success rate achieved during an IVF cycle (Bustillo, 1997).

Several factors are used to predict the probability of success during an IVF-ET. These factors include the age of the patient, the reason for infertility, the endometrial thickness and the average embryo morphology score (Roseboom et al., 1995; Check et al., 1991; Copperman et al., 1995). A large retrospective review by Hu et al. (1998) looked at the statistical threshold for the number of embryos transferred in an attempt to achieve an optimal pregnancy rate, while simultaneously limiting the number of multiple gestations [HU, 118]. They described a mean cumulative embryo score (MCES) to determine the optimal number of embryos to transfer. They based this transfer number on the patient's age and embryo quality. The incidence of multiple gestations after IVF depends upon both maternal age and the number of embryos transferred.

It is recommended to transfer up to four poor quality, two fair quality, or two good quality embryos in women who are less than 35 years old. This will yield a PR of approximately 35% with little to no risk of having triplets. To achieve a maximum PR of approximately 50% one needs to transfer five poor-quality, three to four fair-quality, or three to four good-quality embryos. This leads to a higher-order multiple conception rate of up to 22%. As mentioned, these recommendations will vary depending on the maternal age.

CONCLUSIONS

This chapter has attempted an overview of the factors involved in IVF and ET. Fortunately, the field historically has been very dynamic. Research has led the techniques of IVF-ET a long way, with the changes ranging from varying methods and location of ET to different timing of ET. Techniques to improve the deleterious factors that affect IVF-ET continue to emerge, such as treatment for endometriosis, hydrosalpinx, and cervical infections. There is no doubt that IVF-ET remains a dilemma; however, with the plentitude of research going on in this area, this dilemma in medicine will one day be unravelled.

REFERENCES

Agarwal, S.K. et al. (1996). 'Cornual pregnancies in patients with prior salpinnegectomy undergoing *in vitro* fertilization and embryo transfer', *Fertil. Steril.*, **65**: 659.

American Society for Reproductive Medicine/Society for Assisted Reproductive Technology Registry (1994). 'Assisted reproductive technology in the United States and Canada: 1994 results', *Fertil. Steril.*, **66**: 697.

Arrive, L. et al. (1989). 'Pelvic endometriosis: MR imaging', *Radiology*, **171**: 687.

Atri, M. et al. (1994). 'Accuracy of endovaginal sonography for the detection of fallopian tube blockage', *J. Ultrasound Med.*, **13**: 429.

Azem, F. et al. (1995). 'Transfer of six or more embryos improves success rates in patients with repeated *in vitro* fertilization failures', *Fertil. Steril.*, **63**: 1043.

Badaway, S.Z.A. et al. (1988). 'Cumulative pregnancy rates in infertile women with endometriosis', *J. Reprod. Med.*, **33**: 757.

Badaway, S.Z.A. et al. (1988). 'Cumulative pregnancy rates in infertile women with endometriosis', *J. Reprod. Med.*, **33**: 757.

Barbieri, R.L. et al. (1986). 'Elevated serum concentrations of CA-125 in patients with advanced endometriosis', *Fertil. Steril.*, **45**: 630.

Bavister, B.D. (1995). 'Culture of preimplantation embryos: Facts and artifacts', *Hum. Reprod. Update*, **1**: 91.

Beck, P. et al. (1990). 'Survival of the cornual pregnancy in a heterotopic gestation after *in vitro* fertilization and embryo transfer', *Fertil. Steril.*, **53**: 732.

Ben Rafail-Z, et al. (1995). 'The use of fibrin sealant in *in vitro* fertilization and embryo transfer', *Int. J. Fertil. Menopausal. Stud.*, **40**(6): 303.

Berkowitz, R.L. et al. (1996). 'The current status of multifetal pregnancy reduction', *Am. J. Obstet. Gynecol.*, **174**: 1265.

Bolton, V.N. et al. (1989). 'Development of spare human preimplantation embryos *in vitro*: an analysis of the correlation among gross morphology, cleavage rates and development to the blastocyst', *J. In Vitro Fertil. Emrbyo. Transfer*, **6**: 30.

Bonnicksen, A. (1989). *In vitro Fertilization*. Columbia University Press, New York, p. 151.

Braude, P. et al. (1988). 'Human gene expression first occurs between the four and eight cell stages of preimplantation development', *Nature*, **332**: 459.

Bronson, R. (1997). 'Embryo transfer and multiple gestation: How should the number of embryos transferred to the uterus following *in vitro* fertilization be determined to avoid the risk of multiple gestation?' *Hum. Reprod.*, **12**: 1605.

Bustillo, M. (1997). 'Imposing limits on the number of oocytes and embryos transferred: Is it necessary/wise or naughty/nice?' *Hum. Reprod.*, **12**: 1616.

Buttram, V.C. Jr. and J.W. Betts (1979). 'Endometriosis', *Curr. Probl. Obstet. Gynecol.*, **11**: 11.

Callahan, T.L. et al. (1994). 'The economic impact of multiple-gestation pregnancies and the contribution of assisted-reproduction techniques to their incidence', *N. Engl. J. Med.*, **331**: 244.

Candiani, G.B. et al. (1991). 'Mild endometriosis and infertility: A critical review of epidemiologic data, diagnostic pitfalls, and classification limits', *Obstet. Gynecol. Survey.*, **46**: 1991.

Carrillo, A.J. et al. (1998). 'Improved clinical outcomes for *in vitro* fertilization with delay of embryo transfer from 48 to 72 hours after oocytes retrieval: Use of glucose and phosphate-free media', *Fertil. Steril.*, **69**(2): 329.

Chacho, K.J. et al. (1986). 'Peritoneal fluid in patients with and without endometriosis: Prostanoids and macrophages and their effect on the spermatozoa penetration assay', *Am. J. Obstet. Gynecol.*, **154**: 1290.

Check, J.H. et al. (1991). 'Influence of endometrial thickness and echo patterns on pregnancy rates during *in vitro* fertilization', *Fertil. Steril.*, **56**: 1173.

Chen, C. et al. (1998). 'Cornual pregnancy after IVF-ET', *J. Reprod. Med.*, **43**: 393.

Claman, P. et al. (1987). 'The impact of embryo quality and quantity on implantation and the establishment of viable pregnancies', *J. In Vitro Fert. Embryo. Transfer*, **4**: 218.

Cohen, J. et al. (1990). 'Impairment of the hatching process following IVF in the human and improvement of implantation by assisting hatching using micromanipulation', *Hum. Reprod.*, **5**: 7

Conaghan, J. et al. (1993). 'Effects of pyruvate and glucose on the development of human preimplantation embryos *in vitro*', *J. Reprod. Fertil.*, **99**: 87.

Copperman, A.B. et al. (1995). 'Cumulative number and morphological score of embryos resulting in success: Realistic expectations from *in vitro* fertilization embryo transfer', *Fertil. Steril.*, **64**: 88.

Cramer, D.W. (1993). 'Epidemiology of endometriosis', *New Engl. J. Med.*, **328**: 1759.

______(1985). 'Epidemiology of endometriosis', in E.A. Wilson (Ed). *Endometriosis*, Alan R. Liss Inc., New York, p. 5.

Croxatto, H.B. et al. (1978). 'Studies on the duration of egg transport by the human oviduct II: Ovum location at various intervals follow luteinizing hormone peak', *Am. J. Obstet. Gynecl.*, **132**: 629.

Crvendovic, G. et al. (1995). 'Right-sided interstitial (cornual) pregnancy', *J. Ultrasound Med.*, **14**: 329.

Damewood, M.D. and S.G. Meng (1990). 'Personnel and the organization of the IVF team', in M.D. Damewood (ed.) *The Johns Hopkins Handbook of in vitro Fertilization and Assisted Reproductive Technologies*, Little Brown and Company, Boston, p. 39.

David, A. (1969). 'Human hydrosalpinx: Histologic study and chemical composition of fluid', *Am. J. Obstet. Gynecol.*, **105**: 400.

Dawson, K.J. et al. (1995). 'Delaying transfer to the third day post-insemination, to select non-arrested embryos, increases development to the fetal heart stage', *Hum. Reprod.*, **10**: 177.

Diedrich, K. Van der Ven, et al. (1989). 'Establishment of pregnancy related to embryo transfer techniques after *in-vitro* fertilization', *Hum. Reprod.*, **4** (Suppl): 111.

Doody, M.C. et al. (1988). 'Linear regression analysis of ultrasound follicular growth series: Evidence for an abnormality of follicular growth in endometriosis patients', *Fertil. Steril.*, **49**: 47.

Dor, J. et al. (1991). 'The incidence of combined intrauterine and extrauterine pregnancy after *in vitro* fertilization and embryo transfer', *Fertil. Steril.*, **55**: 833.

Drake, T.S. et al. (1980). 'Peritoneal fluid volume in endometriosis', *Fertil. Steril.*, **34**: 280.

Drake, T.S. et al. (1981). 'Peritoneal fluid thromboxane B2 and 6-ketoprostaglandin E-1 alpha in endometriosis', *Am. J. Obstet. Gynecol.*, **140**: 401.

Edwards, R.G. et al. (1984). 'Factors influencing the success of *in vitro* fertilization for alleviating human infertility', *J. In vitro Fertil. Embryo. Transfer*, **1**: 13.

Elsner, C.W. et al. (1997). 'Multiple pregnancy rate and embryo number transferred during *in vitro* fertilization', *Am. J. Obst. Gynecol.*, **177**: 350.

Fayez, J.A. et al. (1988). 'Comparison of different modalities of treatment for minimal and mild endometriosis', *Am. J. Obstet. Gynecol.*, **159**: 927.

Fedele, L. et al. (1992). 'Buserelin acetate versus expectant management in the treatment of infertility associated with minimal or mild endometriosis: A randomized clinical trial', *Am. J. Obstet. Gynecol*, **166**: 1345.

Fernandez, H. et al. (1991). 'Controlled ovarian hyperstimulation as a risk factor for ectopic pregnancy', *Obstet. Gynecol.*, **78**: 656.

Fluker, M.R. et al. 'A prospective randomized comparison of zygote intrafallopian transfer and *in vitro* fertilization-embryo transfer for nontubal factor infertility', *Fertil. Steril.*, **60**: 515.

Fong, C. et al. (1998). 'Blastocyst transfer after enzymatic treatment of the zona pellucida: Improving *in vitro* fertilization and understanding implantation', *Hum. Reprod.*, **13**: 2926.

Friedman, H. et al. (1985). 'Endometriosis detection by US with laparascopic correlation', *Radiology*, **157**: 217.

Gardner, D.K. et al. (1996). 'Environment of the preimplantation human embryo *in vivo*: Metabolite analysis of oviduct and uterine fluids and metabolism of cumulus cells', *Fertil. Steril.*, **65**: 349.

Giorgetti, C. et al. (1995). 'Embryo score to predict implantation after *in vitro* fertilization: Based on 957 single embryo transfers', *Hum. Reprod.*, **10**: 2427.

Giudice, L.C. (1994). 'Growth factors and growth modulators in human uterine endometrium: Their potential relevance to reproductive medicine', *Fertil. Steril.*, **61**: 1.

Groutz, A. et al. 'Comparison of transmyometrial and transcervical embryo transfer in patients with previously failed *in vitro* fertilization—embryo transfer cycles and/or cervical stenosis', *Fertil. Steril.*, **67**: 1073.

Halme, J. et al. (1984). 'Accentuated cyclic activation of peritoneal macrophages in patients with endometriosis', *Am. J. Obstet. Gynecol.*, **148**: 85.

Harper, M.J. (1994). 'Gamete and zygote transport', in E. Knobil and J.D. Neill (ed.) *The physiology of reproduction*, Raven Press, New York, **1**: 123.

Hewitt, J. et al. (1985). 'Bilateral tubal ectopic pregnancy following *in vitro* fertilization and embryo replacement', *Br. J. Obstet. Gynaecol.*, **92**: 850.

Hill, G.A. et al. (1986). 'Enlargement of hydrosalpinges during ovarian stimulation protocols for *in vitro* fertilization and embryo replacement', *Fertil. Steril.*, **45**: 883.

Hu, Y. (1998). 'Maximizing pregnancy rates and limiting higher order multiple conceptions by determining the optimal number of embryos to transfer based on quality', *Fertil. Steril.*, **69**: 650.

Huisman, G.J. et al. (1994). 'A comparison of *in vitro* fertilization results after embryo transfer after two, three and four days of embryo culture', *Fertil. Steril.*, **61**: 970.

Human Fertilization and Embryology Authority (1996). *Fifth Annual Report.* Human Fertilization and Embryology Authority, London.

Ishimaru, T. and H. Masuzaki (1991). 'Peritoneal endometriosis: Endometrial tissue implantation as its primary etiologic mechanism', *Am. J. Obstet. Gynecol.*, **165**: 210.

Jansen, R.P.S. and P. Russel (1986). 'Nonpigmented endometriosis: Clinical, laparoscopic and pathologic definition', *Am. J. Obstet. Gynecol.*, **155**: 1154.

Jenkins, S. et al. (1986). 'Endometriosis: Pathogenetic implications of the anatomic distribution', *Obstet. Gynecol.*, **67**: 335.

Jones, H.W.J. (1995). 'Twins or more', *Fertil. Steril.*, **63**: 701.

Kauma, S. (1997). 'Discussant for: "Multiple pregnancy rate and embryo number transferred during *in vitro* fertilization",', *Am. J. Obstet. Gynecol.*, **177**: 355.

Khaldoun, S. et al. (1998). 'Is bedrest following embryo transfer necessary?' *Fertil. Steril.*, **69**: 478.

Leeton, J.F. (1984). 'Embryo transfer', in A. Trounson and C. Wood (eds.) *In vitro Fertilization and Embryo Transfer*, Churchill Livingstone, Edinburgh, 197.

Lessey, B.A. et al. (1992). 'Integrin adhesion molecules in the human endometrium. Correlation with the normal and abnormal menstrual cycle', *J. Clin. Invest.*, **90**: 188.

Levran, D. et al. (1998). 'Zygote intrafallopian transfer may improve pregnancy rate in patients with repeated failure of implantation', *Fertil. Steril.*, **69**: 26.

Liu, D.T.Y. and A. Hitchcock (1986). 'Endometriosis: Its association with retrograde menstruation, dysmenorrhea, and tubal pathology', *Br. J. Obstet. Gynaecol.*, **93**: 859.

Loke, Y.W. et al. (1989). 'Laminin in human trophoblast decidual interaction', *Hum. Reprod.*, **4**: 453.

Luke, B. and L.G. Keith (1992). 'The contribution of singletons, twins and triplets to low birth weight, infant mortality and handicap in the United States', *J. Reprod. Med.*, **37**: 661.

Mansour, R.T. et al. (1991). 'Fluid accumulation of the uterine cavity before embryo transfer: A possible hindrance for implantation', *J. In Vitro Fertil. Emrbyo. Transf.*, **8**: 157.

Marcus, S.F. and P.R. Brinsden (1995). 'Analysis of the incidence and risk factors associated with ectopic pregnancy following *in vitro* fertilization and embryo transfer', *Hum. Reprod.*, **10**: 199.

Marshal, R.J. and S.G. Braye (1987). 'Immunohistochemical demonstration of a1-antitrypsin and a1-antichymotrypsin in normal human endometrium', *Int. J. Gynecol. Pathol.*, **6**: 49.

Martin, P.M. and H.G. Welch (1998). 'Probabilities for singleton and multiple pregnancies after *in vitro* fertilization', *Fertil. Steril.*, **70**: 478.

Mathur, S. et al. (1982). 'Autoimmunity to endometrium and ovary in endometriosis', *Clin. Exp. Immunol.*, **50**: 259.

Molloy, D et al. (1990). 'Multiple-sited (heterotropic)

pregnancy after *in vitro* fertilization and gamete intrafallopian transfer', *Fertil. Steril.*, **53**: 1068.

Mori, H. et al. (1992). 'Expression of interleukin-1 (IL-1) beta messenger ribonucleic (mRNA) and IL-1 receptor antagonist mRNA in peritoneal macrophages from patients with endometriosis', *Fertil. Steril.*, **57**: 535.

Mukherjee, T. (1996). 'Hydrosalpinx fluid has embryotoxic effects on murine embryogenesis: A case for prophylactic salpingectomy', *Fertil. Steril.*, **66**: 851.

Oehninger, S. et al. (1989). 'Effects of the severity of tubo-ovarian disease and previous tubal surgery on the results of *in vitro* fertilization and embryo transfer', *Fertil. Steril.*, **51**: 126.

Olive, D.L. and A.F. Haney (1986). 'Endometriosis associated infertility: A critical review of therapeutic approaches', *Obstet. Gynecol. Survey*, **41**: 538.

Olive, D.L. and K.L. Lee (1986). 'Analysis of sequential treatment protocol for endometriosis associated infertility', *Am. J. Obstet. Gynecol.*, **154**: 613.

Olive, D.L. and L.B. Schwartz (1993). 'Endometriosis', *New Engl. J. Med.*, **328**: 1759.

Pavic, N. et al. (1986). 'Interstitial pregnancy following bilateral salpingectomy and *in vitro* fertilization-embryo transfer', *Fertil. Steril.*, **46**: 701.

Pittaway, D.E. (1990). 'The use of serial CA-125 concentrations to monitor endometriosis in infertile women', *Am. J. Obstet. Gynecol.*, **163**: 1032.

Pool, T.B. et al. (1998). 'Oocytes and embryo culture: Basic concepts and recent advances', in J. May (ed.) *Infertility and Reproductive Medicine Clinics of North America*, Saunders, Philadelphia.

Puistola, V. et al. (1989). 'The human embryo produces basement membrane collagen (type IV collagen) degrading protease activity', *Hum. Reprod.*, **4**: 309.

Queenan, J. et al. (1987). 'Regulation of urokinase-type plasminogen activator production by cultured human cytotrophoblasts', *J. Biol. Chem.*, **262**: 10903.

Quinn, P. et al. (1995). 'Successful human *in vitro* fertilization using a modified human tubal fluid medium lacking glucose and phosphate ions', *Fertil. Steril.*, **63**: 922.

Renato, F. et al. (1998). 'Microbial flora of the cervix assessed at the time of embryo transfer adversely affect *in vitro* fertilization outcome', *Fertil. Steril.*, **70**: 866.

Rezai, N. et al. (1987). 'Cul-de-sac fluid in women with endometriosis: Fluid volume, protein and prostanoid concentration during the periovulatory period—days thirteen to eighteen', *Fertil. Steril.*, **48**: 29.

Ribic-Pucelj, M. et al. (1995). 'Risk factors for ectopic pregnancy after *in vitro* fertilization and embryo transfer', *J. Assist. Reprod. Genet.*, **12**: 594.

Rock, J.A. et al. (1982). 'Cul-de-sac fluid in women with endometriosis: Fluid volume and prostanoid concentration during the proliferative phase of the cycle–days eight to twelve', *Fertil. Steril.*, **37**: 747.

Roseboom, T.J. et al. (1995). 'The probability of pregnancy after embryo transfer is affected by the age of the patient, cause of infertility, number of embryos transferred and the average morphology score, as revealed by multiple logistic regression analysis', *Hum. Reprod.*, **10**: 3035.

Sampson, J.A. (1927). 'Peritoneal endometriosis due to the menstrual dissemination of endometrial tissue into the peritoneal cavity', *Am. J. Obstet. Gynecol.*, **14**: 422.

Scholtes, M.C.W. and G.H. Zeilmaker (1996). 'A prospective, randomized study of embryo transfer results after three or five days of embryo culture in *in vitro* fertilization', *Fertil. Steril.*, **65**: 1245.

Schoolcraft, W.B. et al. (1994). 'Assisted hatching in the treatment of poor prognosis *in vitro* fertilization candidates', *Fertil. Steril.*, **62**: 551.

Schulman, J.D. (1984). 'Delayed expulsion of transfer fluid after IVF-EF (letter)', *Lancet*, **i**: 44.

______(1986). 'Delayed expulsion of transfer fluid after IVF-ET', *Lancet*, **1**: 44.

Sehsagiri, P.B. and B. Bavister (1991). 'Glucose and phosphate inhibit repiration and oxidative metabolism in cultured hamster eight-cell embryos: Evidence for the "Crabtree effect"', *Mol. Reprod. Dev.*, **30**: 105.

Society for Assisted Reproduction Technology (SART) and The American Fertility Society Medical Research International (1992). '*In vitro* fertilization-embryo transfer in the United States: 1990 results from the IVF-ET Registry', *Fertil. Steril.*, **57**: 15.

Society for Assisted Reproductive Technology and The American Society for Reproductive Medicine (1996). 'Assisted reproductive technology in the United States and Canada: 1994 results generated from the American Society for Reproductive Medicine/ Society for Assisted Reproductive Technology Registry', *Fertil. Steril.*, **66**: 697.

Staessen, C. (1992). 'The relationship between embryo

quality and the occurrence of multiple pregnancies', *Fertil. Steril.*, **57**: 626.

Staessen, C. et al. (1992). 'The relationship between embryo quality and the occurrence of multiple pregnancies', *Fertil. Steril.*, **57**: 626.

Suginami, H. (19991). 'A reappraisal of the coelomic metaplasis theory by reviewing endometriosis occurring in unusual sites and instances', *Am. J. Obstet. Gynecol.*, **165**: 214.

Tan, S.L. et al. (1990). 'Surgical techniques of oocyte collection and embryo transfer', *Br. Med. Bull.*, **46**: 628.

Tanbo, T. et al. (1990). 'Assisted fertilization in infertile women with patent fallopian tubes: A comparison of *in vitro* fertilization, gamete intrafallopian transfer and tubal embryo stage transfer', *Hum. Reprod.*, **5**: 266.

Telford, N.A. et al. (1990). 'Transition from maternal to embryonic control of early mammalian development: A comparison of several species', *Mol. Reprod. Dev.*, **26**: 90.

Toner, J.P. et al. (1993). 'Basal follicle stimulating hormone level and age affect the chance for and outcome of pre-embryo cryopreservation', *Fertil. Steril.*, **59**: 664.

Toth, T.L. et al. (1992). 'Embryo transfer to the uterus or the fallopian tube after *in vitro* fertilization yields similar results', *Fertil. Steril.*, **52**: 1110.

Ueki, M. (1991). 'Histologic study of endometriosis and examination of lymphatic drainage in and from the uterus', *Am. J. Obstet. Gynecol.*, **165**: 201.

van Os, H.C. et al. (1989). 'The influence of the interval between *in vitro* fertilization and embryo transfer and some other variables on treatment outcome', *Fertil. Steril.*, **2**: 360.

Van Voorhis, B.J. et al. (1995). 'Tubal versus uterine transfer of cryopreserved embryos: A prospective randomized trial', *Fertil. Steril.*, **63**: 578.

Visser, D.S. et al. (1993). 'Multiple attempts at embryo transfer: Effect on pregnancy outcome in an IVF and ET program', *J. Assist. Reprod. Genet.*, **10**: 37.

Wegmann, T.G. et al. (1989). 'The role of M-CSF and GM-CSF in fostering placental growth, fetal growth and fetal survival', *Transplant. Proc.*, **21**: 566.

Witkin, S.S. et al. (1994). 'Unsuspected Chlamydia trachomatis infection and *in vitro* fertilization outcome', *Am. J. Obstet. Gynecol.*, **171**: 1208.

Yovitch, J.L. et al. (1998). 'The relative chance of pregnancy following tubal or uterine transfer procedures', *Fertil. Steril.*, **49**: 858.

Zeyneloglu, H.B. et al. (1998). 'Adverse effects of hydrosalpinx on pregnancy rates after *in vitro* fertilization-embryo transfer', *Fertil. Steril.*, **70**: 492.

15

Failures and Successes of In Vitro Fertilization and Embryo Transfer

Sozos J. Fasouliotis and Joseph G. Schenker

INTRODUCTION

It is estimated that about one in six couples suffers from problems of infertility at some time in their lives (Shushan et al., 1995). While the prevalence of infertility has remained constant over the last two to three decades, the number of individuals seeking medical care for infertility has increased markedly (Chandra and Mosher, 1994). On the basis of the 1988 National Survey of Family Growth data (Wilcox and Mosher, 1993), 43% of the women in the United States characterized as having impaired fecundity had obtained some type of infertility service, and 24% of these women had received specialized treatment services. The emergence of new techniques to alleviate infertility has affected dramatically the terms and issues surrounding infertility. Couples considered sterile only a few years ago can currently acquire assistance to conceive. *In vitro* fertilization (IVF), initially developed for women suffering from mechanical infertility, currently is used for a wide range of indications and has become an acceptable tool in the treatment of subfertile couples. Current practices differ remarkably from those initially used two decades ago. Indeed, the advances in basic research and the practical applications of the research that has been performed since the first successful IVF in 1978 (Steptoe and Edwards, 1978) have given rise to hitherto unthinkable strategies for achieving human reproduction. Innovations in gonadotrophin preparations, techniques for culturing gametes and embryos, sperm and embryo cryopreservation techniques, endocrine assays, ultrasound imaging and laparoscopic surgery all have contributed to the evolution of assisted reproductive technology (ART). Many causes of infertility are now treatable with the application of one of the ART methods.

Nonetheless, considerable uncertainty exists regarding the comparative effectiveness of available ARTs, as well as the likelihood of success of particular treatments in couples with particular clinical characteristics (Steinberg et al., 1998). In addition, people are often faced with a confusing variety of treatments, technical jargon, clinics, statistical probabilities and worrisome financial decisions (Goldfarb et al., 1997).

During the last few years, most countries started to be concerned about the registration of their *In Vitro* Fertilization and Embryo Transfer (ET) activity, in order to increase the peer control of this procedure. The number of the registered centres increased during the years as a consequence of this social pressure. Although the registries of all countries do not include all the existing units around the world, it is assumed that the main activity and results in this field of infertility treatment are adequately expressed through their activity (Ezra and Schenker, 1993). In this chapter, we review the available data regarding the effect of patient and embryo variables, the procedure-related pregnancy and perinatal outcome, and the general and specific complications related to pregnancy after assisted conception.

APPRAISAL OF CONVENTIONAL *IN VITRO* FERTILIZATION AND EMBRYO TRANSFER

Although current ART practices typically involve the induction of development follicles using gonadotrophins, followed by a retrieval of the eggs that emerge from this process, patients can undergo an IVF cycle without ovarian stimulation. In IVF, oocyte harvesting, performed either vaginally, with ultrasound guidance or laparoscopically, is followed by oocyte insemination and, if fertilization occurs, embryo transfer. Gamete Intrafallopian Transfer (GIFT) and Zygote Intrafallopian Transfer (ZIFT) soon followed the advent of IVF. Gamete intrafallopian transfer, which involves the transfer of gametes to the fallopian tube immediately after oocyte retrieval, was proposed as an alternative to IVF that would allow for *in vivo* fertilization in patients with at least one functional fallopian tube (Asch et al., 1986). Zygote intrafallopian transfer typically involves the laparoscopic transfer of a fertilized oocyte, or zygote, to the fallopian tube the day following oocyte retrieval. It was developed not only to capitalize on the increased pregnancy rates achieved with GIFT, but also to permit confirmation of oocyte fertilization before the tubal transfer (Devroey et al., 1986).

RESULTS

In an era of fiscal restraint, it is imperative that expensive therapies such as IVF be assessed objectively (Van Voorhis et al., 1997). It is also critical that patients, physicians and governing bodies evaluate objectively the success of continuing treatment. Choosing the best methodology for assessing the success of IVF-ET is a challenging problem. Numerous methods have been used to compute the success of IVF, and although each method can be informative, the lack of standardization is confusing. Standardization is essential so that results may be compared among IVF centres (Yuzpe et al., 1989).

In recent years, infertility treatment by assisted reproduction has often been performed repeatedly due to a relatively low success rate per cycle. It has, therefore, proved the importance of estimating the couple's expected pregnancy rate (PR) after a defined number of treatment cycles (Hull et al., 1992; Check et al., 1994).

Alsalili et al. (1995), by using life table analysis, reported on the cumulative pregnancy rates and pregnancy outcome after IVF in a large series of 5,209 cycles in 2,391 couples over a 10-year period. They reported a 20% conception rate of embryo transfers and 22% multiple pregnancies. The cumulative pregnancy rate for the various causes of infertility, following six cycles, was estimated to be 65% for idiopathic, 63% for multifactorial, 60% for endometriosis, 55% for tubal, and 40% for male. They concluded that the infertility factor (with the exception of the male factor) did not influence the results.

In another study from Israel (Dor et al., 1996), the authors examined 951 couples who had completed 2,252 IVF treatment cycles during the period 1984–1992. It was found that the cumulative pregnancy rate showed a constant rise during the six initial IVF treatment cycles, reaching 56%, and plateaued in the subsequent three cycles (63%). Various infertility factors did not influence this rate; however, women ≥40 years of age had a significantly lower cumulative pregnancy rate.

While the study of the French National Registry (FIVNAT, 1993) showed no change in the pregnancy rate in repeated cycles, the study of Kovacs (1996) revealed cumulative pregnancy rates of 56.4% and 76% after 5 cycles, reaching 78.9% and 89.8% after 10 cycles, for IVF and GIFT, respectively.

Nevertheless, in recent years, there have been dramatic changes in clinical and laboratory protocols, including the introduction of gonadotrophin-releasing hormone analogues, purified forms of gonadotrophins, ready-to-use and high-quality culture media, and methods for treating male infertility. These, along with many other modifications, have significantly increased the actual pregnancy and birth rates to such an extent that they are no longer comparable to the older figures that constitute part of those cumulative rates (Lewin and Schenker, 1998). Registries containing data regarding the content and outcome of care offer tremendous potential benefits to patients, providers and society as a whole. To realize those potential benefits, including continuous improve-

Table 15.1. United Kingdom: IVF Clinical and Live Birth Rates, 1.1.1985 to 31.3.1996

	1985	1986	1987	1988	1989	1990	1991	1992	1993	1994–5
Pregnancy rate (%)	11.2	9.9	12.5	12.9	15.4	17.3	17.8	16.9	18	17.9
Birth rate (%)	8.6	8.6	9.1	9.1	11.1	12.5	13.8	12.7	14.2	14.5

ment in the quality of the care patients receive, participation in the registry must be easy; the data captured must be relevant, reliable and unselected; and analyses of the data must be performed in a clinically and statistically meaningful way.

Currently, the most extensive data available to date is the 1995 ART World Collaborative Report (de Mouzon and Lancaster, 1997), which comprises data from 775 clinics in 45 countries. In addition, data retrieved from the report of ART activities as prepared by the American Society for Reproductive Medicine (ASRM/SART Registry, 1998), as well as by the Human Fertilization and Embryology Authority (HFEA, 1997) in the United Kingdom, will be also presented.

In a survey of the world results of IVF-ET during the years 1985–1989, the pregnancy rate and live birth rate per treatment cycle were only about 14% and 11%, respectively (Ezra and Schenker, 1993). Current surveys indicate significantly improved results. This steady, though rather slow, rise in success is seen in the reports of the HFEA (1997), where the clinical pregnancy and live birth rates per treatment cycle rose from 11.2% and 8.6% respectively, in 1985, to 17.9% and 14.5%, respectively, in 1995 (see Table 14.1). However, significant variations are often observed among countries, which can be attributed to the heterogeneity of IVF units in terms of activity range, research efforts and success rates (De Mouzon and Lancaster, 1997).

In the 1995 reports regarding standard IVF (Table 15.2), pregnancy rates per retrieval were about 30%,

Table 15.2: Reported Outcomes for Standard IVF Procedures in 1995

Variable	World Report	ASRM/SART	HFEA*
Started cycles	127,641	36,035	36,994
Cancellations (%)	10.9	16.1	NA
No. of oocyte pick-ups	113,732	30,223	NA
No. of transfers	96,605	27,125	30,354
No. of transfers per retrieval (%)	85.2	89.7	NA
No. of pregnancies	23,888	8,299	6,827
Pregnancy loss (%)	29.0	18.6	18.8
No. of deliveries	16,951	6,754	5,542
Deliveries per retrieval (%)	14.9	22.3	21.0
Singleton pregnancies (%)	70.9	64.1	68.0
Twin pregnancies (%)	24.7	29.6	27.8
Triplets pregnancies (%)	4.1	6.4	4.1
Higher-order pregnancies (%)	0.2	0.6	0.1
Ectopic pregnancies per total pregnancies (%)	3.6	2.6	2.5

Note: NA= not available

* Includes fresh and frozen embryo transfers

whereas deliveries per retrieval varied from 15%–22.3%, depending on the country studied. Pregnancy loss, estimated to be about 18% in the US and UK, also seemed to fluctuate greatly among the reports of the various clinics. The rate of ectopic pregnancies per pregnancy achieved reached about 3.0%, and the incidence of multiple pregnancies remained still high (~ 30%–35%), the majority of which consisted of twins (~ 25%–30%), with triplets and higher-order pregnancies appearing at a much lower frequency (6% and 0.1%, respectively).

Gamete Intrafallopian Transfer (GIFT) is currently applied in a much smaller number of cases. According to the 1995 ART World Report (de Mouzon and Lancaster, 1997), of the total 8,938 cycles of GIFT reported, 7,956 retrievals (89% of cycles) resulted. A total of 6,685 transfers were performed, or 84% of retrievals resulted in a transfer of gametes. A total of 2,489 clinical pregnancies were established, with a clinical pregnancy rate of 27.8% per initiated cycle, 31.3% per retrieval, and 37.2% per gamete transfer. Of these pregnancies, 1,930 were reported as deliveries, or 21.6% deliveries per initiated cycle, 24.2% per retrieval, and 28.9% per gamete transfer. Of the clinical pregnancies identified, 77.5% overall went to delivery. Ectopic pregnancies represented 3.7% of all pregnancies. Of the delivered pregnancies, 67.3% were singletons, 26.8% twins, 5.4% triplets, and 0.5% higher-order multiples.

Zygote Intrafallopian Transfer (ZIFT), according to the ASRM/SART Registry report (1998), consisted of a total number of procedures at initiation of 1078 cycles, with 941 retrievals (12.7% of cycles cancelled), and 863 transfers resulting in 91.7% transfers per retrieval. As a result, 322 clinical pregnancies were established, and 263 delivered, with an overall success rate of 24.4% deliveries per initiated cycle, 27.9% per retrieval, and 30.5% per zygote transfer. Of the 263 delivered pregnancies, 68.8% were singletons, 25.9% twins, 4.5% triplets, and 0.8% quadruplets. In addition, 12 ectopic pregnancies were reported, or 1.4% of transfers and 3.6% of all pregnancies.

Summarizing the 1995 ART World Report (de Mouzon and Lancaster, 1997), there seems to be an increase in the number of programmes reporting, and an increase in the number of cycles of ART, with an increased probability of success, compared to the 1993 ART World Report. However, considerable variations between countries and centres continue to exist. Also, the incidence of multiple pregnancies and preterm births has not shown any decrease.

Factors Influencing IVF Outcome

A number of factors have been suggested to influence pregnancy rates in IVF, either positively or negatively (Minaretzis et al., 1998). An evaluation of the strength of each factor in increasing or decreasing pregnancy rates would provide the basis for the development of a flexible individualized IVF approach and improve patient counselling. This potentially can offer the best chance of success in each cycle to each couple.

Advanced Age

Demographic changes, coupled with the need to postpone childbearing in favour of pursuing a career, contribute to the increasing number of women wishing to conceive towards the end of their reproductive period. Unfortunately, such aspirations are often met with disappointment due to the natural decline in PR with age (Tarin et al., 1998).

Age is known to be the most important factor affecting the outcome of fertility treatment, and especially IVF (Hull et al., 1992; Roseboom et al., 1995). In particular, advancing age has been associated with reduced fecundity, both *in vivo* and *in vitro*. The results of donor insemination programmes support a natural decline in fecundity with advancing age (Van Noord-Zaadstra et al., 1991). These findings are also supported by studies of both involving IVF-ET and GIFT. Piette et al. (1990) showed a significant decrease in the assisted reproduction outcome from 37 years of age, while others found a decline after 35 years(Segal and Casper, 1990; Kenny, 1994). *In vivo*, there is a further decline in fertility between 40 and 44 years, and fertility rates become negligible between 45 and 49 years of age, with only 2%–5% of women having successful pregnancies (Wood et al., 1992). Also, the 'take-home baby' rate in women older than 40 years in ART programnes has been shown to be extremely low due to a reduced conception rate and an increase in pregnancy wastage (Bopp et al., 1995).

Templeton et al. (1996), in an analysis of all IVF treatment cycles and outcomes registered for the years 1991–1994 by the HFEA, found an overall live birth rate of 13.9% per cycle treatment . The highest live birth rates were in the age-group of 25–30 years, whereas compared with a predicted live birth rate of 17% per cycle started at age 30, the success rates at ages 40 and 45 were only 7% and 2%, respectively. They proposed that the effect of age can be overcome to a great extent by the use of donated eggs.

In a retrospective study of 779 patients undergoing ART, the results for women of 40 and above were compared with those for women between 36 and 39 years of age and those younger than 36 years (Dew et al., 1998). The pregnancy rate, pregnancy outcome, fertilization rate and ovarian response to stimulation diminished with increasing age. Despite a fertilization rate of 34%, there were no live births in women older than 42 years. Al-Shawaf et al. (1992) and Bopp et al. (1995) also found that women older than 43 years are unlikely to benefit from IVF or GIFT, with no live births being achieved, whereas Abdalla et al. (1993) had a 55% miscarriage rate in women aged 40 to 44 years, and a 100% miscarriage rate in women between 45 and 49 years.

The decrease in fertility with ageing has been attributed mainly to decreased oocyte quality; however, other factors have also been proposed, like a decrease in uterine receptivity and advanced paternal age (see analysis under Oocyte Donation).

Although it is a difficult ethical decision, it may be suggested that women of advanced age (usually older than 45) should be advised against proceeding with infertility treatment, in view of the disappointing results achieved in this age-group, unless oocyte donation is available. However, enforcing an age limit embraces great difficulties, as couples are often desperate to have a child no matter how low their chances (Eisenberg and Schenker, 1997).

Cause of Infertility

The cause of infertility appears to have a limited effect on the probability of pregnancy and live birth following conventional IVF. The HFEA report for 1997 presents similar results for the various causes of female infertility (see Table 14.3). Templeton et al. (1996), after adjusting for age and the duration of infertility, also showed that there was no significant overall effect of female causes on the live birth rate per treatment cycle.

The impact of IVF-ET as a treatment modality on the various causes of infertility has also been investigated (Shushan et al., 1995). *In vitro* fertilization is obviously not the first therapeutic option for patients with an ovulatory defect, i.e. polycystic ovarian disease (PCOD). Nevertheless, it can happen that a patient with these characteristics has failed after the application of the usual therapeutic options for the syndrome, or simply that she should undergo IVF because of an associated factor such as tubal pathology or male-factor infertility (Shulman and Dor, 1997).

Early reports concerning the results obtained with ART in PCOD patients, though based on small non-controlled series, revealed improved success rates in subfertile women with PCOD who were

Table 15.3: IVF Clinical and Live Birth Rate for Female Causes of Infertility (HFEA, 1997)

Factor	No. of cycles	% of all cycles	Clinical pregnancy rate (%)	Live birth rate (%)
Tubal Disease	14, 667	39.6	16.9	13.3
Endometriosis	3,663	9.9	18.6	15.0
Unexplained	15,627	42.2	19.0	15.9
Others	5,887	15.9	20.6	16.4

Note: % are of number of treatment cycles

resistant to other treatments (Dale et al., 1991). Homburg et al. (1993) have also shown that IVF is a successful treatment alternative for these patients. The pregnancy rate per ET was 23%, with a cumulative conception and live birth rates of 82% and 69%, respectively, after six cycles.

Tubal disease is one of the major causes of female infertility, and IVF-ET was initially introduced as a method to overcome tubal infertility. Tubal disease includes an array of disorders, including blockage, both proximally and distally, peritubal adhesions and hydrosalpinx. Severe tubal disease, specifically distal tubal obstruction leading to hydrosalpinx, is associated with a poor fertility prognosis.

During the last few years, many investigators have reported that the PR after only one or two IVF-ET treatments may be equal to the result after a first attempt at surgical repair (Abyholm et al., 1991), and in many centres, IVF-ET has become the preferred method for the treatment of women who have failed to conceive due to tubal damage. Soliman et al. (1993), in a randomized clinical trial, demonstrated a significant beneficial effect of IVF treatment in patients with bilateral severe tubal disease and reported that IVF increases the likelihood of pregnancy by 40% in women with severe tubal disease.

The presence of hydrosalpinx has a negative effect on IVF-ET by decreasing the pregnancy rates and implantation rates, compared with patients undergoing IVF-ET for tubal disease but without hydrosalpinx (Zeyneloglu et al., 1998). Hydrosalpingeal fluid has been demonstrated to be embryotoxic to developing embryos, thus leading to increased early pregnancy losses (Schenk et al., 1996). Poor endometrial receptivity has also been demonstrated in the presence of hydrosalpinges (Lessey et al., 1994). Removal of the hydrosalpinges leads to improved IVF-ET rates; thus salpingectomy has been recommended for patients with hydrosalpinx who will be undergoing IVF-ET (Nackley and Muasher, 1998).

Over the past decade, infertility associated with endometriosis has been an expanding indication for pursuing IVF. Of the available data regarding the impact of varying degrees of endometriosis on the outcome of IVF, conclusions have ranged from impaired outcome with increasing severity (Dmowski et al., 1995) to comparable results with different stages (Geber et al., 1995; Oliveness et al., 1995). Also, Pal et al. (1998) analysed the results of 81 IVF cycles being performed in 61 patients with a primary diagnosis of endometriosis, and concluded that the outcome of IVF-ET is not affected by the increasing severity of endometriosis.

The efficacy and cost-effectiveness of alternative treatments for unexplained infertility were recently evaluated (Guzick et al., 1998). Whereas the combined pregnancy rates per initiated cycle were low when no treatment was applied (1.3%–4.1%), they increased considerably when clomiphene citrate was associated with IUI (8.3%). However, the application of IVF or GIFT led to pregnancy rates of 20.7% and 27%, respectively. They concluded that clomiphene citrate with IUI is a cost-effective treatment for unexplained infertility, and in cases where this fails, menotropins with IUI and assisted reproduction are efficacious options.

Success Rate with Repeated Cycles of IVF-ET

It is essential to counsel couples who have failed one or more cycles of ART to be able to provide a reasonably precise estimate of the negative impact, if any, of a previous attempt. Table 14.4 shows the results from various studies published in the literature that have numerical data, tabulated for repeat cycles. With one exception (Hershlag et al., 1991), the results are remarkably consistent despite varying outcome measures and design, showing a modest reduction of successful outcome with increasing previous cycle failures. Factors other than the fertility potential of the remaining couples could influence success with repeat cycles. Couples with a lower prognosis could elect to stop therapy, or could be actively discouraged or even refused treatment. Land et al. (1997) examined this effect. Although based on a relatively small number of pregnancies, the decline at cycle 3 was 24% compared with no decline in uncorrected rates in their programme. In contrast, Haan et al. (1991) examined this same issue for their programme and con-

Table 15.4: Repeated IVF Outcomes According to Cycle Rank

	Cycle rank				
Study	1	2	3	4	>4
Guzick et al. (1986) (no. of pregnancies/no. of retrievals) (%)	53/394 (13.5)	25/183 (13.7)	15/85 (17.6)	6/44 (13.6)	8/49 (16.3)
Hershlag et al. (1991) (no. of pregnancies/no. of cycles) (%)	75/571 (13)	36/338 (11)	12/173 (7)	4/93 (4)	2/82 (2)
Tan et al. (1992) (no. of births/no. of treatment cycles) (%)	290/2,735 (10.6)	131/1,267 (10.3)	50/497 (9.1)	22/238 (9.2)	11/171 (6.4)
FIVNAT (1993) (no. of pregnancies/no. of retrievals) (%)	4,869/25,666 (18.3)	2,563/15,021 (17.1)	1,523/8,576 (17.8)	816/4,846 (17.8)	1,006/6,209 (16.2)
Templeton et al. (1996) (no. of births/no. of retrievals) (%)	2,918/18,239 (16.0)	1,169/8,123 (14.4)	467/3,706 (12.6)	86/864 (10.0)	101/1,084 (9.3)
Meldrum et al. (1998) (no. of births / no. of retrievals) (%)	652/2,414 (27)	260/948 (27.4)	92/394 (23.4)	23/143 (16.1)	22/143 (15.4)

cluded that the prognosis was the same for couples who did or did not return for repeat cycles.

Several investigators have mentioned the improved prognosis that is often achieved by modifying clinical management (i.e. for stimulation, hCG timing, semen preparation, and transfer method based on experience obtained in the previous cycle) (Meldrum et al., 1998). Women having repeated cycles are usually older than those having their first cycle. In the French National Registry, when the results were corrected for age, there was no longer any significant decline with cycle rank (FIVNAT, 1993).

It may thus be concluded that there is only a modest decline of success with repeated IVF cycle attempts, part of which results from the older age of cycle repeaters. Any selection of patients with a better prognosis for repeat cycles may be counterbalanced by modifying the treatment of repeaters, and better overall results will be obtained by general improvements in programmes with lower results and by systematic improvements in IVF techniques.

Number of Embryos Transferred

A key element pivotal to the potential success to be anticipated from any single IVF attempt is how many embryos to transfer. Ideally, uterine or tubal transfer of a single embryo generated *in vitro* would be optimal if implantation per embryo were as high as 50%. Unfortunately, implantation rates for IVF embryos hover around 10% to 12%, and in severe specific cases may be even lower. As a consequence it is routine for IVF clinics to transfer, on an average, three to four embryos, if available, to help boost the chances of transferring at least one embryo that will implant and go to term, and thus raise the average term pregnancy rates per IVF cycle initiated (Elsner et al., 1997).

The transfer of multiple embryos results in a higher pregnancy rate (Walters et al., 1996). Data retrieved from the HFEA report (1997) reveals that three embryos were replaced in 54.9% of the 30,354 cycles of IVF reported between January 1995 and March 1996. The clinical pregnancy rate was increased if more than one embryo was replaced. The pregnancy rate per cycle was 8.4% (278 out of 3,306) after replacing a single embryo, 20.2% (2,097 out of 10,376) after two embryos, and 26.6% (4,346 out of 16,672) after three embryos. This trend towards a higher pregnancy rate has also been shown by other studies. Elsner et al. (1997), in a retrospective study, reported an increase in the pregnancy rate per embryo transfer from 9.7% after replacing a single embryo, to 28.4% after two embryos and 37.3% after three embryos.

However, a serious consequence of increasing the number of embryos transferred is a concordant increase in the incidence of multiple pregnancies. Currently, multiple pregnancy rates in most IVF programmes are still ~30%, despite the technological developments achieved in assisted reproduction (Coetsier and Dhont, 1998).

The replacement of two and three embryos, or even more embryos is associated with a significantly increased risk of a multiple birth. The chance of a triplet or quadruplet pregnancy is almost 6% after the replacement of three embryos (Table 15.5). Recognizing the detrimental effects of multiple pregnancies on both fetal and maternal outcomes, recommendations have been presented by the British Fertility Society (BFS) and the ASRM relating to the number of embryos which should be transferred after IVF treatment. The ASRM recommends transferring between three and five embryos for IVF, with more for GIFT transfer, whereas the BFS recommends a maximum of two (Murdoch, 1998). The European Society for Human Reproduction and Embryology (ESHRE) Capri Workshop (1996) recommended either two or three embryos, depending on female's age. Other investigators suggested the transfer of one embryo (Coetsier and Dhont, 1998). However, it seems unrealistic to expect that centres will adopt a one-embryo transfer policy with the current technology.

Most investigators stress the need for further research into laboratory aspects reflecting embryo quality, such as prolonged *in vitro* culture, embryo co-culture techniques, or embryo biopsy (Bronson et al., 1997). Only new developments in these areas would produce a scientific basis robust enough to justify the elective transfer of one single embryo.

Blastocyst Culture And Transfer

Human preimplantation embryos conceived through IVF are routinely transferred to the uterus on day 2 or 3, around the four- to eight-cell stage of development and resultant implantation rates of 10–20% are routinely reported. *In vivo,* the four- to eight-cell embryo resides in the fallopian tube; it is, therefore, plausible that the premature exposure of cleavage-stage embryos to the uterus after

Table 15.5. Single and Multiple Pregnancy Rates by the Numbers of Embryos Transferred

	No. of embryos replaced		
	One	Two	Three
Singleton			
HFEA (1997)	265 (95.3)	1,587 (75.7)	2,630 (67.1)
Elsner et al. (1997)	22 (100)	97 (85)	164 (66)
Twin			
HFEA (1997)	10 (3.6)	505 (24.1)	1,163 (26.8)
Elsner et al. (1997)	0	17 (15)	74 (30)
Triplets or quadruplets			
HFEA (1997)	3 (1.1)	5 (0.2)	253 (5.8)
Elsner et al. (1997)	0	0	10 (4)

Table 15.6. Comparison of Reported Outcomes for ICSI Procedures in 1995

Variable	World Report	ASRM/SART	HFEA
Started cycles	19,318	5,638	5,209
Cancellations (%)	4.4	3.7	NA
No. of oocyte pick-ups	18,471	5,428	NA
No. of transfers	16,683	5,248	4,848
No. of transfers per retrieval (%)	90.3	96.7	NA
No. of pregnancies	4,067	1,659	1,207
Pregnancy loss (%)	32.2	18.6	15.3
No. of deliveries	2,756	1,350	1,022
Deliveries per retrieval (%)	14.9	24.9	NA
Singleton pregnancies (%)	72.4	62.4	NA
Twin pregnancies (%)	24.3	30.8	NA
Triplets pregnancies (%)	3.2	6.2	NA
Higher-order pregnancies (%)	0.1	0.3	NA
Ectopic pregnancies per total pregnancies (%)	1.2	1.0	1.2

Note: NA= not available

* Includes fresh and frozen embryo transfers

day-2 and day-3 transfers compromises embryo development and viability. In other mammalian species, the transfer of cleavage-stage embryos to the uterus does not result in high pregnancy rates, compared with embryos transferred at the blastocyst stage (Bavister, 1995).

Blastocyst transfer may prove beneficial in patients with repeated implantation failure, patients with uterine abnormalities that preclude multiple pregnancies thus requiring more careful selection of the single embryo; patients suspected of defects in oocyte quality thus requiring embryos to be assessed for a more extended period of *in vitro* development; patients needing embryo biopsy for genetic selection; and patients undergoing replacement of supernumerary embryos frozen at the blastocyst stage (Bavister and Boatman, 1998). Animal experiments indicate high implantation, pregnancy, and live birth rates when following blastocyst transfer (Trounson et al., 1994; Hasler et al., 1995). These observations indicate that human IVF-ET may be improved dramatically if embryos are grown under improved conditions to the blastocyst stage before transfer.

Data to date on the replacement of human blastocysts on day 5 of development in culture, indicate that such embryos have a high implantation rate. For good-quality eight-cells and for expanded blastocysts, implantation rates of 18% and 35%, respectively, have been reported (Scholtes and Zeilmaker, 1996). Gardner et al. (1998) evaluated the implantation rates achieved by the transfer of blastocysts on day 5, compared with embryos transferred on day 3. Implantation was significantly increased when embryos were transferred on day 5, compared with those transferred on day 3 (45.5% and 21%, respectively). The ongoing PR for embryos transferred either on day 3 or day 5 was equivalent, although significantly fewer embryos were transferred on day 5, thus minimizing thus the risk of multiple gestation.

Fong et al. (1997) reported the first delivery of a normal healthy baby after the transfer of blastocysts with the zonae completely removed with pronase. The same group (Fong et al., 1998) studied blastocyst transfer after enzymatic treatment of the zona pellucida in a larger group of patients, and reported clinical PR per cycle/transfer and implantation rates of 55% and 33%, respectively. The safety of the method is mentioned, as no congenital anomalies have been observed on regular ultrasound monitoring and no reproductive losses had been observed up to 22 weeks of gestation.

The main problem with blastocyst transfer in human IVF involves the optimal culture conditions that are needed for embryos to grow *in vitro* up to the blastocyst stage. Improved culture media formulations and co-culture systems that can yield blastulation rates as high as 55%–60% are now available (Bongso et al., 1995; Gardner et al., 1998; Jones et al., 1998). Studies on how co-culture systems produce their positive effects will provide the necessary clues for producing even better cell-free culture media formulations in the future. The application of such defined systems should not only significantly reduce the variability between IVF programmes, but will also increase the overall efficiency of human IVF.

Obstetrical And Perinatal Outcome Of IVF Pregnancies

In the evaluation of the outcome of pregnancies after IVF, although parameters such as age, cause of infertility, laboratory technique, multiple pregnancy and preterm labour are taken into consideration, there is always a problem of comparison with natural conception, in which issues such as the cause of infertility cannot be properly matched, and certainly no matching can be found for a pregnancy resulting from cryopreserved embryos. Another problem is the number of embryos that reach the uterus in IVF cycles as compared to natural ones, as well as the very high hormonal levels commonly existing at the beginning of IVF pregnancies. As a result, data retrieved from the literature reveal conflicting results regarding the rate of obstetric complications during IVF pregnancies.

The expected preterm delivery, low birth weight and perinatal mortality rates in singletons in the general population are 5.2%, 4.8% and 7.1%, respectively (Aytoz et al., 1998). Studies evaluating IVF-ET reported that pregnancies achieved by ART are subject to major problems, such as prematurity, low birth weight and an increased perinatal mortality, mainly because of prematurity (Rufat et al., 1994). Others have reported that even if singletons are considered separately, the prematurity rate is twice that for the general population, and the low birth weight and perinatal mortality rates are three times those for the general population (Saunders et al., 1988). In a case-control study of singleton pregnancies obtained by IVF-ET, the preterm delivery rate was significantly higher in the IVF-ET group than in the controls (Verlaenen et al., 1995).

Olivennes et al. (1993) reported similar rates of prematurity, low birth weight and perinatal mortality in IVF-ET pregnancies and in pregnancies obtained after ovarian hyperstimulation. However, the frequencies of prematurity and low birth weight were significantly higher in these two groups than in cases of spontaneous singleton pregnancy. They concluded that the increased risk was linked not to the IVF-ET method itself, but to population characteristics and to underlying infertility. However, the same investigators reported a similar perinatal outcome for twin pregnancies after spontaneous conception and after IVF-ET (Olivennes et al., 1996).

Tanbo et al. (1995), in a retrospective study, evaluated the maternal and perinatal outcome in 355 singleton pregnancies after ART, with a control group of 644 women. Obstetric complications (premature delivery, low birth weight, pregnancy-induced hypertension, placenta previa) were observed with greater frequency in the former group. The rate of elective caesarean sections was also higher in the IVF group.

The Hadassah IVF Group evaluated the obstetric outcome of 260 singleton IVF pregnancies, in comparison with 260 matched natural singleton pregnancies as controls (Reubinoff et al., 1997). No significant difference was found between these groups in the incidence of most obstetric complications, including antenatal bleeding, placenta previa, hypertension, gestational diabetes mellitus, preterm premature rupture of membranes, and preterm premature uterine contractions. Spontaneous onset of delivery was less frequent among IVF patients, and normal vaginal delivery was experienced by fewer patients in the IVF group due to the high caesarean section rate (both elective and emergency) in the IVF group (41.9%), similar to that reported in other centres (Friedler et al., 1992), compared to the control group (15.5%). While the incidence of preterm delivery (<37 weeks) was comparable, there was a nonsignificant trend of increased prematurity rate among IVF pregnancies.

Since the first pregnancy following human IVF turned out to be an ectopic pregnancy (Steptoe and Edwards, 1976), the world literature has recognized the high incidence of ectopic pregnancies in assisted conception, which averages 5% of IVF pregnancies (Marcus et al., 1995).

Heterotopic pregnancy, which is defined as coexistent intrauterine and ectopic gestations, is more common following IVF and the transfer of multiple embryos. While spontaneous heterotopic pregnancy is extremely rare, its occurrence being 1 per 30,000 pregnancies, 1%–3% of ART gestations reportedly present with this serious complication (Lewin and Schenker, 1998). This rate is expected to increase in the future with the rising incidence of pelvic inflammatory disease and greater use and accessibility of ART.

The perinatal mortality rate for IVF pregnancies in 1995 was 22.6/1,000 (HFEA, 1997), whereas in the general population during the same interval, it reached about 8.7/1,000, which is similar to that seen with IVF single births. However, the rate rises to 46.8/1,000 for IVF twins and 82.6/1,000 for IVF triplets (Lieberman, 1998). This increase in the perinatal mortality rate following IVF treatment is likely to be due to the increased incidence of preterm birth associated with multiple pregnancies. Thus, multiple pregnancies, which reach an incidence of about 30% in most IVF programmes, continue to represent a major issue in IVF-ET treatments, also contributing significantly to an increase in the health service cost (Mugford and Henderson, 1995). Over and above the increased risk of fetal and neonatal death, the increased possibility of disability should be borne in mind (Doyle, 1996), as it is known that the risk of cerebral palsy, blindness, learning and behavioural disorders is increased with the birth of premature babies.

Multifetal gestation is correlated with an increased frequency of maternal complications and higher perinatal morbidity and mortality. The major maternal complications include pre-eclampsia, postpartum haemorrhage, antepartum anaemia, hydramnios, urinary tract infections and an increased incidence of caesarean sections. The neonatal prematurity rate is highly complicated by the respiratory distress syndrome, intraventricular haemorrhage and fetal growth retardation. There is also an increased socio-economic strain on the family, especially if some children who survive are severely handicapped (Gonen et al., 1990).

Faced with the prospect of a multiple pregnancy, some couples may contemplate embryo reduction. This procedure has proved to be an efficient and safe way to improve the outcome of multifetal pregnancies, especially those with four or more fetuses, and likely those with three fetuses. As the experience from the procedure continuously increases, it seems that reduction of triplets to twins can be offered to women with satisfactory results. Reduction of twins or higher gestations to singletons has not yet been established and is applied only when medical reasons are indicated (Fasouliotis and Schenker, 1997).

Congenital Malformations And Long-Term Follow-Up Of IVF Children

Considerable attention has been given to the incidence of major congenital abnormalities in children conceived by IVF; in some women embryos have been implanted after cleavage, while in others the embryos have been frozen before use. The incidence of major congenital malformations in both has been reported to be similar to that in population-based estimates (Tan et al., 1992). Data from the register of IVF and GIFT pregnancies in Australia and New Zealand suggest, however, a higher incidence of transposition of the great vessels and spina bifida in newborn infants conceived by IVF than in the general population (Lancaster, 1987). Moreover, a survey of all children born after assisted conception, including IVF, has shown an increased incidence of congenital malformations (Cohen et al., 1988).

In general, prospective follow-up studies comparing IVF pregnancies with appropriate controls, rather than with population-based norms, have not found an association with congenital malformation (Morin et al., 1989), or with impaired growth and development (Morin et al., 1989; Brandes et al., 1992). The ART World Report, 1995 (de Mouzon and Lancaster, 1997), summarized the malformation rates following IVF as an overall 2.1%, which does not differ from those estimated for the general population.

D'Souza et al. (1997) compared the outcome in 278 IVF children from multiple and singleton births with one another, and with 278 normally conceived control children. The high percentage of preterm deliveries noted (34.9%) was largely due to multiple births and these contributed to neonatal conditions in 45% of all IVF children, compared with only 7.6% among the controls. The types of congenital malformations varied: 3.6% of IVF children and 2.5% of controls had minor congenital malformations, and 2.5% of IVF children and none of the controls had major congenital malformations. There were no significant differences in the prevalence of these conditions in IVF children from singleton and multiple births and, overall, between IVF children and controls. IVF children (2.1%) and 0.4% of the controls had mild/moderate developmental disabilities. They were all from multiple births, including two children with cerebral palsy who were triplets. They concluded that the outcome of IVF treatment leading to multiple births is less satisfactory than that in singletons because of neonatal conditions associated with preterm delivery and disabilities in later childhood. Thus, a reduction of multiple pregnancies by limiting the number of embryos transferred remains a priority (Addor et al., 1998).

Other studies evaluating the follow-up of IVF children reported normal development (Olivennes et al., 1997). Wennerholm et al. (1991), who evaluated infants born after IVF-ET during a 7-year period, reported that after a follow-up of 18 months to 8 years, long-term sequelae were associated with immaturity and low birth weight. No problems were encountered during follow-up in children with an uneventful neonatal period.

MALE INFERTILITY INTRACYTOPLASMIC SPERM INJECTION

Without a doubt, one of the greatest breakthroughs in the field of infertility treatment involves the advent of methods for treating male infertility, and specifically, the introduction of intracytoplasmic sperm injection (ICSI). The concept of microinjecting a single spermatozoon into the perivitelline space or into the ooplasm, in order to achieve a form of fertilization, had earlier been achieved in a few uncontrolled animal studies (Edwards, 1997). The weakness of IVF for the treatment of male infertility lay in dealing with severe oligozoospermia, due to which insufficient spermatozoa of normal physiology and good activity were available to achieve successful fertilization *in vitro*.

Three major variants of microsurgical fertilization have been developed and have undergone wide clinical experience during the last years. There are partial zona drilling (PZD), the creation of an opening through the zona pellucida (ZP), either mechanically or chemically; subzonal sperm injection (SUZI)—insertion of sperm into the perivitelline space; and finally, intracytoplasmic sperm injection. Experience with PZD and SUZI has revealed that these approaches increase the fertilization rate but, at the same time, are associated with losses due to oocyte trauma, high rate of polyspermic fertilization and low rates of normal cleavage (Garrissi et al., 1990).

Intracytoplasmic sperm injection with spermatozoa from ejaculated sperm or, later on with epididymal or testicular spermatozoa, has essentially replaced these latter two techniques as it has been proven to be more successful in facilitating fertilization and producing pregnancy (Tsirigotis and Craft, 1995). The introduction of ICSI (Palermo et al., 1992) has resulted in a great enhancement of fertilization and pregnancy rates in patients with severely reduced sperm quality (Van Steirteghem et al., 1993), also facilitating attempts to retrieve testicular sperm in cases with nonobstructive azoospermia (Lewin et al., 1996). Spermatids can also be used instead of spermatozoa, and a few living human offspring have been born (Tesarik, 1995). Spermatids can be obtained from ejaculates of testis preparations, and can be sucked off Sertoli cell membranes if necessary.

In one of the early studies, van Steirteghem et al. (1993) reported injection of a single spermatozoon into the ooplasm of 1,409 oocytes, leading to a fertilization rate of 64.2%. Total and clinical PRs of 49.6% and 39.2%, respectively, per ET were achieved. Retrieving data from the 1995 ART World Report (de Mouzon and Lancaster, 1997), a tenfold increase in the number of the ICSI cycles performed is noted, compared to the same report regarding treatments in 1993, evidencing the establishment of ICSI as a reliable and efficient method for alleviating male infertility. Table 15.4 provides an analysis of the ICSI results as presented by a large series in 1995.

The introduction of ICSI as a novel solution for male infertility has raised new concerns regarding possible congenital malformations in the offspring. These concerns focus on the fact that spermatozoa from poor-quality sperm samples are used, including severe morphological pathology, immotile sperm and sperm with normal parameters but lacking fertilizing ability. Thus, it is important to compare the outcome of ICSI pregnancies, the rate of major and minor congenital malformations, and the karyotypes of children with those resulting from IVF.

Wisanto et al. (1995), who evaluated the outcome of 424 pregnancies resulting from ICSI, considered that the comparison of pregnancy outcomes after ICSI and IVF was not straightforward, as ICSI patients represent an almost homogeneous group in which the majority of the female partners are usually fertile, whereas in conventional IVF, the group of patients is more heterogeneous, with both male and female factors represented. In their study, early pregnancy loss occurred in 99 cases (23.3%), similar to the 18%–24% reported after IVF (Table 15.2), and in agreement with other studies evaluating the IVF and ICSI procedures (Wennerholm et al., 1996). The incidence of ectopic pregnancy was low (0.9%), smaller than that which is usually found in IVF cycles, which supports the idea of tubal damage as the underlying cause in the pathogenesis of ectopic pregnancy after IVF (Wisanto et al., 1995). Complications in ICSI pregnancies, as reported by a large series in the literature, are presented in Table 15.7. The rate of these complications among singletons was similar in ICSI pregnancies and in the general population. The incidence of multiple pregnancies is similar among IVF and ICSI pregnancies, reaching about 30% (Govaerts et al., 1996), whereas the rates of caesarean section are found to be higher both in ICSI and IVF than in the general population (Govaerts et al., 1998). Summarizing these series, it may be concluded that the pregnancy characteristics and perinatal outcome after ICSI show no increase in the number of pathologies in comparison with IVF.

Aytoz et al. (1998) described the outcome of pregnancies obtained after ICSI and the impact of the origin and quality of the sperm used on this outcome. The study involved pregnant patients conceived after microinjection of ejaculated sperm (n=1,427), epididymal sperm (n=79), and

Table 15.7. Complications Reported in ICSI and Spontaneous Pregnancies

No. of cases (%) for singletons

	Wisanto et al. (1995)	Wennerholm et al. (1996)	Govaerts et al. (1998)	General population
Prematurity	7.6	9.3	6.7	7.3
Birth weight <2500g	10.3	6.4	5.0	6.1
SGA	4.4	9.0	1.5	5.0
Hypertension	14.6	9.0	9.0	7.4

testicular sperm (n=93). The obstetric outcome of ICSI pregnancies as a whole was similar to that of conventional IVF pregnancies; however, the rates of preterm deliveries, low and very low birth weight, multiple pregnancies and early perinatal morbidity were higher after ICSI than after natural conception. The rates of subclinical pregnancy, ectopic pregnancy and abortions did not differ in relation to the origin and quality of sperm. In the ejaculated-sperm group, the rate of intrauterine death was higher in the severely defective sperm group than in the better-quality sperm groups, which may be attributed to the poor-quality sperm and its genetic content, as it is known that intrauterine growth retardation and late fetal loss may be associated with placenta-confined mosaicism and uniparental disomy (Wolstenholme et al., 1994).

An important debate about ICSI infants is the risk of congenital malformations. The rates of congenital malformations in ICSI infants reported by several authors are summarized in Table 15.8. The overall frequency of anomalies in these children seems to be similar to the frequency of those arising in IVF or after natural conception (Bonduelle et al., 1995; Wisanto et al., 1995).

In't-Veld et al. (1995) reported a high incidence of sex-chromosome aberrations in a small number of prenatal diagnostic tests, performed for advanced maternal age. Whereas results from other investigators were less striking, ground for concern have been set (Liebaers et al., 1995).

Table 15.8. Incidence of Congenital Malformations in ICSI Neonates

	Major malformations	Minor malformations
Wisanto et al. (1995) (n=923)	3.3	20.5
Palermo et al. (1996) (n=578)	1.6	1.0
Wennerholm et al. (1996) (n=210)	1.0	1.8
Govaerts et al. (1998) (n=141)	0	2.8

Bonduelle et al. (1998) reported 18 (1.66%) cases of *de novo* chromosomal aberrations in 1,082 prenatal tests performed in pregnancies after ICSI, nine (0.83%) of which were sex-chromosomal aberrations and another nine (0.83%) were autosomal aberrations (trisomies and structural). This increase in the incidence of sex-chromosomal aberrations was considered to be statistically significant compared with that described in the literature (Nielsen and Wohlert, 1991). An increased percentage of *de novo* chromosomal aberrations may result from the ICSI procedure itself, or it may be linked to a defined subgroup of males with impaired semen samples (Bonduelle et al., 1998). Other groups have also reported a much higher incidence of chromosomal anomalies after ICSI (In't-Veld et al., 1995; van Opstal et al., 1997).

Bowen et al. (1998) evaluated the medical and developmental outcome at 1 year for children conceived by ICSI, compared with children conceived by conventional IVF and natural conception. Children conceived by ICSI were found to have an increased incidence of mild delays on the Bayley mental development index (MDI), which assesses memory, problem-solving ability and language skill. There was no difference between the groups in the children's performance on the psychomotor development index (PDI), which assesses motor skills. As a result of these findings, the authors supported the need for ongoing developmental follow-up of children conceived by ICSI to verify whether they are at increased risk of intellectual impairment or learning difficulties at the school age.

OOCYTE DONATION

More than a decade ago, the first pregnancies after oocyte donation in women with primary ovarian failure were reported (Lutjen et al., 1984). Since then, oocyte donation has been widely used to alleviate infertility. Initially, this treatment was intended for women with ovarian failure. Subsequently, oocyte donation has been extended to other forms of infertility, including menopausal omen, patients with retained ovarian function who ave repeated IVF failures, or patients with a ge- tic trait precluding the use of their own oocytes.

ESULTS

he majority of publications that deal with oocyte onation focus on PR per embryo transfer as the ain outcome measure. A recent study from Israel cluded 423 oocyte recipients who underwent ,001 oocyte donation cycles (Yaron et al., 1998). 'he donors were all healthy women, less than 34 ears old, who underwent IVF themselves. In 873 ycles (87.2% of initial cycles), fertilization occurred nd embryo transfer was performed, resulting in 94 clinical pregnancies, thus yielding an overall linical pregnancy rate of 22.2% per embryo transfer. 'regnancy rates declined significantly with an ncrease in the number of previous attempts, and vith increasing age of the recipient (36.8%/embryo ransfer in patients ≤30 compared to 17.8% in atients >40 years old). A significant increase in he PR was noted with a greater number of embryos ransferred, which, on the other hand, was also ssociated with a significant increase in multiple pregnancy. The overall 'take-home-baby' rate was 36.6% per patient, 15.5% per treatment cycle, 38.3% per patient undergoing embryo transfer and 17.8% per embryo transfer cycle.

Other oocyte donation programmes have reported PRs as high as 56% (Navot et al., 1991), and 67% (Paulson et al., 1990). These series, however, were comparatively small and included predominantly young amenorrhoeic patients. Subsequent studies that included older patients were somewhat less successful, with a PR of 39% (Antinori et al., 1993). The recent ASRM report (ASRM/SART Registry, 1998) reveals an overall clinical PR of 43.3% per ET and a delivery rate of 36% per transfer. However, other recent, large series reported pregnancy rates as low as 20% per ET (Pados et al., 1994).

FACTORS AFFECTING THE SUCCESS RATE OF OOCYTE DONATION

The relatively low PR achieved by oocyte donation (OD) is unlikely to be due to incompetence, but may be the result of certain factors related to patient selection, like the heterogeneity of the population which includes patients who may have decreased endometrial receptivity, including those of advanced age and patients with an abnormal karyotype; the inclusion of a greater proportion of patients who have repeatedly failed previous embryo transfer cycles; and the use of only anonymous donors, undergoing IVF themselves, who also, in fact, are 'subfertile'.

The age of the recipient and the possible influence of this factor on success rates in OD remains an issue of debate. Some authors claim that the age-related decline in the PR is exclusively attributable to the ageing oocytes (Navot et al., 1991). Guanes et al. (1996) in a prospective study assessing the effects of age on uterine perfusion, using OD as a model, concluded that uterine ageing does not appear to be a factor influencing the poor reproductive performance of women with advancing age. Sauer et al. (1992) found no difference in conception rates after OD in women <40 years old (32.6% per ET) compared with those >40 years old (34.5% per ET). They, too, inferred that the underlying problem with pregnancy establishment in older women was related to the ageing oocyte rather than to age-related endometrial changes. Paulson et al. (1997) retrospectively analysed the outcome of 418 consecutive embryo transfer cycles among 276 recipients of OD and did not find an age-related decrease in the PR. Similar results were reached by Abdalla et al. (1997) in a study of 104 cycles of OD.

On the other hand, others suggest that an age-related decline in endometrial receptivity may also play an important role in the decrease in implantation rates with age. Such age-related changes may be attributed to a decrease in uterine perfusion, the presence of fewer oestradiol receptors on the endometrial cell surface, an increase in the collagen content, and a reduced number of stromal cells in the endometrium (Lewin and Schenker, 1998). Moreover, clinical studies comparing OD in younger and older women have also indicated that there is an age-related decline in the PR (Cano et al., 1995). Yaron et al. (1998) provided further support to the contention that there is an age-related decrease in endometrial receptivity, contributing to the higher rate of implantation failure in older women, as their analysis showed a significant age-related decrease in the PR.

In cases of OD, oocyte quality does not seem to influence the outcome, and especially embryo quality, as the donated oocytes are retrieved from young healthy patients undergoing IVF, and are randomly distributed to the recipients. However, advanced paternal age may have an influence on embryo quality, as it is known that new dominant mutations, many of which are embryologically lethal, are more common in men of advanced age.

The effect of the duration of oestrogen provision for endometrial preparation on the PR in OD programmes has also been studied. The majority of the studies show that the endometrium is tolerant to varying durations of oestradiol stimulation with regard to clinical outcome following OD, and that varying the durations of oestradiol treatment for as long as five weeks has no significant effect on PR (Yaron et al., 1998). A significant increase in the PR in oocyte donation programmes has also been noted by increasing the number of embryos transferred. However, this is also accompanied by a significant increase in the overall rate of multiple pregnancies.

Obstetric And Perinatal Outcome In Oocyte Donation Programmes

First-trimester bleeding is a common complication in OD pregnancies. It has been shown to occur in 35%–70% of such patients (Pados et al., 1994). It has been assumed that this tendency is associated with multiple implantation and early fetal loss (Shaw and Sauer, 1995), and possibly with the endometrial preparation therapy.

The multiple pregnancy rate varies between 20%–60% (Legro et al., 1995; Shaw and Sauer, 1995), and depends highly on the numbers of embryos transferred. Programmes transferring only two embryos report a decline in the incidence of multiple pregnancies, to about 20%. The incidence of monochorionic twins does not seem to vary from that in conventional IVF.

The most conspicuous pregnancy complication in recipients of donated eggs is pregnancy-induced hypertension (PIH), which seems to occur with an unexpectedly high frequency, varying from 20%–50% (Serhal and Craft, 1989; Sauer et al., 1995). This high incidence of PIH in oocyte recipients has been explained by the advanced age of the mothers, the high rate of primiparity and multiple gestations (Pados et al., 1994), and immune system related factors, possibly an altered or inadequate immunoprotection of the fetoplacental unit in oocyte recipients (Serhal and Craft, 1987).

A high percentage of caesarean sections is usually described (50%) which may only partially be explained by advanced maternal age and multiple gestations. Undoubtedly, patients' and physicians' anxiety may also contribute to the high percentage of elective caesarean sections (Pados et al., 1994; Tanbo et al., 1995).

A recent study (Soderstrom-Antilla et al., 1998) compared the obstetric and perinatal outcome of 51 oocyte donation pregnancies (61 infants) with that of a control group of standard IVF patients (97 pregnancies, 126 infants). In the oocyte recipients, first-trimester bleeding (53%) occurred significantly more often than in IVF mothers (31%, P<0.01). Pregnancy-induced hypertension was observed in 31% of oocyte recipients, compared with 14% of IVF mothers. There was no difference in the duration of the pregnancies, preterm delivery rate, or birth weight between the two groups. Perinatal mortality was, however, 3.3% in the OD group and 0% in the IVF group. The authors concluded that OD pregnancies are associated with an increased risk compared with IVF pregnancies, but the complications are usually manageable and most oocyte recipients experience a good pregnancy outcome. In general, the obstetric outcome in pregnancies resulting from oocyte donation is favourable and the indication for oocyte donation treatment does not seem to have significant effects on pregnancy outcomes. Nevertheless, advanced recipient age seems to correlate with increased risks of early abortion and PIH, which underscores the need for adequate patient selection.

CRYOPRESERVATION OF EMBRYOS

Human embryo cryopreservation offers several useful clinical applications to assisted reproduction technology patients. These include the replacement of an optimal number of embryos, thus preventing the risk of high-order pregnancies and allowing the patient to pursue several consecutive non-stimulated thaw cycles. In the light of the latter consideration, it significantly reduces the risk of ovarian hyperstimulation syndrome (OHSS), or offers the opportunity for embryo transfer in a future cycle in the presence of OHSS. It is also often cost-saving for the patient to undergo one or more thaw cycles before needing to face the expense of a medicated cycle again. Storage also gives couples time to decide what should happen to embryos not required for their own treatment. Such embryos may be donated to another couple, or for research, or may be allowed to perish (Fasouliotis and Schenker, 1996). The first pregnancy from a frozen-thawed human embryo transfer that was reported in Australia in 1983 ended in the delivery of a stillborn female child, after premature rupture of the membranes at 23 weeks of gestation (Trounson and Mohr, 1983), whereas the first live births took place in the same year in the Netherlands. Since then, several thousand children have been born following frozen-thawed embryo transfers and the technique is now an established clinical practice at many centres around the world.

Results

Human embryo cryopreservation is considered to be effective in increasing the pregnancy rate achieved with ART per initiated cycle. *In vitro* fertilization centres practising cryopreservation suggest that the transfer of cryopreserved embryos has increased the ongoing PR per retrieval by approximately 6% (Kohn et al., 1993; Van Voorhis et al., 1995). As many frozen embryos remain unutilized in embryo banks, it is estimated that the ultimate increase in deliveries per retrieval will be even more substantial after their transfer to the uterus.

Current methods of cryopreservation retain the viability of >70% of frozen embryos (Horne et al., 1997), whereas the ongoing pregnancy rates maintained vary between 12% and 39% per embryo transfer (Ludwig et al., 1998). The success rate is increased at medical centres where a large number of embryos is transferred in the majority of the replacement cycles.

Experience from cycles with threatened OHSS, in which all embryos have been frozen and transferred in a subsequent cycle, has been reported. A pregnancy rate of 38.6% was achieved by Shaker et al. (1996), whereas Tiitinen et al. (1995), in another study among 23 patients at increased risk of OHSS, reported 15 clinical pregnancies after transfer of two to three frozen-thawed embryos in natural cycles, with a 32.6% pregnancy and 22.7% implantation rate. In 96 patients, after transfer of frozen-thawed embryos, a pregnancy rate of 25.2% per transfer, with a cumulative pregnancy rate of 40.6% was reported by Pattinson et al. (1994). The rate of pregnancy loss is also similar between frozen-thawed ET cycles and fresh IVF-ET cycles, approaching 20% (FIVNAT, 1996), whereas the rate of ectopic pregnancies per ET is estimated to be 0.6% in the former and 0.9% in the latter group (ASRM/SART Registry, 1998).

A lower incidence of multiple gestation (13%) is mentioned for the cryopreserved group, compared to 30% following IVF/GIFT procedures, which may be attributed to the smaller number of embryos transferred in a frozen-thawed ET cycle compared to a fresh IVF-ET (Wang et al., 1994).

Factors Affecting The Success Rate Of Embryo Cryopreservation

It is becoming increasingly clear that factors which have an impact on fresh embryo transfer have a comparable effect on the transfer of frozen-thawed embryos. Patient age, at the time of freezing, influences the pregnancy outcome. This is probably due to the poor quality of oocytes collected from older women, principally because of aneuploidy (Toner et al., 1993). The number of embryos transferred and the quality of embryos also have a comparable impact on the outcome, whether fresh or frozen-thawed embryos are transferred (Tucker et al., 1995). Endometrial preparation using a number of different regimens before frozen-thawed embryo transfer appears to confer no advantage over the natural cycle. In our clinic's experience with 381 frozen-thawed cycles during the years 1991–1993, the implantation rates, clinical pregnancy rates and spontaneous miscarriage rates were found to be similar, whether the cycle was natural, artificial (GnRH-agonist downregulation with oestrogen supplementation), or stimulated (GnRH-agonist downregulation with hMG plus hCG) (Fasouliotis and Schenker, 1996).

The developmental stage at cryopreservation has not been conclusively shown to influence successful pregnancy outcome. Freezing embryos at the one-cell stage alleviates the need to select embryos on the basis of early development, and certain programmes strongly promote cryopreservation at this stage, whereas others prefer to freeze embryos at the second day of development at the two-cell to four-cell stage (van Steirteghem and van den Abbeel, 1993). Blastocyst freezing should minimize the impact of cryoinjury, since damage to the trophectoderm of the blastocyst would probably have little effect on the outcome if it occurs during cryopreservation. Experience from 500 thaws of blastocyst shows an implantation rate of 13.4%, very similar to the 11.2% reported for transfer of early-stage pre-embryos (Kaufmann et al., 1995)

Outcome In Children From Cryopreserved Embryos

Cryopreservation and thawing involve important cellular changes, but until recently, there were no reports of adverse effects in mammalian pre-embryos. Previous studies in animals suggest that freezing is not mutagenic, and the background radiation of frozen pre-embryos does not produce abnormal offspring (Whittingham et al., 1977). A recent French investigation of adult mice obtained by transfer of cryopreserved pre-embryos indicated certain differences in morphological and behavioural features (Dulioust et al., 1995). The authors concluded that embryo cryopreservation, without being severely detrimental, might have certain adverse effects on the offspring.

The frequency of chromosomal abnormalities and congenital malformations in newborn babies conceived after the transfer of cryopreserved thawed embryos or fresh embryos has been studied. Rizk et al. (1991) reported Edward's syndrome in a fetus following cryopreservation. However, in a large retrospective study comparing the outcome of 283 births conceived following cryopreservation with 961 births from fresh embryos with respect to birth characteristics and perinatal mortality, a major malformation was reported in only 1% in the former group, compared to 3% in the latter (Wada et al., 1994). According to the authors, a possible explanation for the reduction in the incidence of congenital malformations could be related to the freezing-thawing technique. Since some embryos are lost during the freezing-thawing procedure, the technique may eliminate defective embryos. Other studies that followed reinforced the conclusion that cryopreservation of human embryos does not increase the incidence of congenital malformations (Sutcliffe et al., 1995; Wennerholm et al., 1997). The perinatal outcome and follow-up of 82 children aged 1–9 years, conceived from cryopreserved embryos was reported by Olivennes et al. (1996), who concluded that the medical and surgical illness, as well as principal acquisitions for children <5 years old and the scholastic performance of older children, did not show pathological features.

SURROGATE PREGNANCIES

A surrogate mother is defined as a woman who carries a fetus and bears a child on behalf of another person or persons, having agreed to surrender the child to this person or those persons at birth or shortly thereafter. There are three forms of surrogacy: partial-natural, partial and complete. Surrogate motherhood may be utilized in cases of uterine infertility or in cases of severe maternal disease during pregnancy (Schenker, 1992). Described first by Utian's group (Utian et al., 1985), the procedure engendered complex ethical, social, moral and legal controversy, and has not received as wide an acceptance as egg donor-recipient pregnancy (Schenker, 1997). The administration of this type of programme demands considerable input and communication between psychologist, reproductive endocrinologist, obstetrician and lawyer. Reports regarding the outcome of surrogate pregnancies are scarce in the literature. However, analysing the existing data, it is deduced that carrier gestation offers a satisfactory solution to childlessness caused by uterine or major medical factors. Specifically, Marrs et al. (1993) described 45 couples who had 81 cycles of ET to a carrier. An average of 3.4 embryos were transferred and a clinical pregnancy was obtained in 19, leading to 15 deliveries (33.3% success per patient). The mean age of the mothers was 38.8 years. There was no difference in PRs in zygote tubal transfers or uterine ET.

Meniru and Croft (1997) reported results of carrier gestation in 16 cases in which hysterectomy had been performed. A total of 11 patients completed 16 cycles of embryo replacement with 6 pregnancies occurring thereby, giving a pregnancy rate of 37.5% (6/16) per patient and embryo transfer of 27.3% (6/22) per cycle of treatment commenced. Two women later miscarried, three have given birth to twins and the remaining host has delivered a male infant. The commissioning mother's age was closely related to the occurrence and continuation of pregnancy in the host. They concluded that hysterectomized women demonstrate varying patterns of response to assisted conception treatment, but gestational surrogacy generally appears to be a feasible option, especially in younger patients. The series of carrier gestation reported by Serafini et al. (1994) covered 91 prospective genetic parenting mothers <39 years of age and 35 mothers >40 years of age. The younger women had greater numbers of oocyte retrieved, but the average numbers of fresh embryos transferred were similar, with 3.7 for the younger group versus 3.4 for the older. They reported 55 ongoing pregnancies, 14 spontaneous abortions, and 67 non-pregnant women in the 136 retrieval cycles for women <40, in which there were 121 fresh and 46 thawed cycles of embryo transfer.

Corson et al. (1998) evaluated the results of a gestational carrier programme in terms of pregnancy rates in fresh and cryopreserved cycles. The population of genetic mothers included 75 women with uterine or medical reasons for unsuccessful gestation. There were 37 established pregnancies for 36 genetic mothers over 120 cycles of fresh and 24 frozen cycles of embryo replacement to a carrier, for a 49.3% success rate per couple. None of the nine patients >40 were successful in 26 cycles of fresh and 1 cycle of frozen ET. For the 64 patients <40 years of age who underwent egg retrieval and replacement, a pregnancy rate of 56.3% was achieved with a cycle rate of 30.8%. The implantation rate for fresh transfer cycles was 0.13, with a mean of 2.5 embryos, compared with 0.26 and 2.7, respectively, for thawed transfers.

Infants delivered through the application of a surrogate pregnancy do not seem to carry an increased risk of congenital anomalies. Petrozza et al. (1997) evaluated the inheritance pattern of congenital absence of the uterus and vagina in affected women undergoing surrogacy IVF with this disorder. A total of 162 IVF cycles were performed, and 34 live-born children were delivered (half female). No congenital anomalies were found, except for one male child with a middle ear defect and hearing loss.

PERINATAL COSTS OF IVF-ART

The past decade has witnessed an explosion in the availability of ART throughout the world, providing an unquestionable benefit to many infertile couples. However, as in other areas of human endeavour, the costs associated with these acknowledged benefits must be accounted for as well.

The costs associated with ART depend on several factors, including the specific ART technique that is employed, the phase of treatment for which costs are examined (i.e., an IVF cycle versus the time from the initiation of ART treatment to delivery), patient eligibility criteria, the number of attempts per patient, and the perspective from which costs are estimated (Porreco, 1998). The cost of IVF treatment resulting in a successful delivery increases with the number of cycles initiated, ranging from $66,667 when an initial cycle results in a live birth to $114,286 when six cycles are required (Neumann et al., 1994). For patients with a more favourable prognosis (i.e., tubal disease), the costs have ranged from $50,000 per delivery resulting from the first cycle to $72,727 for delivery resulting from the sixth cycle. Analogous costs were $160,000 and $800,000, respectively, when the woman was older and male infertility was present.

As would be expected, maternal and neonatal complications, as well as multiple births, increase costs. Golfarb et al. (1996) estimated the cost for a successful birth among singleton and twin pregnancies in their practice to be approximately $40,000, whereas the costs for a successful birth among their triplet and quadruplet pregnancies were approximately $340,000.

IVF is funded differently in various countries (Mor-Yosef, 1995). In Belgium, Holland, Denmark, France, Spain, Norway, Israel and Italy, there is limited or full state insurance for IVF. Although 13 states in the United States have laws governing insurance coverage for the treatment of infertility, only 6 states stipulate that insurance carriers must cover IVF, and in states where coverage exists, it ranges from 100% coverage for the diagnosis and treatment of infertility to coverage for only one out-patient cycle of IVF (Steinberg et al., 1998).

CONCLUSION

Assisted reproductive technology is currently used for a wide range of indications and has become an acceptable tool in the treatment of subfertile couples. However, an ongoing controversy regarding the effectiveness of ART, and especially on the costs of ART compared with conventional treatment for various conditions that cause subfertility, still remains an issue of debate.

REFERENCES

Abdalla, H.I. et al. (1993). 'Age, pregnancy, and miscarriage: Uterine versus ovarian factors', *Hum. Reprod.*, **8**: 1512–7.

______(1997). 'Age of the uterus does not affect pregnancy or implantation rates: A study of egg donation in women of different ages sharing oocytes from the same donor', *Hum. Reprod.*, **12**: 827–9.

Abyholm, T. et al. (1991). 'The first attempt at IVF treatment: Results and requirements for a satisfactory success rate', *Eur. J. Obstet. Gynecol. Reprod. Biol.*, **38**: 125–32.

Addor, V. et al. (1998). 'Impact of infertility treatments on the health of newborns', *Fertil. Steril.*, **69**: 210–15.

Al-Shawaf, T. et al. (1992). 'The influence of ovarian response on gamete intra-fallopian transfer outcome in older women', *Hum. Reprod.*, **7**: 1106–10.

Alsalili, M. et al. (1995). 'Cumulative pregnancy rates and pregnancy outcome after *in vitro* fertilization: > 5000 cycles at one center', *Hum. Reprod.*, **10**: 470–74.

American Society for Reproductive Medicine/ Society for Assisted Reproductive Technology Registry (1998). 'Assisted reproductive technology in the United States and Canada: 1995 results generated from the American Society for Reproductive Medicine/Society for Assisted Reproductive Technology Registry', *Fertil. Steril.*, **69**: 389–98.

Antinori, S. et al. (1993). 'Oocyte donation in menopausal women', *Hum. Reprod.*, **8**: 1487–90.

Asch, R.H. et al. (1986). 'Preliminary experiences with gamete intrafallopian transfer (GIFT)', *Fertil. Steril.*, **45**: 366–71.

Aytoz, A. et al. (1998). 'Outcome of pregnancies after intracytoplasmic sperm injection and the effect of sperm origin and quality on this outcome', *Fertil. Steril.*, **70**: 500–505.

Bavister, B.D. (1995). 'Culture of preimplantation embryos: Facts and artifacts', *Hum. Reprod. Update*, **1**: 91–148.

Bonduelle, M. et al. (1995). 'Comparative follow-up study of 130 children born after ICSI and 130 children born after IVF', *Hum. Reprod.*, **10**: 3327–31.

______(1998). 'Incidence of chromosomal aberrations in children born after assisted reproduction through intracytoplasmic sperm injection', *Hum. Reprod.*, **13**: 781–2.

Bongso, A. et al. (1995). 'Co-culture techniques for blastocyst transfer and embryonic stem cell production', *Assist. Reprod. Rev.*, **5**: 106–14.

Bopp, B.L. et al. (1995). 'Success rates with gamete intrafallopian transfer and *in vitro* fertilization in women of advanced maternal age', *Fertil. Steril.*, **63**: 1278–83.

Bowen, J.R. et al. (1998). 'Medical and developmental outcome at 1 year for children conceived by intracytoplasmic sperm injection', *Lancet*, **351**: 1529–34.

Brandes, J.M. et al. (1992). 'Growth and development of children conceived by *in vitro* fertilization', *Pediatrics*, **90**: 424–9.

Bronson, R. (1997). 'How should the number of embryos transferred to the uterus following *in vitro* fertilization be determined to avoid the risk of multiple gestation?' *Hum. Reprod.*, **12**: 1605–7.

Cano, F. et al. (1995). 'Effect of aging on the female reproductive system: Evidence for a role of uterine senescence in the decline in female fecundity', *Fertil. Steril.*, **64**: 584–9.

Chandra, A. and W.D. Mosher (1994). 'The demography of infertility and the use of medical care for infertility', *Study Design and Statistics for Infertility Research*, **5**: 283–96.

Check, J.H. et al. (1994). 'Comparison of the cumulative probability of pregnancy after *in vitro* fertilization-embryo transfer by infertility factor and age', *Fertil. Steril.*, **61**: 257–61.

Cohen, J. et al. (1988). 'Pregnancy outcomes after *in vitro* fertilization: A collaborative study on 2342 pregnancies', *Ann. N. Y. Acad. Sci.*, **541**: 1–6.

Coetsier, T. and M. Dhont (1998). 'Embryo transfer and multiple gestation: Avoiding multiple pregnancies in *in vitro* fertilization: Who's afraid of single embryo transfer?' *Hum. Reprod.*, **13**: 2663–4.

Corson, S.L. et al. (1998). 'Gestational carrier pregnancy', *Fertil. Steril.*, **69**: 670–74.

Dale, P.O. et al., '*In vitro* fertilization in infertile women with the polycystic ovarian syndrome', *Hum. Reprod.*, **6**: 238–41.

De Mouzon, J. and P. Lancaster (1997). 'World Collaborative Report on IVF: Preliminary Data for 1995', *J. Assist. Reprod. Genet.*, **14**: (Suppl.), 251S–265S.

Devroey, P. et al. (1986). 'Pregnancy after translaparoscopic zygote intrafallopian transfer in a patient with sperm antibodies', *Lancet*, **1329**.

Dew, J.E. et al. (1998). 'The influence of advanced age on the outcome of assisted reproduction', *J. Assist. Reprod. Genet.*, **15**: 210–14.

Dmowski, W.P. et al. (1995). 'The effect of endometriosis, its stage and activity, and of autoantibodies on *in vitro* fertilization and embryo transfer success rates', *Fertil. Steril.*, **63**: 555–62.

Dor, J. et al. (1996). 'Cumulative pregnancy rate following *in vitro* fertilization: the significance of age and infertility aetiology', *Hum. Reprod.*, **11**: 425–8.

Doyle, P. (1996). 'The outcome of multiple pregnancy', *Hum. Reprod.*, **11**: (Suppl. 1), 110–20.

D'Souza, S.W. et al. (1997). 'Children conceived by *in vitro* fertilization after fresh embryo transfer', *Arch. Dis. Child.*, **76**: F70–F74.

Dulioust, E. et al. (1995). 'Long-term effects of embryo freezing in mice', *Proc. Natl. Acad. Sci.*, **92**: 589–93.

Edwards, R.G. (1997). 'Recent scientific and medical advances in assisted human conception', *Int. J. Dev. Biol.*, **41**: 255–62.

Eisenberg, V.H. and J.G. Schenker (1997). 'Pregnancy in the older woman: Scientific and ethical aspects', *Int. J. Gynecol. Obstet.*, **56**: 163–9.

Elsner, C.W. et al. (1997). 'Multiple pregnancy rate and embryo number transferred during *in vitro* fertilization', *Am. J. Obstet. Gynecol.*, **177**: 350–57.

ESHRE Capri Workshop (1996). 'Infertility revisited: The state of the art today and tomorrow', *Hum. Reprod.*, **11**: 1779–1807.

Ezra, Y. and J.G. Schenker (1993). 'Appraisal of *in vitro* fertilization', *Eur. J. Obstet. Gynecol. Reprod. Biol.*, **48**: 127–33.

Fasouliotis, S.J. and J.G. Schenker (1996). 'Cryopreservation of embryos: Medical, ethical and legal issues', *J. Assist. Reprod. Genet.*, **13**: 756–61.

______(1997). 'Multifetal pregnancy reduction: A review of the world results for the period 1993–1996', *Eur. J. Obstet. Gynecol. Reprod. Biol.*, **75**: 183–190.

FIVNAT, (1993). 'French National IVF Registry: Analysis of 1986 to 1990 data', *Fertil. Steril.*, **59**: 587–95.

______(1996). 'Bilan des transferts d'embryons congeles de 1987 a 1994', *Contracept. Fertil. Sexual.*, **24**: 700–705.

Fong, C.Y. et al. (1997). 'Ongoing normal pregnancy after transfer of zona-free blastocysts: Implications for embryo transfer', *Hum. Reprod.*, **12**: 557–60.

______(1998). 'Blastocyst transfer after enzymatic treatment of the zona pellucida: Improving *in vitro* fertilization and understanding implantation', *Hum. Reprod.*, **13**: 2926–32.

Friedler, S. et al. (1992). 'Births in Israel resulting from *in vitro* fertilization and embryo transfer 1982–1989: National Registry of the Israeli Association for Fertility Research', *Hum. Reprod.*, **7**: 1159–63.

Gardner, D.K. et al. (1998). 'Culture and transfer of human blastocysts increases implantation rates and reduces the need for multiple embryo transfers', *Fertil. Steril.*, **69**: 84–8.

Garrissi, G.J. et al. (1990). 'Clinical evaluation of three approaches to micromanipulations-assisted fertilization', *Fertil. Steril.*, **54**: 671–7.

Geber, S. et al. (1995). 'Results of IVF in patients with endometriosis: The severity of the disease does not affect the outcome or the incidence of miscarriage', *Hum. Reprod.*, **10**: 1507–11.

Goldfarb, J.M. et al. (1996). 'Cost-effectiveness of *in vitro* fertilization', *Obstet. Gynecol.*, **87**: 18–21.

______(1997). 'Factors influencing patients' decision not to repeat IVF', *J. Assist. Reprod. Genet.*, **14**: 381–4.

Gonen, R. et al. (1990). 'The outcome of triplet, quadruplet and quintuplet pregnancies managed in a perinatal unit: Obstetrics, neonatal and follow-up data', *Am. J. Obstet. Gynecol.*, **2**: 454–9.

Govaerts, I. et al. (1996). 'Is intracytoplasmic sperm injection a safe procedure? What do we learn from early pregnancy data in ICI?' *Hum. Reprod.*, **11**: 440–43.

______(1998). 'Comparison of pregnancy outcome after intracytoplasmic sperm injection and *in vitro* fertilization', *Hum. Reprod.*, **13**: 1514–8.

Guanes, P.P. et al. (1996). 'Age does not affect uterine resistance to vascular flow in patients undergoing oocyte donation', *Fertil. Steril.*, **66**: 265–70.

Guzick, D.S. et al. (1986). 'Cumulative pregnancy rates for *in vitro* fertilization', *Fertil. Steril.*, **46**: 663–7.

______(1998). 'Efficacy of treatment for unexplained infertility', *Fertil. Steril.*, **70**: 207–13.

Haan, G., Bernardus et al. (1991). 'Selective drop-out in successive *in vitro* fertilization attempts: the pendulum danger', *Hum. Reprod.*, **6**: 939–43.

Hasler, J.F. et al. (1995). 'Production, freezing and transfer of bovine IVF embryos and subsequent calving results', *Theriogenology*, **43**: 141–52.

Hershlag, A. et al. (1991). 'Heterogeneity of patient populations explains differences in *in vitro* fertilization programs', *Fertil. Steril.*, **56**: 913–7.

Homburg, R. et al. (1993). '*In vitro* fertilization and embryo transfer for the treatment of infertility associated with polycystic ovary syndrome', *Fertil. Steril.*, **60**: 858–63.

Horne, G. et al. (1997). 'A prospective evaluation of cryopreservation strategies in a two-embryo transfer programme', *Hum. Reprod.*, **12**: 542–7.

Hull, M.G.R. et al. (1992). 'Expectations of assisted conception for infertility', *Br. Med. J.*, **304**: 1465–9.

Human Fertilization and Embryology Authority. (1997). Sixth Annual Report, 1997.

In't-Veld, P. et al. (1995). 'Sex chromosomal abnormalities and intracytoplasmic sperm injection', *Lancet*, **346**: 773.

Jones, G.M. et al. (1998). 'Evolution of a culture protocol for successful blastocyst development and pregnancy', *Hum. Reprod.*, **13**: 169–77.

Kaufmann, R.A. et al. (1995). 'Co-cultured blastocyst cryopreservation: Experience of more than 500 transfer cycles', *Fertil. Steril.*, **64**: 1125–9.

Kenny, D.T. (1994). 'The impact of maternal age on clinical pregnancy and spontaneous abortion in women undergoing gamete *in vitro* fertilization and gamete intra-fallopian transfer', *Aust. N. Z. J. Obstet. Gynecol.*, **34**: 443–8.

Kohn, J.A. et al. (1993). 'The efficacy and efficiency of an *in vitro* fertilization program including embryo cryopreservation: A cohort study', *Hum. Reprod.*, **8**: 247–52.

Kovacs, G.T. (1996). 'The likelihood of pregnancy with IVF and GIFT in Australia and New Zealand', *Med. J. Aust.*, **158**: 805–7.

Lancaster, P.A.L. (1987). 'Congenital malformations after *in vitro* fertilization', *Lancet*, **2**: 1392–3.

Land, J.A. et al. (1997). 'Patient drop-out in an assisted reproductive technology program: Implications for pregnancy rates', *Fertil. Steril.*, **68**: 278–81.

Legro, R.S. et al. (1995). 'Multiple implantation after oocyte donation: A frequent but inefficient event', *Fertil. Steril.*, **63**: 849–53.

Lessey, B.A. et al. (1994). 'Effect of hydrosalpinges on markers of uterine receptivity and success in IVF', Presented at the 50th annual meeting of the American Fertility Society 1994, American Fertility Society, program supplement, S45.

Lewin, A. and J.G. Schenker (1998). 'Conception following assisted reproduction techniques', in A. Kurjak (ed.) *Textbook of Perinatal Medicine.*, Parthenon Publishing Group, Carnforth, 204–225.

Lewin, A. et al. (1996). 'Delivery following intracytoplasmic injection of mature sperm cells recovered by testicular fine needle aspiration in a case of hypergonadotropic azoospermia due to maturation arrest', *Hum. Reprod.*, **11**: 769–771.

Liebaers, I. et al. (1995). 'Sex chromosome abnormalities and intracytoplasmic sperm injection', [Letter to the editor], *Lancet*, **346**: 1095.

Lieberman, B. (1998). 'Embryo transfer and multiple gestation: An embryo too many?' *Hum. Reprod.*, **13**: 2664–6.

Ludwig, M. et al. (1998). 'Safety of embryo cryopreservation: Statistical facts and artefacts. No impacts of cryopreservation and thawing on embryo developmental potential—one more example for the problems of retrospective, non-controlled data', *Hum. Reprod.*, **13**: 786–7.

Lutjen, P. et al. (1984). 'The establishment and maintenance of pregnancies using *in vitro* fertilization and embryo donation in a patient with primary ovarian failure', *Nature*, **307**: 174–5.

Marcus, S.F. et al. (1995). 'The prediction of ectopic pregnancy after IVF-ET', *Hum. Reprod.*, **10**: 2165–8.

Marrs, R.P. et al. (1993). 'The use of surrogate gestational carriers for assisted reproductive technologies', *Am. J. Obstet. Gynecol.*, **168**: 1858–63.

Meldrum, D.R. et al. (1998). 'Success rate with repeated cycles of *in vitro* fertilization-embryo transfer', *Fertil. Steril.*, **69**: 1005–9.

Meniru, G.I. and I.L. Craft (1997). 'Experience with gestational surrogacy as a treatment for sterility resulting from hysterectomy', *Hum. Reprod.*, **12**: 51–54.

Minaretzis, D. et al. (1998). 'Multivariate analysis of factors predictive of successful live births after *in vitro* fertilization (IVF) suggests strategies to improve IVF outcome', *J. Assist. Reprod. Genet.*, **15**: 365–71.

Morin, N.C. et al. (1989). 'Congenital malformations and psychosocial development in children conceived by *in vitro* fertilization', *J. Pediatr.*, **115**: 222–7.

Mor-Yosef, S. (1995). 'Cost effectiveness of *in vitro* fertilization', *J. Assist. Reprod. Genet.*, **12**: 524–30.

Mugford, M. and J. Henderson (1995). 'Resource implications of multiple births', in H.R. Ward and M. Whittle (eds.), *Multiple Births.*, *RCOG*, London, pp. 334–45.

Murdoch, A.P. (1998). 'Embryo transfer and multiple gestation: How many embryos should be transferred?' *Hum. Reprod.*, **10**: 2666–70.

Nackley, A.C. and S.J. Muasher (1998). 'The significance of hydrosalpinx in *in vitro* fertilization', *Fertil. Steril.*, **69**: 373–84.

Navot, D. et al. (1991). 'Poor oocyte quality rather than implantation failure as a cause of age-related decline in female fertility', *Lancet*, **337**: 1375–7.

Neumann, P.J. et al. (1994). 'The cost of a successful delivery with *in vitro* fertilization', *N. Engl. J. Med.*, **331**: 239–43.

Nielsen, J. and M. Wohlert (1991). 'Chromosome abnormalities found among 34910 newborn children: Results from a 13-year study in Arhus, Denmark', *Hum. Genet.*, **87**: 81–3.

Olivennes, F. et al. (1993). 'The increased risk of complication observed in singleton pregnancies resulting from *in vitro* fertilization does not seem to be related to the IVF method itself', *Hum. Reprod.*, **8**: 1297–300.

______(1995). 'Endometriosis: A stage by stage analysis—the role of *in vitro* fertilization', *Fertil. Steril.*, **64**: 392–8.

______(1996). 'Perinatal outcome of twin pregnancies obtained after *in vitro* fertilization: Comparison with twin pregnancies obtained spontaneously or after ovarian stimulation', *Fertil. Steril.*, **66**: 105–9.

______(1996). 'Perinatal outcome and follow-up of 82 children aged 1-9 years conceived from cryopreserved embryos', *Hum. Reprod.*, **11**: 1565–8.

______(1997). 'Follow-up of a cohort of 422 children aged 6 to 13 years conceived by IVF', *Fertil. Steril.*, **67**: 284–9.

Pados, G. et al. (1994). 'The evolution and outcome of pregnancies from oocyte donation', *Hum. Reprod.*, **9**: 538–42.

Pal, L. et al. (1998). 'Impact of varying stages of endometriosis on the outcome of *in vitro* fertilization-embryo transfer', *J. Assist. Reprod. Genet.*, **15**: 27–31.

Palermo, G. et al. (1992). 'Pregnancies after intracytoplasmic injection of single spermatozoa into an oocyte', *Lancet*, **340**: 17–8.

Palermo, G.D. et al. (1996). 'Evolution of pregnancies and initial follow-up of newborns delivered after intracytoplasmic sperm injection', *J. Am. Med. Assoc.*, **276**: 1893–7.

Pattinson, H.A. et al. (1994). 'Outcome of thaw embryo transfer after cryopreservation of all embryos in patients at risk of ovarian hyperstimulation syndrome', *Fertil. Steril.*, **62**: 1192–6.

Paulson, R.J. et al. (1990). 'Embryo implantation after human *in vitro* fertilization: Importance of endometrial receptivity', *Fertil. Steril.*, **53**: 870–74.

______(1997). 'Cumulative conception and live birth rates after oocyte donation: Implications regarding endometrial receptivity', *Hum. Reprod.*, **12**: 835–9.

Petrozza, J.C. et al. (1997). 'Congenital absence of the uterus and vagina is not commonly transmitted as a dominant genetic trait: Outcomes of surrogate pregnancies', *Fertil. Steril.*, **67**: 387–9.

Piette, C. et al. (1990). '*In vitro* fertilization: Influence of women's age on pregnancy rates', *Hum. Reprod.*, **5**: 56–9.

Porreco, R.P. (1998). 'Perinatal costs of assisted reproductive technology', *Obstet. Gynecol. Surv.*, **53**: 393–4.

Reubinoff, B. et al. (1997). 'Is the obstetrical outcome of *in vitro* fertilized singleton gestations different from natural ones? A controlled study', *Fertil. Steril.*, **67**: 1077–83.

Rizk, B. et al. (1991). 'Edward's syndrome after the replacement of cryopreserved-thawed embryos', *Fertil. Steril.*, **55**: 208–10.

Roseboom, T.J. et al. (1995). 'The probability of pregnancy after embryo transfer is affected by the age of the patients, cause of infertility, number of embryos transferred and the average morphology score, as revealed by multiple logistic regression analysis', *Hum. Reprod.*, **10**: 3035–41.

Rufat, P. et al. (1994). 'Task force report on the outcome of pregnancies and children conceived by *in vitro* fertilization', *Fertil. Steril.*, **61**: 324–30.

Sauer, M.V. et al. (1992). 'Reversing the natural decline in human infertility: An extended clinical trial of oocyte donation to women of advanced reproductive age', *J. Am. Med. Assoc.*, **268**: 1275–9.

______(1995). 'Pregnancy in women 50 or more years of age: Outcomes of 22 consecutively established pregnancies from oocyte donation', *Fertil. Steril.*, **64**: 111–5.

Saunders, D.M. et al. (1988). 'The Australian Register: Current research and future role—a preliminary report', Ann. N.Y. *Acad. Sci.*, **541**: 7–12.

Schenk, L.M. et al. (1996). 'Embryotoxicity of hydrosalpinx fluid', Presented at the 43rd annual meeting of the Society of Gynecologic Investigators 1996, *J. Soc. Gynecol. Invest.*, 88A.

Schenker, J.G. (1992). *The surrogate mother*, Harefuah, **123**: 330–33.

______(1997). 'Assisted reproduction practice in Europe: Legal and ethical aspects', *Hum. Reprod. Update*, **3**: 173–84.

Scholtes, M. and G. Zeilmaker (1996). 'A prospective randomized study of embryo transfer results after 3 or 5 days of embryo culture in *in vitro* fertilization', *Fertil. Steril.*, **65**: 1245–8.

Segal, S. and R.F. Casper (1990). 'The response to ovarian hyperstimulation and *in vitro* fertilization in women older than 35 years', *Hum. Reprod.*, **5**: 225–7.

Serafini, P. et al. (1994). 'In vitro fertilization surrogacy', *Assist. Reprod. Rev.*, **4**: 155–61.

Serhal, P.F. and I.L. Craft (1987). 'Immune basis for pre-eclampsia: Evidence from oocyte recipients', *Lancet*, **2**: 744.

______(1989). 'Oocyte donation in 61 patients', *Lancet*, **1**: 1185–7.

Shaker, A.G. et al. (1996). 'Comparison of intravenous albumin and transfer of fresh embryos with cryopreservation of all embryos for subsequent transfer in prevention of ovarian hyperstimulation syndrome', *Fertil., Steril.*, **65**: 992–6.

Shaw, K.J. and M.V. Sauer (1995). 'Obstetric care of surrogates and recipients of donor oocytes', *Semin. Reprod. Endocrinol.*, **13**: 237–43.

Shulman, A. and J. Dor (1997). '*In vitro* fertilization treatment in patients with polycystic ovaries', *J. Assist. Reprod. Genet.*, **14**: 7–9.

Shushan, A. et al. (1995). 'Subfertility in the era of assisted reproduction: Changes and consequences', *Fertil. Steril.*, **64**: 459–69.

Soderstrom-Anttila, V. et al. (1998). 'Obstetric and perinatal outcome after oocyte donation: Comparison with *in vitro* fertilization pregnancies', *Hum. Reprod.*, **13**: 483–90.

Soliman, S. et al. (1993). 'A randomized trial of *in vitro* fertilization versus conventional treatment for infertility', *Fertil. Steril.*, **59**: 1239–44.

Steinberg, E.P. et al. (1998). 'Profiling assisted reproductive technology: Outcomes and quality of infertility management', *Fertil. Steril.*, **69**: 617–23.

Steptoe, P.C. and R.G. Edwards (1976). 'Reimplantation of a human embryo with subsequent tubal pregnancy', *Lancet*, **1**: 880–82.

______(1978). 'Birth after reimplantation of a human embryo', *Lancet*, 366.

Suttcliffe, A.G. et al. (1995). 'Minor congenital, major congenital malformations and development in children conceived from cryopreserved embryos', *Hum. Reprod.*, **10**: 3332–7.

Tan, S.L. et al. (1992). 'Obstetric outcome of *in vitro* fertilization pregnancies compared with normally conceived pregnancies', *Am. J. Obstet. Gynecol.*, **167**: 778–84.

______(1992). 'Cumulative conception and live birth rates after *in vitro* fertilization', *Lancet*, **339**: 1390–94.

Tanbo, T. et al. (1995). 'Obstetric outcome in singleton pregnancies after assisted reproduction', *Obstet. Gynecol.*, **86**: 188–92.

Tarin, J.J. et al. (1998). 'Long-term effects of delayed parenthood', *Hum. Reprod.*, 2371–6.

Templeton, A. et al. (1996). 'Factors that affect outcome of *in vitro* fertilization treatment', *Lancet*, **348**: 1402–6.

Tesarik, J. (1995). 'Viable embryos from injection of round spermatids into oocytes', N. Engl. *J. Med.*, **333**: 525.

Tiitinen, A. et al. (1995). 'The effect of cryopreservation in prevention of ovarian hyperstimulation syndrome', *Br. J. Obstet. Gynecol.*, **102**: 326–9.

Toner, J.P. et al. (1993). 'Basal follicle-stimulating hormone level and age affect the chance for and outcome of pre-embryo cryopreservation', *Fertil. Steril.*, **59**: 664–7.

Trounson, A. and L. Mohr (1983). 'Human pregnancy following cryopreservation, thawing and transfer of an eight-cell embryo', *Nature*, **305**: 707–9.

Trounson, A. et al. (1994). 'Current status of IVM/IVF and embryo culture in human and farm animals', *Theriogenology*, **41**: 57–66.

Tsirigotis, M. and I.L. Craft (1995). 'Sperm retrieval methods and ICSI for obstructive azoospermia', *Hum. Reprod.*, **10**: 758–60.

Tucker, M.J. et al. (1995). 'Cryopreservation of human embryos and oocytes', *Curr. Opin. Obstet. Gynecol.*, 7: 188–92.

Utian, W.H. et al. (1985). 'Successful pregnancy after *in vitro* fertilization and embryo transfer from an infertile woman to a surrogate', *N. Engl. J. Med.*, **313**: 1351–2.

Van Noord-Zaadstra, B.M. et al. (1991). 'Delaying childbearing: Effect of age on fecundity and outcome of pregnancy', *Br. Med. J.*, **302**: 1361–5.

Van Opstal, D. et al. (1997). 'Determination of the parent of origin in nine cases of prenatally detected chromosome aberrations found after intracytoplasmic sperm injection', *Hum. Reprod.*, **12**: 682–6.

Van Steirteghem, A.C. et al. (1993). 'High fertilization and implantation rates after intracytoplasmic sperm injection', *Hum. Reprod.*, **8**: 1061–8.

Van Steirteghem, A.C. and A. Van den Abbeel (1993). 'Freezing of embryos: Early versus late stages', *J. Assist. Reprod. Genet.*, **10**: 185–6.

Van Voorhis, B.J. et al. (1995). 'The efficacy and cost effectiveness of embryo cryopreservation compared with other assisted reproductive techniques', *Fertil. Steril.*, **64**: 647–50.

______(1997). 'Cost-effectiveness of infertility treatments: A cohort study', *Fertil. Steril.*, **67**: 830–36.

Verlaenen, H. et al. (1995). 'Singleton pregnancy after *in vitro* fertilization: Expectations and outcome', *Obstet. Gynecol.*, **86**: 906–10.

Wada, I. et al. (1994). 'Birth characteristics and perinatal outcome of babies conceived from cryopreserved embryos', *Hum. Reprod.*, **9**: 543–6.

Walters, D.E. (1996). 'The statistical implication of the "number of replacements" in embryo transfer', *Hum. Reprod.*, **11**: 10–12.

Wang, X.J. et al. (1994). 'The contribution of embryo cryopreservation to *in vitro* fertilization/gamete intra-fallopian transfer: 8 years experience', *Hum. Reprod.*, **9**: 103–9.

Wennerholm, U.B. et al. (1991). 'Pregnancy complications and short-term follow-up of infants born after *in vitro* fertilization and embryo transfer (IVF/ET)', *Acta Obstet. Gynecol. Scand.*, **70**: 565–73.

______ (1996). 'Obstetric and perinatal outcome of pregnancies following intracytoplasmic sperm injection', *Hum. Reprod.*, **11**: 1113–19.

______(1997). 'Obstetric and perinatal outcome of children conceived from cryopreserved embryos', *Hum. Reprod.*, **12**: 1819–25.

Wilcox, L.S. and W.D. Mosher (1993). 'Use of infertility services in the United States', *Obstet. Gynecol.*, **82**: 122–7.

Wisanto, A. et al. (1995). 'Obstetric outcome of 424 pregnancies after intracytoplasmic sperm injection', *Hum. Reprod.*, **10**: 2713–8.

Whittingham, D.G. et al. (1977). 'Long-term storage of mouse embryos at –196°C: The effect of background radiation', *Genet. Res.*, **29**: 171–81.

Wolstenholme, J. et al. (1994). 'Confined placental mosaicism, IUGR, and adverse pregnancy outcome: A controlled retrospective U.K. collaborative survey', *Prenat. Diagn.*, **14**: 345–61.

Wood, C. et al. (1992). 'Age and fertility: Results of assisted reproductive technology in women over 40 years', J. *Assist. Reprod. Genet.*, **9**: 482–4.

Yaron, Y. et al. (1998). 'Oocyte donation in Israel: A study of 1001 initiated treatment cycles', *Hum. Reprod.*, **13**: 1819–24.

Yuzpe, A.A. et al. (1989). 'Rates and outcome of pregnancies achieved in the first 4 years of an *in vitro* fertilization program', *Can. Med. Assoc. J.*, **40**: 167–72.

Zeyneloglu, H.B. et al. (1998). 'Adverse effects of hydrosalpinx on pregnancy rates after *in vitro* fertilization-embryo transfer', *Fertil. Steril.*, **70**: 492–99.

16

Cryopreservation of Oocytes, Sperms and Embryos

Josiane Van der Elst

ABOUT CRYOPRESERVATION OF REPRODUCTIVE CELLS AND TISSUES

Preservation of tissues, organs and even the whole body is a challenge to the imagination of man. The possibility of stopping the biological clock of body cells and tissues by cryopreservation can have far-reaching applications in the field of transplantation. In the context of storage of reproductive cells and tissues, the potential of preserving even future generations comes into the scope.

According to our knowledge, the male gamete was the first human reproductive cell to be cryopreserved successfully. By the early sixties, routine cryopreservation of the male gamete had resulted in the establishment of sperm banks. The use of semen from sperm banks was a direct application in the context of autoconservation or donor conservation for artificial insemination. The human oocyte was lacking the direct application for cryopreservation, thus it reduced the interest in this type of research. Nevertheless, some successful attempts had been made to cryopreserve animal oocytes and even ovarian tissue (Chang, 1953; Parrott, 1960). But finally, it was going to be the human embryo and not the human oocyte that was cryopreserved first. For this evolution to occur, the world of reproductive medicine had to wait for the breaktrough in infertility treatment in 1978 by the birth of Louise Brown, the first human test-tube baby. By this accomplishment, the pioneers of *in vitro* fertilization (IVF) (Steptoe and Edwards, 1978; Edwards et al., 1980) made it possible for the first time in man's written history to collect human oocytes and fertilize them outside a women's body, leading to the creation of human embryos *in vitro*. It was the increasing efficiency of IVF treatments by the introduction of ovarian stimulation that forced embryologists to find a destiny for good quality embryos supernumerary to those needed for replacement. Embryo cryopreservation was welcomed as an elegant solution to the dilemma caused by the creation of supernumerary embryos. Though embryo cryopreservation was considered a beneficiary add-on facility to IVF treatment, ethical objections were raised such that in certain countries embryo cryopreservation was discouraged or even prohibited by law. This attitude towards human embryo cryorespervation, in turn, renewed the interest in cryopreservation of the human oocyte. Cryopreservation of the mature human oocyte as collected during IVF cycles has, however, been less successful than expected. The latest developments in oocyte cryopreservation are, therefore, to freeze immature oocytes and even ovarian tissue. Equally so, evolution in the treatment of male infertility has introduced the cryopreservation of male reproductive tissue. In particular, the collection of spermatozoa from testicular biopsies in azoospermic men has led to the issue of cryopreservation of testicular spermatozoa and tissue.

This chapter will examine the cryopreservation of oocytes, sperm cells and embryos. Emphasis will be laid on the evolution of the strategies of cryopreservation existing now and those in future. Less attention will be paid to the technology of cryopreservation as extensive reviews are available on scientific cryobiological principles of oocyte, sperm and embryo cryopreservation (Mazur, 1970;

1984; 1990; Leibo, 1977; Ashwood-Smith, 1986; Bernard and Fuller, 1996; Karow and Critser, 1997; Nugent et al., 1997; Van der Elst et al., 1997b; Newton, 1998).

CRYOPRESERVATION OF OOCYTES

Attempts to cryopreserve animal oocytes and ovarian tissue had already been made in the fifties and sixties (Smith and Parkes, 1951; Chang, 1953; Lin et al., 1957; Sherman and Lin, 1958; Parkes, 1958; Parrott, 1960), but due to the lack of clinical application, this line of research was abandoned.

It was the advent of *in vitro* fertilization that opened the window for cryopreservation of human oocytes and embryos. By the introduction of ovarian stimulation schedules in IVF treatments, a number of embryos are created in excess of the number of embryos needed for replacement. In this respect, embryo cryopreservation is still an elegant solution to prevent high-rank transfers leading to multiple pregnancies (Van den Abbeel et al., 1988). Moreover, cryopreservation of supernumerary embryos offers the couple an additional chance for transfer within the frame of one IVF treatment. However, embryo cryopreservation raised legal, moral and ethical objections in some countries. This, in turn, stimulated the research on oocyte cryopreservation.

Based on the techniques of human embryo cryopreservation, human oocyte cryopreservation was started. The success rates were unexpectedly low and only a few pregnancies were reported (Chen, 1986, 1988; van Uem et al., 1987; Al-Hasani et al., 1987; Kolodziej et al., 1991), of which only five live births ensued. The survival of oocytes after freezing-thawing was highly variable and often dramatically lower than for embryos; the fertilization rate was disappointingly low; and the genetic normality of the resulting human embryos was questionable (Al-Hasani et al., 1987). Due to the inefficiency and the possible genetic risk, the technique was abandoned.

In the years following the adverse experience with human oocyte freezing, research was done on animal and human oocyte cryopreservation to discover why the results were so poor. It was shown that the cryopreservation of oocytes can interfere with the stability of the microtubules of the meiotic spindle carrying the oocyte's chromosomes, as well as with the actin filaments co-managing polar body extrusion (Magistrini and Szöllösi, 1980; Johnson and Pickering, 1987; Pickering and Johnson, 1987; Sathananthan et al., 1988; Van der Elst et al.,1988; Pickering et al., 1990; Aigner et al., 1992; Vincent and Johnson, 1992). The genetic constitution of embryos resulting from cryopreserved oocytes was reported to be abnormal by induction of aneuploidy (Kola et al., 1988) or polyploidy (Al-Hasani et al.,1987; Glenister et al., 1987; Carroll et al., 1989; Bouquet et al., 1992; Van der Elst et al., 1993a). Furthermore, the freezing procedure was shown to induce hardening of the zona pellucida, making fertilization by conventional IVF more difficult (Johnson et al., 1988; Johnson, 1989; Trounson and Kirby, 1989; Vincent et al., 1990; Hunter et al., 1991; Pickering et al., 1991; Bernard et al., 1992; George and Johnson, 1993). In addition, it was shown that mouse oocytes can be parthenogenetically activated by the cryoprotective agent 1, 2-propanediol (Shaw and Trounson, 1989; Van der Elst et al., 1992).

On the basis of this research outcome, protocols for human oocytes have been fine-tuned and a workable strategy for human oocytes was proposed by Gook et al. (1993, 1994, 1995). Cryopreservation of the human oocyte with 1,2-propanediol was advocated and linked to the use of intracytoplasmic sperm injection (ICSI), (Gook et al., 1995; Kazem et al., 1995), which helped to obtain high levels of fertilization and embryo cleavage rates with no apparent genetic risk. Taking into account these guidelines, successful pregnancies following oocyte cryopreservation have been obtained recently (Tucker et al., 1996; Porcu et al., 1997, 1998; Borini et al., 1998; Polak de Fried et al., 1998). It remains questionable, however, as to whether equal chances can be offered to a couple by oocyte cryopreservation rather than by managing a fresh replacement cycle combined with a cycle of transfer of cryopreserved embryos.

As an outgrowth of the problems encountered in the freezing of mature oocytes, another line of research into the cryopreservation of immature oocytes in the germinal vesicle stage has been settled upon as a rescue scenario. It was estimated that cryopreservation could hence be done in a less sensitive stage in terms of spindle damage and genetic risk since in the immature oocyte, chromosomes are decondensed and protected within a nuclear membrane. Indeed, the absence of a meiotic spindle carrying the chromosomes, which had clearly been a target for damage in cryopreservation of mature oocytes, was thought to solve the problem of spindle damage and the associated genetic risk. Research on cryopreservation of immature mouse oocytes has proved that it is feasible to carry out cryopreservation of germinal-vesicle, stage oocytes-followed by *in vitro* maturation, *in vitro* fertilization, embryo development and even the production of live offspring, be it with low efficiency (Schroeder et al., 1990; Van der Elst et al., 1992, 1993b). Also, for human immature oocytes, the technique was less successful than expected. The cryopreservation of human immature oocytes has been shown to be problematic in terms of survival and maturation to the MII stage (Mandelbaum et al., 1988; Toth et al., 1994; Son et al., 1996). A pregnancy obtained from a cryopreserved human *in vitro* matured oocyte is still unknown. A handful of pregnancies were made possible from non-frozen *in vitro* matured oocytes derived from fresh ovarian biopsies, collected during IVF treatment cycles or collected from unstimulated ovaries (Cha and Chian, 1998). It is clear that the effect of *in vitro* maturation of human oocytes on embryonic and fetal development has to be sorted out before the combination with cryopreservation can be considered again.

The latest development in human oocyte cryopreservation is to freeze ovarian cortical tissue containing the store of primordial follicles. This is looking back to the experiments of the fifties and sixties again, since cryopreservation of ovarian sections with the birth of a live young was already reported then (Parrott, 1960). Cryopreservation of ovarian tissue was started by oncologists to preserve the fertility of young patients undergoing sterilizing anti-cancer treatment. Since cryopreservation of mature oocytes and of embryos would require ovarian stimulation and since embryo cryopreservation is not even an option for children or young women without a partner, it was left to investigate the possibility of cryopreserving ovarian tissue.

Cryopreservation of ovarian cortical tissue, followed by orthotopic transplantation, has already led to pregnancies in mice (Parrott, 1960; Cox et al., 1996; Gunasena et al., 1997), sheep (Gosden et al., 1994a) and rats (Aubard et al., 1998). Follicular development was observed in ovine and feline (Gosden et al., 1994b) and cryopreserved marmoset tissue (Candy et al., 1995) after xenografting in SCID mice. Cryopreservation of human ovarian cortical tissue has shown that morphologically normal follicles are present in the thawed tissue (Hovatta et al., 1996). Xenografting of frozen-thawed human ovarian cortical tissue under the kidney capsule of immunodeficient SCID mice has shown that follicle survival after transplantation can be obtained (Newton et al., 1996). Recently, it has been shown by Oktay et al. (1998) that gonadotrophic stimulation of human xenografts in hypogonadal mice can lead to the growth of follicles to the antral stage.

Taking into account the physical constraints in transplantation in small animals (Oktay et al., 1998) and the concern of transmitting malignant cells (Shaw et al., 1996), *in vitro* culture and growth of follicles has a promising future (Nayudu and Osborn, 1992; Spears et al., 1994; Cortvrindt et al., 1996 a,b; Eppig and O'Brien, 1996). Extensive reviews of ovarian tissue transplantation have been published recently by Nugent et al. (1997) and Newton et al. (1998), in which strategies for the use of frozen-banked tissue for assisted reproduction are being explored thoroughly.

CRYOPRESERVATION OF SPERM CELLS

The concept of sperm banking is not new and had already been forwarded by Mantagazza (1866), while the first report on the maintenance of the motility of human spermatozoa after exposure to low temperature goes back to the birth of the American nation (Spallanzani, 1776). Almost two hundred years later, in 1949, to be precise the way to successful cryopreservation of sperm cells was discovered rather accidentally. Polge et al. (1949) found that glycerol had a beneficial effect on fowl sperm cryopreservation, in particular in terms of motility preservation. Bunge and Sherman (1953) were the first to report normal offspring of human sperm that had been stored on dry ice. The first birth after deep freezing of human sperm with glycerol and storage in liquid nitrogen was described by the same group (Perloff et al., 1964). Gradually, human sperm banks arose around the world: CECOS (Centre d'Etude et de Conservation du Sperme) in France in 1973, American Association of Tissue Banks in the United States in 1976 and many others since then (Sherman, 1979). Frozen human sperm can be frozen either for autoconservation or as donor sperm. Autoconservation is done where future fertility may have to be ensured in case of men who have to undergo sterilizing anti-cancer therapies, or in case of sterilization by vasectomy. The clinical use of frozen instead of fresh donor semen was increased when concern was raised about the possibility of infecting patients with hepatitis B or human immunodeficiency virus during artificial insemination with fresh semen. Cryopreservation of the sperm allowed for a quarantine period of 6 months, during which screening of the donor for infectious diseases can be done. Furthermore, the arrival of IVF in 1978 created new facilities for sperm banking: in case of large variation in sperm quality, in case of problem in semen collection on the day of oocyte retrieval, or even in case of the husband's absence during treatment (Mahadevan et al., 1983). In recent years, the tremendous impact of intracytoplasmic sperm injection (ICSI) (Palermo et al., 1992; Van Steirteghem et al., 1993), on IVF decreased the demand for donor semen, since even for men with oligo-astheno-teratozoospermia, it is possible to use their own genetic material. Further, the ultimate hope of fathering a genetically-own-child for men who were azoospermic became possible by the introduction of techniques for the recovery of spermatozoa from the epidydimis and the testis (Schoysman et al., 1993a,b; Tournaye et al., 1994; Devroey et al., 1996). As an outgrowth of these surgical sperm collection techniques, residual cells may be frozen to avoid repeated surgery in a following treatment (Nagy et al., 1995; De Croo et al.,1998). So, a new specialisation in sperm banking is arising.

The technology of freezing human sperm cells has not changed much over the past half-century. The standard liquid nitrogen vapour freezing, using glycerol as a cryoprotective agent, that was introduced by Sherman (1954), is still used today, of course with some modifications. The technique consists in placing straws horizontally in the vapour phase above the liquid nitrogen surface and eventually lowering them in this phase, prior to plunging them into liquid nitrogen. During the years, the addition of buffers and so-called extenders, like egg-yolk, have been introduced and this has been found to improve sperm cryosurvival (Behrman et al., 1969; Mahadevan and Trounson, 1983; Jeyendran et al., 1984). Controlled-rate freezing of sperm was introduced in the 1980s but it is still debatable whether programmed freezing is really beneficial to human spermatozoa. It is not excluded that low-quality sperm samples or sperm cells of testicular origin might benefit from a programmed slow freezing rate. What has been shown unequivocally is that the prefreeze addition and post-thaw removal of cryoprotective agents should be done in a step-wise, and preferably drop-wise, manner to minimize osmotic injury (McLaughlin et al., 1990; Gao et al., 1992, 1993; Verheyen et al., 1993).

The difficulty with sperm cryopreservation has also been to define the parameter to evaluate freezing thawing efficiency. The process of cryopreservation definitely has an effect on sperm quality. Post-thaw motility and morphology are generally regarded as sensitive quality parameters to evaluate freezing-thawing damage (Serres et al., 1980; Mahadevan and Trounson, 1984; Cross and Hanks, 1991; Gao et al., 1993; Verheyen et al., 1993). Studies comparing the outcome of IUI or IVF with frozen and fresh sperm present conflicting results, but suggest that the post-thaw loss of motility of a substantial amount of spermatozoa from a normospermic sample does not reduce the chances of fertilization or pregnancy, since sufficient numbers of sperm cells show the required characteristics after thawing (Englert et al., 1989).

The use of spermatozoa from oligo-asthenoteratozoospermic samples or the use of sperm cells of testicular origin may, however, require a more fine-tuned approach to cryopreservation. When applying cryopreservation on testicular spermatozoa that have very limited motility, it is difficult to distinguish dead from live spermatozoa after thawing based on the recovery of motility. In the case of testicular spermatozoa, the use of biopsy freezing has begun (Salzbrunn et al., 1996; Schulze et al., 1998). Results regarding the clinical use of frozen versus fresh testicular sperm for ICSI are still scarce. Most publications deal with case-reports and the experiences described in the present retrospective studies are conflicting (Gil-Salom et al., 1996; De Croo et al., 1998).

CRYOPRESERVATION OF EMBRYOS

In the early days of the introduction of IVF, cryopreservation of embryos was not an option to consider. The efficiency of IVF was not very high and the one ovulatory oocyte bulging from the surface of the ovary could be retrieved with the new revolutionary technique of laparoscopy, introduced by the late Patrick Steptoe. It was only after ovarian stimulation was introduced that the efficiency of IVF increased unquestionably, by increasing the number of available oocytes. The availability of surplus oocytes also led to the creation of embryos supernumerary to the ones to be selected for transfer. Experience with successful cryopreservation of the mouse embryo (Whittingham et al., 1972) was then applied to supernumerary human embryos originating from IVF treatment cycles. The first pregnancy achieved after transfer of a frozen-thawed human embryo was reported by Trounson and Mohr (1983). The first childbirth originating from cryopreserved embryos was that of twins born in the Netherlands on Boxing Day, 1983 (Zeilmaker et al., 1984). Since then, many centres have tried to extend their IVF programme by including cryopreservation of embryos. Over the years, researchers have learnt that cryopreservation is not to be taken lightly. It is a delicate issue and the success of the technique is highly determined by respecting the essence of details in a protocol. Wherever embryo cryopreservation has been regarded as an add-on facility, considered to be less important than the fresh cycle, success has not been reached. Moreover, cryopreservation should be regarded as a surplus chance for the couple within the frame of one IVF treatment cycle.

Successful cryopreservation of two-pronuclear or multicellular embryos, with different cryoprotectants according to different freezing protocols, was reported by various centres around the globe during the eighties and nineties (Trounson and Mohr, 1983; Zeilmaker et al., 1984; Cohen et al., 1985, 1986, 1988; Fehilly et al., 1985; Lassalle et al., 1985; Marrs et al., 1987; Mohr et al., 1985; Frydman et al., 1986; Testart et al., 1986, 1987a, b; Van Steirteghem et al., 1987; Mandelbaum et al., 1988; Van den Abbeel et al., 1988; Camus et al., 1989; Fugger et al., 1991; Schalkoff et al., 1993; Veeck et al., 1993; Van der Elst et al., 1995, 1996, 1997). Today, the decision of which protocol to use is largely dictated by a centre's transfer policy, or by the moral or legal guidelines of the centre. Generally, embryo transfer is done on day 2 or 3, following oocyte pick-up (OPU). When the policy is to cryopreserve multicellular embryos, freezing is done on the day of transfer or the consecutive day, but preferably not beyond day three. When freezing of multicellular embryos is not done or not allowed for legal, moral or ethical reasons, the option is to freeze two-pronuclear embryos on day 1, following OPU. The problem associated with this policy is that the number of embryos to be left in culture for guaranteeing transfer of fresh embryos has to be reflected on. The advantage is that two-pronuclear embryos tend to survive freezing better than multicellular embryos do. With multicellular embryos, one has an idea of the developmental potential, but the best embryos have already been selected for fresh transfer.

Crucial to embryo cryopreservation is the management of selection criteria before freezing and following thawing. Before freezing, the morphology of the embryo, as described by cell stage and degree of fragmentation, is a good indicator of the probability of cryosurvival of multicellular embryos; following thawing, the 24-h developmental potential has proved to be a very helpful indicator of viability (Van der Elst et al., 1997a). For 2PN embryos, survival is more easily defined as it concerns a unicellular system, and cleavage following thawing is the paramount parameter to judge viability.

With the gradual introduction of day-5 blastocyst culture in programmes of assisted reproduction as an alternative to day-2 or day-3 transfers (Gardner and Lane, 1997), the freezing of blastocysts will have to be developed as another approach of cryopreservation. In a report from the eighties by Fehilly et al. (1985), the cryopreservation of human blastocysts compared favourably to that of cleavage-stage embryos. The pregnancy rate per transfer was 53% in the blastocyst freezing group versus 24% per transfer in the group where cleavage-stage embryos had been frozen. In another report from the eighties (Cohen et al., 1985), two pregnancies were obtained from 11 frozen-thawed blastocyst replacements. More recent reports of larger series show conflicting findings—from no pregnancies at all (Troup et al., 1991) to low (Nakayama et al., 1995) and promising pregnancy rate results (Hartshorne et al., 1991; Ménézo et al., 1992; Olivennes et al., 1994; Kaufman et al., 1995). In order to optimize blastocyst freezing, the prefreezing culture media as well as the freezing media and protocols used will have to be adequately chosen.

Another recent development in the cryopreservation of embryos is the freezing of embryos in the frame of an IVF treatment cycle, involving preimplantation genetic diagnosis. In order to increase the benefit of a PGD-cycle, it is imperative to cryopreserve the supernumerary nonaffected embryos. The influence of the biopsy procedure on the survival of cryopreserved embryos has been studied in the model of the mouse embryo. Varying results have been obtained. Wilton et al. (1989) reported high implantation rates after ultra-rapid freezing of biopsied 4-cell mouse embryos. Liu et al. (1993) carried out a study in which it was demonstrated that biopsy of up to two blastomeres from mouse eight-cell embryos was not detrimental for cryosurvival, blastocyst formation and live offspring. Other authors did find an effect of freezing on the survival and/or blastocyst formation rates of biopsied mouse embryos (Krzyminska and O'Neill, 1991; Thompson et al., 1995).

Results on the combination of biopsy and cryopreservation of human embryos are scarce. A very recent report by Joris et al. (1998) has shown that biopsying embryos for preimplantation diagnosis interferes with the success of cryopreservation. The authors analysed the cryosurvival of human multicellular embryos developed from abnormally fertilized oocytes and found that drilling itself had a negative impact on survival which was strengthened by the biopsy procedure.

FUTURE STRATEGIES

The concept of combining cryopreservation of reproductive tissues with autotransplantation holds great promise for the future, particularly for preserving fertility in patients undergoing foreseeable depletion of their store of germ cells (Nugent et al., 1997).

A major task for the future will also be the long-term follow-up of children originating from cryopreserved gametes, embryos or tissues. Workers in the field of reproductive medicine must be aware of the tremendous impact assisted reproduction has had in the field of human procreation during the final decades of the last century. It is with a spirit of endeavour, but also of caution, that we should enter the millennium.

REFERENCES

Aigner, S. et al. (1992). 'The influence of slow and ultrarapid freezing on the organization of the meiotic spindle of the mouse oocyte', *Hum. Reprod.*, 7: 857–64.

Al-Hasani, S. et al. (1987). 'Cryopreservation of human oocytes', *Hum. Reprod.*, **2**: 695–700.

Ashwood-Smith, M.J. (1986). 'The cryopreservation of human embryos', *Hum. Reprod.*, **1**: 319–32.

Aubard, Y. et al. (1998). 'Conservation of the follicular population in irradiated rats by the cryopreservation and orthotopic autografting of ovarian tissue', *Eur. J. Obstet. Gynecol. Reprod. Biol.*, **79**: 83–7.

Behrman, S.J. and D.R. Ackerman (1969). 'Freeze preservation of human sperm', *Am. J. Obstet. Gynecol.*, **103**: 654.

Bernard, A. and B.J. Fuller (1996). 'Cryopreservation of human oocytes: A review of current problems and perspectives', *Hum. Reprod. Update.*, **2**: 193–207.

Bernard, A. et al. (1992). 'Fertilisation and embryonic development of human oocytes after cooling', *Hum. Reprod.*, 7: 1447–50.

Borini, A. et al. (1998). 'Pregnancies after oocyte freezing and thawing: Preliminary data', *Hum. Reprod.*, **13** (Abstract book 1): 124–5.

Bouquet, M. et al. (1992). 'The incidence of chromosomal abnormalities in frozen-thawed mouse oocytes after *in vitro* fertilization', *Hum. Reprod.*, 7: 76–80.

Bunge, R.G. and J. K. Sherman (1953). 'Fertilizing capacity of frozen human spermatozoa', *Nature* (London), **172**: 767

Camus, M. et al. (1989). 'Human embryo viability after freezing with dimethylsulfoxide as a cryoprotectant', *Fertil. Steril.*, **51**: 460–65.

Candy C.J. et al. (1995). 'Follicular development in cryopreserved marmoset ovarian tissue after transplantation', *Hum. Reprod.*, **10**: 2334–8.

Carroll, J. et al. (1989). 'Increase in digyny explains polyploidy after *in vitro* fertilization of frozen-thawed mouse oocytes', *J. Reprod. Fert.* **85**: 489–94.

Cha, K.-Y. and R.C. Chian (1998). 'Maturation *in vitro* of immature human oocytes for clinical use', *Hum. Reprod. Update.*, **4**: 103–20.

Chang, M.C. (1953). 'Storage of unfertilized rabbit ova: Subsequent fertilization and the probability of normal development', *Nature*, **172**: 353–4.

Chen, C. (1986). 'Pregnancy after human oocyte cryopreservation', *Lancet*, **1**: 884–6.

______(1988). 'Pregnancies after human oocyte cryopreservation', *Ann. NY. Acad. Sci.*, **541**: 541–9.

Cohen, J. et al. (1988). 'Cryopreservation of zygotes and early cleaved human embryos', *Fertil. Steril.*, **49**: 283–9.

______(1985). 'Birth after replacement of hatching blastocyst cryopreserved at expanded blastocyst stage', *Lancet*, **i**: 647.

______(1986). 'Factors affecting survival and implantation of cryopreserved human embryos', *J. In Vitro Fertil. Embryo. Transfer*, **3**: 46–52.

Cortvrindt, R. et al. (1996a). '*In vitro* maturation, fertilisation and embryo development of immature oocytes from early preantral follicles of prepubertal mice in a simplified culture system', *Hum. Reprod.*, **11**: 2656–66.

______(1996b). 'A morphological and functional study of the effect of slow freezing followed by complete *in vitro* matuartion of primary mouse ovarian follicles', *Hum. Reprod.*, **11**: 2648–55.

Cox, S.L. et al. (1996). 'Transplantation of cryopreserved fetal ovarian tissue to adult recipients in mice', *J. Reprod. Fertil.*, **107**: 315–22.

Cross, N.L. and S.E. Hanks (1991). 'Effects of cryopreservation on human sperm acrosomes', *Hum. Reprod.*, **6**: 1279–83.

De Croo, I. et al. (1998). 'Fertilization, pregnancy and embryo implantation rates after ICSI with fresh and frozen-thawed testicular spermatozoa', *Hum. Reprod.*, **13**: 1893–7.

Devroey P. et al. (1996). 'Outcome of intracytoplasmic sperm injection with testicular spermatozoa in obstructive and non-obstructive azoospermia', *Hum. Reprod.*, **11**: 1015–18.

Edwards, R.G. et al. (1980). 'Establishing full-term pregnancies with cleaving embryos grown *in vitro*', *Br. J. Obstet. Gynaec.*, **887**: 757–68.

Englert, Y. et al. (1989). 'Is fresh or frozen sperm to be used in *in vitro* fertilization with donor sperm?' *Fertil. Steril.*, **51**: 661–4

Eppig, J. J. and M. J. O'Brien (1996). 'Development *in vitro* of mouse oocytes from primordial follicles', *Biol. Reprod.*, **54**: 197–207.

Fehilly, C.B. et al. (1985). 'Cryopreservation of cleaving embryos and expanded blastocysts in the human: A comparative study', *Fertil. Steril.*, **44**: 638–44.

Frydman, R. et al. (1986). 'Programmed oocyte retrieval during routine laparoscopy and embryo cryopreservation for later transfer', *Am. J. Obstet. Gynecol.*, **155**: 112–7.

Fugger, E.F. et al. (1991). 'Human preimplantation embryo cryopreservation: Selected aspects', *Hum. Repr.*, **6**: 131–5.

Gao, D.Y. et al. (1993). 'Hyperosmotic tolerance of human spermatozoa: Separate effects of glycerol, sodium chloride, and sucrose on spermolysis', *Biol. Reprod.*, **49**: 112–23.

Gao, D.Y. et al. (1992). 'Glycerol permeability of human spermatozoa and its activation energy', *Cryobiology*, **29**: 657–67.

Gardner, D. K. and M. Lane (1997). 'Culture and

selection of viable blastocysts: A feasible proposition for human IVF', *Hum. Reprod. Update.*, **3**: 367–82.

George M. A. and M. H. Johnson (1993). 'Cytoskeletal organisation and zona sensitivity to digestion by chymotrypsin of frozen-thawed mouse oocytes', *Hum. Reprod.*, **8**: 612–20.

Gil-Salom M. et al. (1996). 'Pregnancies after intracytoplasmic sperm injection with cryopreserved testicular spermatozoa', *Hum. Reprod.*, **11**: 1309–13.

Glenister, P.H. et al. (1987). 'Incidence of chromosome anomalies in first-cleavage mouse embryos obtained from frozen-thawed oocytes fertilized *in vitro*', *Gamete. Res.*, **16**: 205–16.

Gook, D.A. et al. (1993). 'Cryopreservation of mouse and human oocytes using 1, 2-propanediol and the configuration of the meiotic spindle', *Hum. Reprod.*, **8**: 1101–9.

______(1994). 'Fertilisation of human oocytes following cryopreservation: Normal karyotypes and absence of stray chromosomes', *Hum. Reprod.*, **9**: 684–91.

______(1995). 'Intracytoplasmic sperm injection and embryo development of human oocytes cryopreserved using 1, 2-propanediol', *Hum. Reprod.*, **10**: 2637–41.

Gosden, R.G. et al. (1994a). 'Restoration of fertility to oophorectomized sheep by ovarian autografts stored at –196°C', *Hum. Reprod.*, **9**: 597–603

Gosden, R.G. et al. (1994b). 'Follicular development of ovarian xenografts in SCID mice', *J. Reprod. Fertil.*, **101**: 619–23.

Gunasena, K. T. et al. (1997). 'Live births after autologous transplant of cryopreserved mouse ovaries', *Hum. Reprod.*, **12**: 101–6.

Hartshorne, G. M. et al. (1991). 'The influence of *in vitro* development upon post-thaw survival and implantation of cryopreserved human blastocysts', *Hum. Reprod.*, **6**: 136–41.

Hovatta, O. et al. (1996). 'Cryopreservation of human ovarian tissue using dimethylsulpoxide and propanediol-sucrose as cryoprotectants', *Hum. Reprod.*, **11**: 1268–72.

Hunter, J.E. et al. (1991). 'Fertilization and development of the human oocyte following exposure to cryoprotectants, low temperatures and cryopreservation: A comparison of two techniques', *Hum. Reprod.*, **6**: 1460–65.

Jeyendran, R.S. et al. (1984). 'Comparison of glycerol and a zwitterion buffer system as cryoprotective media for human spermatozoa', *J. Androl.*, **5**: 1.

Johnson, M.H. (1989). 'The effect on fertilization of exposure of mouse oocytes to dimethylsulphoxide: An optimal protocol', *J. In vitro Fert. Embryo. Trans.*, **6**: 168–75.

Johnson, M.H. and S.J. Pickering (1987). 'The effect of dimethylsulphoxide on the microtubular system of the mouse oocyte', *Development*, **100**: 313–24.

Johnson, M.H. et al. (1988). 'The influence of cooling on the properties of the zona pellucida of the mouse oocyte', *Hum. Reprod.*, **3**: 383–7.

Joris, H. et al. (1998). 'Reduced survival after embryo biopsy and cryopreservation of human embryos obtained after abnormal fertilisation', *Hum. Reprod.*, **13** (Abstract book 1): 61.

Kaufman, R. A. et al. (1995). 'Cocultured blastocyst cryopreservation: Experience of more than 500 transfer cycles', *Fertil. Steril.*, **64**: 1125–9.

Karow, A. M. and J. K. Critser (eds.) (1997). *Reproductive Tissue Banking: Scientific Principles.*, Academic Press, Harcourt Brace and Company, pp. 472.

Kazem, R. et al. (1995). 'Cryopreservation of human oocytes and fertilisation by two techniques: *In vitro* fertilisation and intracytoplasmic sperm injection', *Hum. Reprod.*, **10**: 2650–54.

Kola, I. et al. (1988). 'Vitrification of mouse oocytes results in aneuploid zygotes and malformed fetuses', *Teratology*, **38** 467–74.

Kolodziej, F.B. et al. (1991). 'Cryopreservation of human oocytes and pronuclei embryos—First results. Reproduction in domestic animals', Zuchthygiene, 24 Jahrestagung über Physiologie und Pathologie der Fortpflanzung, 16 Veterinar-Humanmedizinische Gemeinschaftstagung, Leipzig.

Krzyminska, U. and C. O. Neill (1991). 'The effects of cryopreservation and thawing on the development *in vitro* and *in vivo* of biopsied 8-cell mouse embryos', *Hum. Reprod.*, **6**: 832–5.

Lassalle, B. et al. (1985). 'Human embryo features that influence the success of cryopreservation with the use of 1, 2-propanediol', *Fertil. Steril.*, **44**: 645–51.

Leibo, S.P. (1977). 'Fundamental cryobiology of mouse ova and embryos', in K.Eliott and J. Whelan (eds.) *The Freezing of Mammalian Embryos.* Ciba Foundation Symposium no. 52, Elsevier, Amsterdam, pp. 69–92.

Lin, T.P. et al. (1957). 'Survival of unfertilized mouse eggs in media containing glycerol and glycine', *J. Exp. Zool.*, **134**: 275–92.

Liu, J. et al. (1993). 'The *in vitro* and *in vivo* developmental potential of frozen and non-frozen biopsied 8-cell mouse embryos', *Hum. Reprod.*, **8**: 1481–6.

Magistrini, M. and D. Szöllösi (1980). 'Effects of cold and of isopropyl-N-phenylcarbamate on the second meiotic spindle of mouse oocytes', *Eur. J. Cell Biol.*, **22**: 699–707.

Mahadevan, M. and A.D. Trounson (1983). 'Effect of cryoprotective media and dilution methods on the preservation of human spermatozoa', *Andrologia*, **15**: 355–66.

______(1984). 'Effect of cooling, freezing and thawing rates and storage conditions on preservation of human spermatozoa', *Andrologia*, **16**: 52–60.

Mahadevan, M.M. et al. (1983). 'Successful use of semen cryobanking for *in vitro* fertilization', *Fertil. Steril.*, **40**: 340–43.

Mandelbaum, J. et al. (1988). 'Cryopreservation of human embryos and oocytes', *Hum. Reprod.*, **3**: 117–9.

Mantagazza, P. (1866). 'Sullo sperma umano', *Rendic Reale Inst. Lomb.*, **3**: 183.

Marrs, R.P. et al. (1987). 'Successful pregnancies from cryopreserved human embryos produced by *in vitro* fertilisation', *Am. J. Obstet. Gynecol.*, **156**: 1503–8.

Mazur, P. (1970). 'Cryobiology: The freezing of biological systems', *Science*, **168**: 939–49.

______(1984). 'Freezing of living cells: Mechanisms and implications', *Am. J. Physiol.*, **247**: C125-C142.

______(1990). 'Equilibrium, quasi-equilibrium, and nonequilibrium freezing of mammalian embryos', *Cell Biophysics*, **17**: 53–92.

McLaughlin, E.A. et al. (1990). 'A comparison of the freezing of human semen in the uncirculated vapour above liquid nitrogen and in a semi-programmable freezer', *Hum. Reprod.*, **5**: 724–8.

Ménézo, Y. et al. (1992). 'Freezing cocultured human blastocysts', *Fertil. Steril.*, **58**: 977–80.

Mohr, L.R. et al. (1985). 'Deep-freezing and transfer of human embryos', *J. In Vitro Fertil. Embryo. Transfer*, **2**: 1–10.

Nagy, Z.P. et al. (1995). 'Using ejaculated, fresh and frozen-thawed epididymal and testiculat spermatozoa gives rise to comparable results after intracytoplasmic sperm injection', *Fertil. Steril.*, **63**: 808–15.

Nakayama, T. et al. (1995). 'Developmental potential of frozen–thawed human blastocysts', *J. Assist. Reprod. Genet.*, **12**: 239–43.

Nayudu, P. L. and S. M. Osborn (1992). 'Factors influencing the rate of preantral and antral growth of mouse ovarian follicles *in vitro*', *J. Reprod. Fertil.*, **95**: 349–62.

Newton, H. (1998). 'The cryopreservation of ovarian tissue as a strategy for preserving the fertility of cancer patients', *Hum. Reprod. Update.*, **4**: 237–47.

Newton, H. et al. (1996). 'Low temperature storage and grafting of human ovarian tissue', *Hum. Reprod.*, **11**: 1487–91.

Nugent, D. et al. (1997)' Transplantation in reproductive medicine: Previous experience, present knowledge and future prospects', *Hum. Reprod. Update.*, **3**: 267–80.

Oktay, K. et al. (1998). 'Development of human primordial follicles in SCID/hpg mice stimulated with follicle stimulating hormone', *Hum. Reprod.*, **13**: 1133–8.

Olivennes, F. et al. (1994). 'Four indications for embryo transfer at the blastocyst stage', *Hum. Reprod.*, **9**: 2367–73.

Palermo G. et al. (1992). 'Pregnancy after intracytoplasmic injection of a single spermatozoon into an oocyte', *Lancet*, **304**: 17–8.

Parkes, A.S. (1958). 'Factors affecting the viability of frozen ovarian tissue', *J. Endocrinol.*, **17**: 337–46.

Parrott, D.M.V. (1960). 'The fertility of mice with orthotopic ovarian grafts derived from frozen tissue', *J. Reprod. Fertil.*, **1**: 230–41.

Perloff, W.H. et al. (1964). 'Conception with human spermatozoa frozen by nitrogen vapour technique', *Fertil. Steril.*, **15**: 501.

Pickering, S.J. and M.H. Johnson (1987). 'The influence of cooling on the organization of the meiotic spindle of the mouse oocyte', *Hum. Reprod.*, **2**: 207–16.

Pickering, S.J. et al. (1991). 'Cryopreservation of human oocytes: Inappropriate exposure to DMSO reduces fertilization rates', *Hum. Reprod.*, **6**: 142–3.

______(1990). 'Transient cooling to room temperature can cause irreversible disruption of the meiotic spindle in the human oocyte', *Fertil. Steril.*, **54**: 102–8.

Polak de Fried et al. (1998). 'Pregnancy after human donor oocyte cryopreservation and thawing in association with intracytoplasmic sperm injection in a patient with ovarian failure', *Fertil. Steril.*, **69**: 555–7.

Polge, C. et al. (1949). 'Revival of spermatozoa after vitrification and dehydration at low temperatures', *Nature*, **4172**: 666, (1949).

Porcu, E. et al. (1997). 'Birth of a healthy female after intracytoplasmic sperm injection of cryopreserved human oocytes', *Fertil. Steril.*, **68**: 724–6.

Porcu, E. et al. (1998). 'Birth of six healthy children after intracytoplasmic sperm injection of cryopreserved human oocytes', *Hum. Reprod.*, **13** (Abstract book 1): 124.

Salzbrunn, A. et al. (1996). 'A new concept for the extraction of testicular spermatozoa as a tool for assisted fertilization (ICSI)', *Hum. Reprod.*, **11** 752–5.

Sathananthan, A.H. et al. (1988). 'The effects of ultrarapid freezing on meiotic and mitotic spindles of mouse oocytes and embryos', *Gamete. Res.*, **21**: 385–401.

Schalkoff, M.E. et al. (1993). 'A multifactorial analysis of the pregnancy outcome in a successful embryo cryopreservation program', *Fertil. Steril.*, **59**: 1070–4.

Schoysman R. et al. (1993a). 'Succesful fertilization by testicular spermatozoa in an *in vitro* fertilization programme (letter)', *Hum. Reprod.*, **8**: 1339–40.

______(1993b). 'Pregnancy after fertilization with human testicular spermatozoa', *Lancet*, **342**: 1237.

Schroeder, A.C. et al. (1990). 'Developmental capacity of mouse oocytes cryopreserved before and after maturation *in vitro*', *J. Reprod. Fertil.*, **89**: 43–50.

Schulze, W. et al. (1998). 'Cryopreservation of testicular tissue: A highly effective method to provide sperm for successful TESE/ICSI procedures', in D. Kempers et al. (eds.), *Fertility and Reproductive Medicine*, Elsevier Science B. V., pp. 621–6.

Serres, C. et al. (1980). 'Effects of freezing on spermatozoa motility', in G. David and W.S. Price (eds.), *Human artificial insemination and semen preservation*, Plenum Press, NY, pp. 147–61.

Shaw, J.M. and A.O. Trounson (1989). 'Parthenogenetic activation of unfertilized mouse oocytes by exposure to 1, 2-propanediol is influenced by temperature, oocyte age and cumulus removal', *Gamete Res.*, **24**: 269–79.

Shaw, J.M. et al. (1996). 'Fresh and cryopreserved ovarian tissue samples from donors with lymphoma transmit the cancer to graft recipients', *Hum. Reprod.*, **11**: 1668–73.

Sherman, J.K. (1954). 'Freezing and freeze-drying of human spermatozoa', *Fertil. Steril.*, **5**: 357.

______(1979). 'Synopsis of the use of frozen semen since 1964: State of the art of human semen banking', *Fertil. Steril.*, **24**: 397–412.

Sherman, J.K. and T.P. Lin (1958). 'Effect of glycerol and low temperature on survival of unfertilized mouse eggs', *Nature*, **4611**: 785–6.

Smith, A.U. and A.S. Parkes (1951). 'Preservation of ovarian tissue at low temperatures', *Lancet*, **570**.

Son, W. et al. (1996). 'Effects of 1,2-propanediol and freezing-thawing on the *in vitro* developmental capacity of human immature oocytes', *Fertil. Steril.*, **66**: 995–9.

Spallanzani, L. (1776). 'Opuscoli di Fisca. Animale, e Vegetabile', Opusculo II. Osservazioni, e Sperienze Intorno ai Vermicelli Spermatici dell'Uomo e degli Animali. Modena.

Spears, N. et al. (1994). 'Mouse oocytes derived from *in vitro* grown primary ovarian follicles are fertile', *Hum. Reprod.*, **9**: 527–32.

Steptoe, P.C. and R.G. Edwards (1978). 'Birth after the reimplantation of a human embryo', *Lancet*, **ii**: 336.

Testart, J. et al. (1986). 'High pregnancy rate after early human embryo freezing', *Fertil. Steril.*, **46**: 268–72.

______(1987a). 'Human embryo viability related to freezing and thawing procedures', *Am. J. Obstet. Gynecol.*, **157**: 168–71.

______(1987b). 'Factors influencing the success rate of human embryo freezing in an *in vitro* fertilization and embryo transfer program', *Fertil. Steril.*, **48**: 107–12.

Thompson, L. A. et al. (1995). 'A comparison of the effects of different biopsy strategies on the post-thaw survival of 8-cell-stage mouse embryos: Implications for preimplantation diagnosis', *Hum. Reprod.*, **10**: 659–63.

Toth, T. L. et al. (1994). 'Fertilisation and *in vitro* development of cryopreserved human prophase I oocytes', *Fertil. Steril.*, **61**: 891–4.

Tournaye H. et al. (1994). 'Microsurgical epididymal sperm aspiration and intracytoplasmic sperm injection: A new effective approach to infertility as a result of congenital bilateral absence of the vas deferens', *Fertil. Steril.*, **61**: 1045–50.

Trounson, A. and C. Kirby (1989). 'Problems in the cryopreservation of unfertilized eggs by slow cooling in dimethyl sulfoxide', *Fertil. Steril.*, **52**: 778–86.

Trounson, A. and L. Mohr (1983). 'Human pregnancy following cryopreservation, thawing and transfer of an eight-cell embryo', *Nature*, **305**: 707–9.

Troup, S. A. et al. (1991). 'Cryopreservation of human embryos at the pronucleate, early cleavage, or expanded blastocyst stages', *Eur. J. Obstet. Gynecol. Reprod. Biol.*, **38**: 133–9.

Tucker, M. et al. (1996). 'Preliminary experience with human oocyte cryopreservation using 1, 2-propanediol and sucrose', *Hum. Reprod.*, **11**: 1513–5.

Van den Abbeel, E. et al. (1988). 'Hyperstimulation: The need for cryopreservation of embryos', *Hum. Reprod.*, **3**: 53–7.

Van der Elst, J. et al. (1995). 'Prospective randomized study on the cryopreservation of human embryos with dimethylsulfoxide or 1, 2-propanediol protocols', *Fertil. Steril.*, **63**: 92–100.

Van der Elst, J. et al. (1992). '*In vitro* maturation of mouse germinal vesicle-stage oocytes following cooling, exposure to cryoprotectants and ultrarapid freezing: Limited effect on the morphology of the second meiotic spindle', *Hum. Reprod.*, **7**: 1440–46.

______(1993a). 'Association of ultrarapid freezing of mature mouse oocytes with increased polyploidy at the pronucleate stage, reduced cell numbers in blastocysts and impaired fetal development', *J. Reprod. Fert.*, **99**: 25–32.

______(1993b). 'Slow and ultrarapid freezing of fully-grown germinal vesicle-stage mouse oocytes: Optimal survival rate outweighed by defective blastocyst formation', *J. Assis. Reprod. Gen.*, **10**: 202–12.

______(1996). 'Long-term evaluation of implantation of fresh and cryopreserved human embryos following ovarian stimulation with buserelin acetate-HMG or clomiphene citrate-HMG', *Hum. Reprod.*, **11**: 2097–106.

______(1988). 'Effect of 1, 2-propanediol and dimethylsulphoxide on the meiotic spindle of the mouse oocyte', *Hum. Reprod.*, **3**: 960–67.

______(1992). 'Parthenogenetic activation pattern and microtubular organisation of the mouse oocyte after exposure to 1, 2-propanediol', *Cryobiology*, **29**: 549–62.

______(1997a). 'Selective transfer of cryopreserved human embryos with further cleavage after thawing increases delivery and implantation rates', *Hum. Reprod.*, **12**: 1513–21.

Van der Elst, J. et al. (1997b), 'Cryoconservation: Sperms and oocytes', in T Rase, et al. (eds.), *Manual on Assisted Reproduction*, Springer-Verlag, Berlin, Heidelberg, pp. 223-251.

Van Steirteghem, A. et al. (1993). 'High fertilization and implantation rates after intracytoplasmic sperm injection', *Hum. Reprod.*, **8**: 1061–6.

______(1987). 'Cryopreservation of human embryos obtained after gamete intra-Fallopian transfer and/or *in vitro* fertilization', *Hum. Reprod.*, **2** 593–8.

van Uem, J.F. et al. (1987). 'Birth after cryopreservation of unfertilized oocytes (letter)', *Lancet*, **1**: 752–3.

Veeck, L.L. et al. (1993). 'Significantly enhanced pregnancy rates per cycle through cryopreservation and thaw of pronuclear stage oocytes', *Fertil. Steril.*, **59**: 1202–7.

Verheyen, G. et al. (1993). 'Effect of freezing method, thawing temperature and post-thaw dilution/washing on motility (CASA) and morphology characteristics of high-quality human sperm', *Hum. Reprod.*, **8**: 1678–84.

Vincent, C. and M.H. Johnson (1992). 'Cooling, cryoprotectants and the cytoskeleton of the mammalian oocyte', *Oxf. Rev. Reprod. Biol.*, **14**: 73–100.

Vincent, C. et al. (1990). 'The hardening effects of dimethylsulphoxide on the mouse zona pellucida requires the presence of an oocyte and is associated with a reduction in the number of cortical granules present', *J. Reprod. Fertil.*, **89**: 253–9.

Whittingham, D.G. et al. (1972). 'Survival of mouse embryos frozen to –196°C and –269°C', *Science*, **178**: 414.

Wilton, L. J. etal. (1989). 'Successful single-cell biopsy and cryopreservation of preimplantation embryos', *Fertil. Steril.*, **51**: 513–7.

Zeilmaker, G.H. et al. (1984). 'Two pregnancies following transfer of intact frozen-thawed embryos', *Fertil. Steril.*, **42**: 293–6.

17

Preimplantation Genetic Diagnosis

Semra Kahraman

Chromosomal abnormalities are the major cause of pre- and postimplantation embryo loss. It is estimated that approximately half of human embryos are chromosomally abnormal and the majority of them fail to implant (Munne 1994). This is primarily due to numerical chromosomal anomalies, occuring either before or after fertilization. In general, at least 30% of normally developing and 75% of arrested embryos are abnormal at the chromosomal level. About 60% of spontaneously aborted fetuses developing from oocytes fertilized *in vivo* have an abnormal karyotype, most of which are trisomies or polyploidies. After *in vitro* fertilization, the rate of chromosomal anomalies in spontaneous abortions was assumed to be 62% (Plachot et al., 1988).

Preimplantation genetic diagnosis (PGD) is a current diagnostic tool for couples undergoing assisted reproductive techniques. PGD is based on the genetic analysis of one or two cells obtained by blastomere biopsy, and allows for the selection of chromosomally normal embryos to achieve a healthy pregnancy in patients carrying a risk for genetic disease (Lissens and Sermon, 1997). It offers an alternative to current practice, which requires a pregnant women with a fetus at risk of carrying a genetic disease to terminate an established pregnancy.

Many factors have been suggested as contributing to the low success rate of Assisted Reproductive Techniques (ART) in women of advanced maternal age (AMA). These factors can either be endometrial or oocyte related. Defective hormonal milieu, poor uterine flow and inadequate endometrial proliferation cause reduced endometrial receptivity and thus, implantation failure. Alternatively, reduced embryo quality, ageing of oocytes and chromosomal imbalance may explain the low success rate in aged women, indeed 'if oocytes from younger women are donated to the aged women, pregnancy successfully occur' (Navot et al., 1994). Aneuploidy may be a major contributing factor in implantation failure in women of AMA undergoing ART. Therefore, the selection of normal embryos could increase the rate of pregnancy and healthy offspring (Mancuso et al., 1996).

PGD can also provide us with a chromosomal evaluation of embryos, especially in repeated implantation failure which occurs in some young patients even though good quality embryos are transferred more than twice. However, PGD is still under research by several centres for patients with repeated implantation failure (RIF) (Gianaroli et al., 1997c; Grossmann et al., 1998).

Aneuploidy significantly increases with maternal age even in morphologically and developmentally normal embryos. These findings could also explain the increased incidence of spontaneous abortion with advanced maternal age (Munne et al., 1993). The objectives of PGD are to prevent chromosomal disorders to reduce spontaneous abortion due to aneuploidy, and it may improve the effectiveness of ART. Therefore, chromosomal evaluation of oocytes/embryos obtained from women of AMA may provide advantages in analysing chromosomally normal embryos to improve pregnancy rates (Gianaroli et al., 1997 a, b; Munne et al., 1995a).

Aneuploidy screening in women of AMA undergoing ART may be performed for the following indications: aneuploidy or genetic screening in male infertility following intracytoplasmic sperm injection (ICSI); identification of sex in X-linked disease; aneuploidy of translocation carriers; single gene defects.

The idea of PGD is not new: in 1967, Edwards and Gardner succeeded in sexing rabbit embryos at the blastocyst stage and successfully transferred them. They predicted the use of similar technology in humans to avoid genetic disease. However, it took until the 1990s for the first clinical application of PGD to emerge (Handyside et al.,1990). Y chromosome-specific sequences were amplified, using polymerase chain reaction (PCR), to determine the sex of embryos obtained from couples at risk of X-linked diseases. Sexing by PCR has now largely been abandoned in favour of fluorescent *in situ* hybridization (FISH) (Grifo et al., 1992), in which five or more different chromosomes can be detected in a single cell simultaneously; FISH has an advantage over PCR for sexing as it detects the X and Y chromosomes simultaneously, thus, it can determine the sex of the embryo and whether there is aneuploidy of sex chromosomes, allowing for screening of the commonest aneuploidies and trisomies 13,18 and 21. Five or more chromosomes can be detected by FISH at the single-cell level allowing screening for the most common aneuploidies for chromosomes 13, 18, 21 and 22 and the sex chromosomes (Munne, 1994)

Clinical progress with PGD has been slow, partly because of the complexity and diversity of chromosomal and single-gene defects. Only those centres that combine expertise in both reproductive medicine and molecular genetics have been involved. In the future, however, an increasing knowledge of the genetic defects associated with infertility, especially male infertility with the development of (ICSI), will stimulate the development of PGD to avoid transmission of these defects to their offspring (Handyside et al., 1998). Indeed, PGD for cystic fibrosis mutations has already been executed in infertile men with congenital bilateral absence of the vas deference (Liu et al., 1994), as well as Yq deletions and sex chromosomal aneuploidy in Klinefelter's syndrome (Staessen et al., 1997).

Cleavage-stage embryos may not reflect the chromosomal constitution of the embryo due to a high frequency of mosaicism. A polar body biopsy (PBB) may be more reliable for a PGD of common aneuploidies than the cleavage-stage FISH, as the latter has less value due to the high frequency of mosaicism in preimplantation embryos. Maternal age-related aneuploidies originate through non-disjunction during the first, and less frequently, the second meiotic division.

The use of first polar body analysis for aneuploidy detection is an alternative to blastomere analysis, especially since most aneuploidies originate from maternal meiosis I nondisjunctions (Munne et al., 1995b; Verlinsky et al., 1995, 1996). In addition, polar body analysis in combination with blastomere biopsy would allow screening for aneuploidy resulting from the male.

Polar body analysis for PGD is performed for cystic fibrosis, alfa-1 antitripsin deficiency, retinitis pigmentosa, haemophilia A and B, thalassaemia, Alport's, Gaucher's, Tay Sach's and sickle cell disease, long-chain acyl-CoA dehyrogenasedeficiency and chromosomal abnormalities (Verlinsky et al., 1996, 1998).

Genetic analysis of the first polar body should disclose most genetically imbalanced oocytes (Verlinsky et al., 1995). Therefore, first and second polar body analysis could be useful in reducing the age-related risk for trisomy in patients of advanced maternal age. However, it has been stated by Angell (1994) that the mechanism of trisomy formation in man would caution against PGD of chromosome disorders from information on the chromosome constitution of the polar bodies.

First and second polar body biopsy procedures were first developed by Verlinsky et al. (1996). They have shown that a polar body biopsy does not affect fertilization or the viability of the resulting embryos, as well as pre- and postimplantation development. Polar bodies and performing genetic analysis of their DNA make it possible to predict the gene type of the embryos resulting from the corresponding oocytes. This will accordingly involve induction of superovulation to retrieve several follicles, micromanipulation to remove polar bodies, and the subsequent fertilization and transfer of preselected unaffected embryos back to the patient. To avoid an additional biopsy, sampling of both the first and second polar bodies can be done simultaneously, following insemination. After an additional 24 hours in culture, the oocytes are checked for cleavage, and those which result from the embryos whose first polar body is found to be homozygous for the abnormal gene are transferred to the patient to achieve a pregnancy; the second polar body in these cases contains a normal gene. In cases of a heterozygous first polar body, only the embryos resulting from the oocytes whose second polar body contains the abnormal gene are transferred. The affected oocytes subjected to polar body removal (PBR) are followed up by a blastomere biopsy, or by another possible sampling to confirm the diagnosis (Strom et al., 1997). Preimplantation polar body analysis for common aneuploidies can also be performed by the use of a FISH technique and application of specific probes for chromosomes 13, 18 and 21. Studies showed no detrimental effect of the procedures on the developmental potential of the resulting embryos (Verlinsky et al., 1998). No significant decrease was observed in the fertilization rate, and the proportion of cleaving embryos derived from the oocytes subjected to PBR appeared not to differ from that in the control oocytes. No increase was observed in the percentage of polyspermic embryos in the polar body removed oocytes. Approximately 60% of embryos from the PBR oocytes developed to a blastocyst stage and PBR had no effect on the implantation rate or on the outcome of pregnancy following PBR (Verlinsky et al., 1995, 1996).

Translocation carriers having a higher incidence of infertility may produce chromosomally abnormal offspring, and often experience repeated spontaneous abortions. Reproductive problems associated with translocations can be alleviated through preimplantation genetic diagnosis. Normal healthy babies have been born after PGD of X-linked genetic diseases (Handyside et al., 1990; Grifo et al., 1992), single-gene defects (Handyside et al., 1992), aneuploidy (Munne et al., 1995b; Verlinsky et al., 1996), and recently, PGD of translocations (Munne et al., 1998).

Two approaches to PGD of translocations have been used. One is to develop specific probes for each translocation type. The second, useful only for female carriers of translocation(s), is based on the observation that the first polar body chromosomes are at metaphase stage immediately, for a limited period, after oocyte retrieval. Therefore, FISH analysis with chromosome-painting probes can easily be performed.

Around 35 centres worldwide are currently offering PGD clinically. By the end of 1996, almost 600 cycles of PGD following cleavage-stage biopsy had resulted in >100 pregnancies, and nearly 100 babies had been born, giving a pregnancy rate of 26% per embryo transfer. An equal number of cycles, involving polar body biopsy for aneuploidy screening in women of advanced maternal age or after repeated IVF failure, have already been carried out over a shorter period of time, indicating that this may become a major application of PGD (Verlinsky, 1996). Moreover, multicolour FISH may be used to diagnose unbalanced transmission of translocations in embryos from parents carrying a balanced translocation.

The results of PGD were evaluated at Sevgi Hospital Embryology and Genetic Laboratory, between December 1998–June 1999, for third-day embryos obtained from 72 couples with 72 cycles using Ca^{2+}/Mg^{2+}-free medium for advanced maternal age (n=49) and recurrent implantation failure (RIF) with more than two cycles, even though good quality embryos were transferred (n=23). As all males had severe male factor in our study, a blastomere biopsy was performed in preference to PBB to screen for aneuploidy in women of both AMA and RIF, and males with severe male factor. This would allow for screening of aneuploidy as well as for the male. A high frequency of constitutional chromosomal abnormalities may be present in the severely infertile male population; in addition, patients with severe asthenozoospermia may have centriolar defects which can cause impaired cellular division. PGD for women aged between 36–45 years undergoing ART were evaluated by using multiprobe FISH for chromosomes XY, 18, 13 and 21.

From 360 embryos, a successful FISH procedure was carried out on 329 blastomeres (91.3%). Ca^{2+}/Mg^{2+}-free medium was used for biopsy.It has been reported that embryo biopsy is easier to perform in the absence of Ca^{2+}/Mg^{2+} ions (Grifo et al., 1990; Santalo et al., 1996; Dumoulin et al., 1998). No detrimental effect on the viability of biopsied mouse embryos was observed during the limited time of exposure to Ca^{2+}/Mg^{2+}-free medium compared to the control group (Ducibella and Anderson, 1979; Reeve, 1981).

The minimum exposure to Ca^{2+}/Mg^{2+}-free medium was 5 minutes, while the maximum was 10 minutes before biopsy. In 107 embryos, the biopsy procedure lasted less than 3 minutes, whilst in 222 embryos, the duration was longer than 3 minutes. The minimum and maximum lengths of the biopsy procedure were found to be 1 minute 20 seconds and 8 minutes, respectively. No statistically significant difference was found between the rate of normally cleaved and arrested embryos during further development, where the duration of the biopsy was less or more than 3 minutes ($p>0.05$).

Third-day embryos were biopsied with the aim of chromosomal evaluation. AMA and RIF groups with more than two cycles were included. From these two groups, 8 patients had centrally located granular oocytes in their present and previous cycles, and 6 male partners had megalo-pin head sperm, globozoospermic forms and round spermatids in their ejaculates.

Patients signed a consent form before PGD, consenting to the use of their embryos for blastomere biopsy, and in case of pregnancy, amniocentesis. An embryo biopsy was performed at 64–68 hours after injection and only embryos with more than 7–8 blastomeres were selected for biopsy.

Pedigree analysis, family history and the appropriatness of cases for PGD were evaluated. Patients were counselled regarding the advantages of aneuploidy screening. Furthermore, couples were counselled regarding the possible increased risk of sex chromosomal abnormalities in the offspring and the need for follow-up prenatal testing. Males were karyotyped and counselled about the possibility of gonadal mosaicism or Y chromosome deletion/insertion.

The embryos were placed in HEPES-buffered medium without Ca^{2+}/Mg^{2+} ions (EB™-10 medium, Scandinavian IVF Science, Gothenburg, Sweden) before the biopsy procedure. A stimulation protocol was as previously described by Kahraman et al. (1999). Embryos were incubated for 5–10 minutes with EB™-10 medium according to the degree of compaction between the blastomeres. Embryos with compacted blastomeres on the third day were exposed between 5 and 10 minutes to an EB™-10 medium. Granulation of blastomeres were observed in these embryos exposing a relatively longer duration. Each Petri dish contained 10μl EB™-10 medium, covered with sterile equilibrated mineral oil. The first droplet was prepared for, biopsy procedure and the second one was to replace the biopsied blastomere(s) in the same Petri dish.

Three-dimensional partial zona dissection, in the shape of a cross-hatching or V shape, was performed to facilitate the biopsy procedure as originally introduced by Verlinsky's group (Cieslak et al., 1999). A V-shaped assisted hatching was performed in most of the embryos to create a triangular flap opening with a diameter of 25–30 μm to allow the replacement of the blastomere biopsy pipette.

A hand-drawn holding pipette, microneedle and biopsy pipette (Cook, IVF, K-EBPH-3535, Australia) were used for the purpose of the biopsy. A double pipette holder (Narishige HD-21, Japan) was used for the microneedle and biopsy pipette on the same side. The embryo was fixed with the holding pipette and the first partial zona dissection (PZD) was created by passing from the largest perivitelline space at the 12 o'clock position. To create a V-shaped opening, the embryo was rotated until the first slit was visible at the 12 o'clock position. A second cross was performed by entering with a microneedle into the first slit, tangentially through the perivitelline space, and a second zona dissection was performed (Cieslak et al., 1999). The embryo was then released and rotated until the V-shaped opening would be at the 3 o'clock position. The embryo was held by the holding pipette, and the biopsy pipette was inserted to remove one or two blastomeres with a visible nucleus.

Figures 17.1 and 17.2 show the cross-hatching and

blastomere biopsy procedures in a step-by-step manner. In 67.2% of the embryos, the blastomeres were biopsied by pressing the zona pellucida with a biopsy pipette to make the blastomere protrude from the zona opening. In the remaining embryos (32.8%), the blastomeres were biopsied by entering the opening of the zona pellucida with the biopsy pipette.

The biopsy procedure was executed 64–68 hours after insemination, for embryos obtained by ICSI. Only embryos with 7 or more blastomeres were selected for biopsy. Embryos with a poor morphology, with uneven blastomeres and a fragmentation rate of more than 30% were excluded.

The biopsy procedure was performed by the same operator and was observed by a second person on a monitor, connected to a video camera mounted on a microscope. The duration of the biopsy procedure was noted from the beginning (from fixing the embryos with a holding pipette to replacing one biopsied blastomere in a second EB™-10 droplet) to the end. The embryo to be biopsied was placed in a Petri dish in Ca^{2+}/Mg^{2+}-free medium, with a concentration of 2 µl (containing HSA and 100 IU/mL Pc-6 EB™-10 after equilibration at 37°C and 5% CO_2). The number of blastomeres in the beginning of the procedure, biopsied blastomeres, and nuclei, multinucleated blastomeres, damaged blastomeres in the embryo or damaged biopsied blastomeres were recorded. Furthermore, the type of biopsy protrusion or entering the embryo with the biopsy pipette and subsequent development of embryos were observed for 24 more hours to follow their developmental capacity, as well as to allow for a sufficient period for the FISH procedure. Any sign of cell or embryo damage was recorded.

Embryos were classified as 'complex abnormal' when two or more chromosomes had an abnormal count, but were not completely polyploid or haploid.

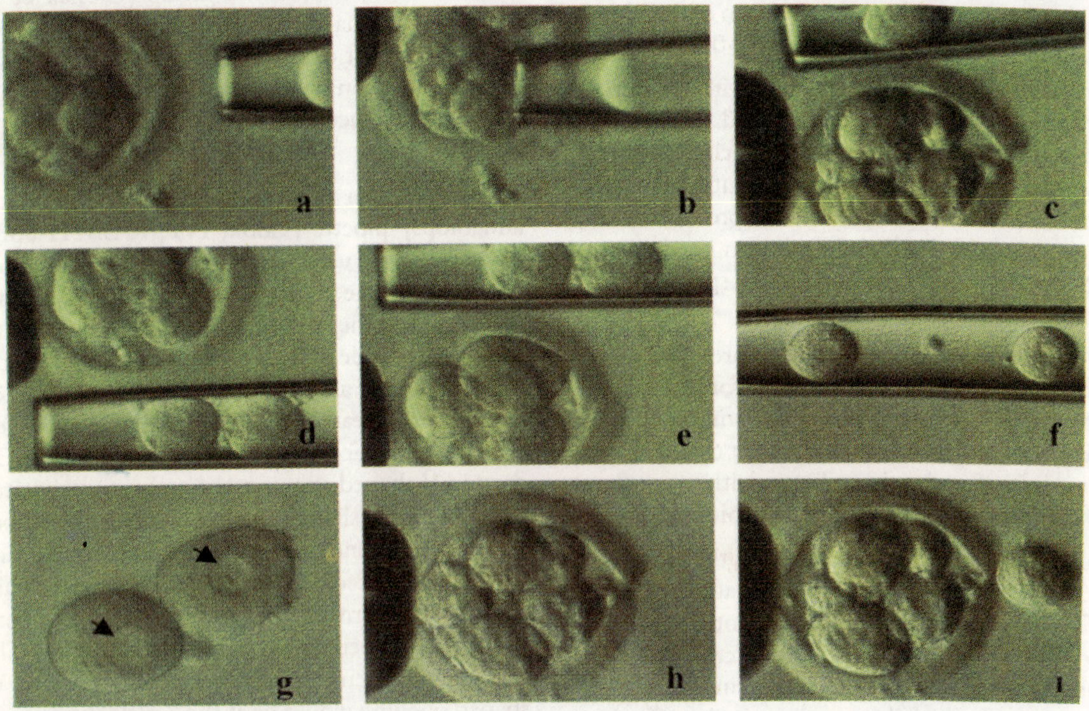

Fig. 17.1. (a) Embryo is fixed with the holding pipette. (b, c) First partial zona dissection is created, bypassing from the largest perivitelline space at the 12 o'clock position. (d) Embryo is rotated until the first slit is visible at the 12 o'clock position. (e, f) A second cross is performed by entering with a microneedle into the first slit tangentially through the perivitelline space. (g, h) A second zona dissection is performed. (i) A cross-shaped opening can be seen.

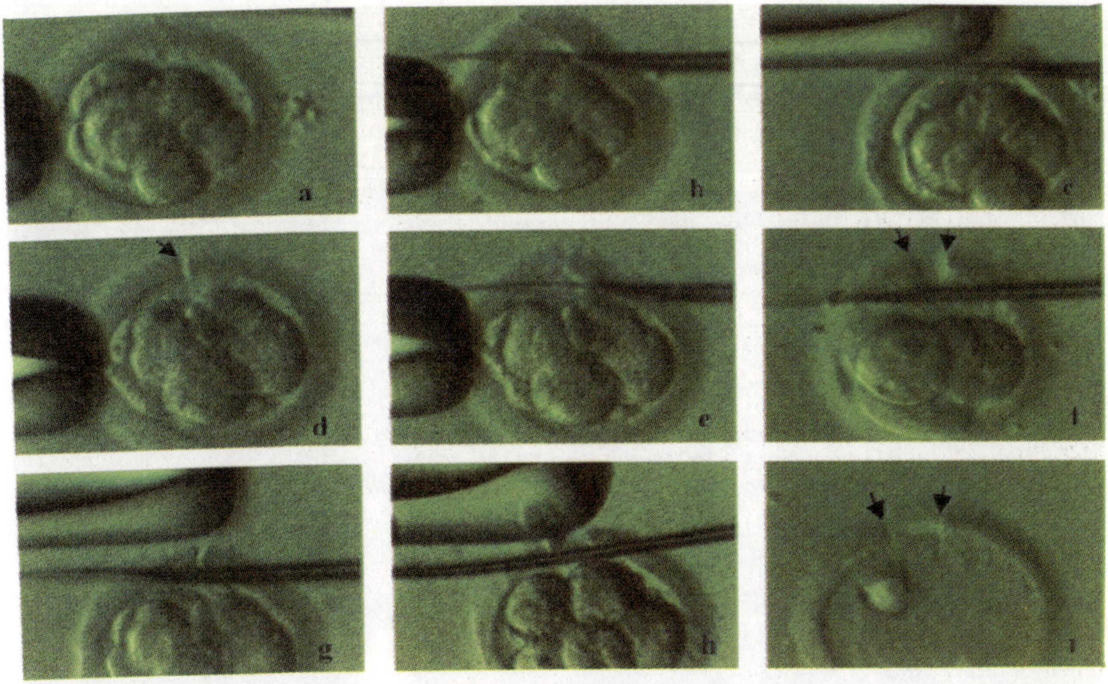

Fig. 17.2. (a) The embryo is then released and rotated until the V-shaped opening is seen at the 3 o'clock position. (b, c, d, e, f, g) The embryo is held by the holding pipette and the biopsy pipette is inserted to remove one or two blastomeres with a visible nucleus. (h, i) Blastomere biopsy by pressing the zona pellucida with a biopsy pipette to make the blastomere protrude from the zona opening.

Statistical analysis was performed using a Student's t-test or a chi-square test, where appropriate.

FLUORESCENCE *IN SITU* HYBRIDIZATION

The isolated blastomeres were analysed with a protocol previously described by Munne et al. (1993), except for the hybridization time as 3 hours. A Nikon E-600 microscope with filters recommended by Vysis for the probe mixture was used.

The scoring criteria described by Munne and Weier (1996) were followed and minor hybridization spots with low fluorescence intensity were not scored. For the multicolour FISH analysis, five DNA probes were used for the simultaneous detection of chromosomes XY, 13, 18 and 21. Figure 17.3 represents a blastomere FISH result with an extra marker of chromosome 13 (trisomy 13). The blastomeres of an abnormal embryo or embryos not being transferred were fixed and evaluated by the FISH procedure to confirm the diagnosis. Figure 17.4 represents a double-nucleated megalo-head spermatozooa diagnosed by the FISH technique.

A successful FISH analysis was realized in 329 out of 360 blastomeres (91.3%). The rates of normal and abnormal chromosomal evaluation of embryos were 58.7% and 41.3%, respectively. In 72.8% of the abnormal embryos (99), aneuploidy was diagnosed. In 5.1% (7) of the embryos, haploidy, in 9.6% (13) polyploidy, and in 12.5% (17) complex aneuploidy were diagnosed. Figures 17.5 and 17.6 show the rates of chromosomally normal and abnormal embryos, and the distribution of chromosomally abnormal embryos. The majority of the abnormal embryos were found to have aneuploidy (72.8%). Polyploidy, complex aneuploidy and haploidy were found to be 9.6%, 12.5% and 5.1%, respectively. Monosomy was diagnosed in 40.8% of the aneuploid embryos, and 43.4% trisomy, 3.9% double monosomy, 3.9% double trisomy and 3.9% trisomy-monosomy were observed. The most significant chromosomal abnormality was found in chromosome 18 (35.3%) in the aneuploid embryo group; secondly, chromosome 21 (27.1%), and thirdly, chromosome 13 (22.4%) were observed.

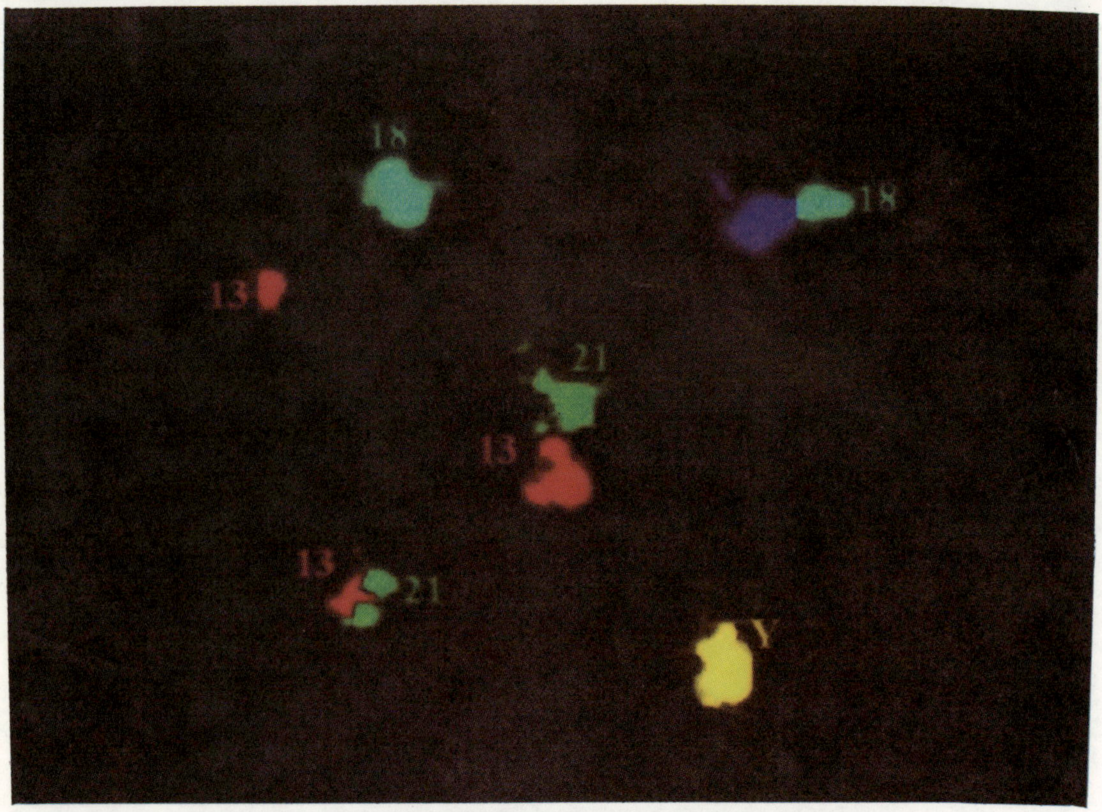

Fig. 17.3. A blastomere FISH analysis with an extra marker of chromosome 13 (trisomy 13)

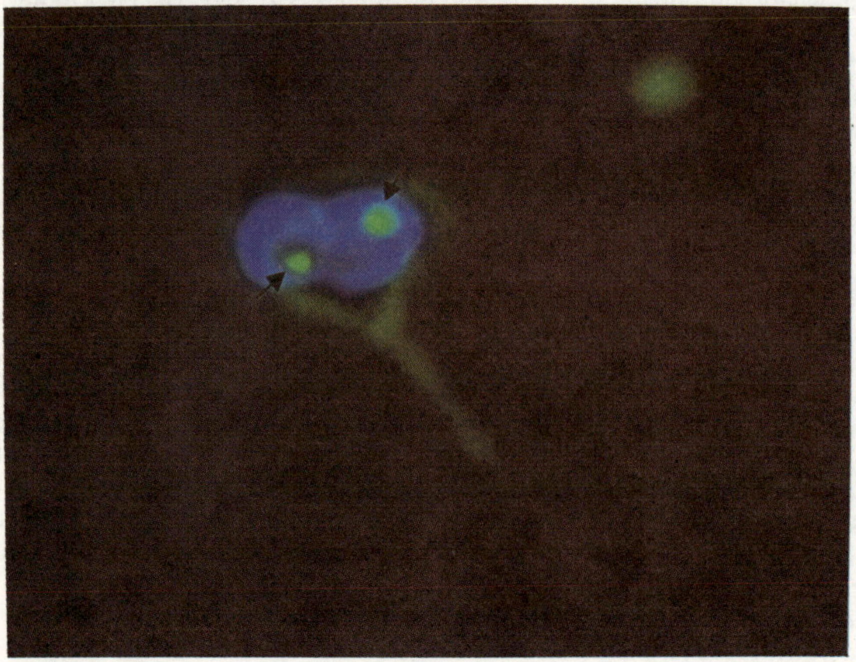

Fig. 17.4. A double-nucleated megalo-head spermatozoon diagnosed with FISH technique

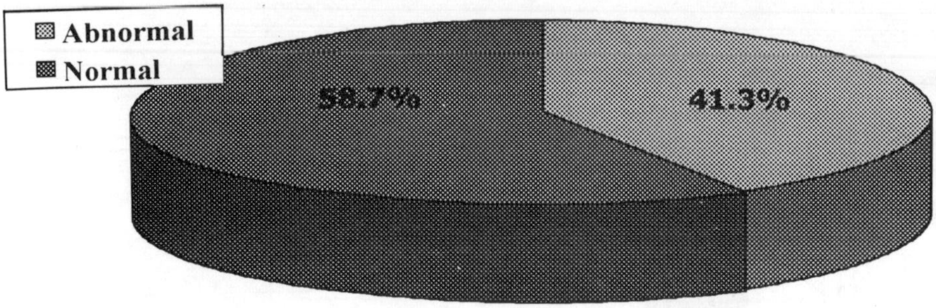

Fig. 17.5. Distribution of the rate of chromosomally normal and abnormal embryos (n = 329)

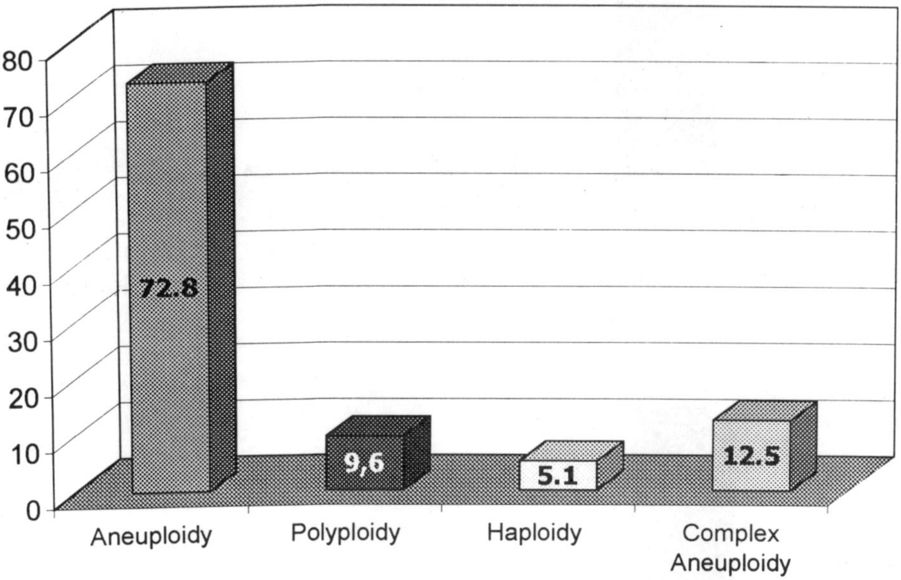

Fig. 17.6. Distribution of the rate of chromosomally abnormal embryos (n=136)

Table 17.1 represents the results of the chromosomal analysis. In the AMA group, the rates of chromosomally abnormal and normal embryos were 40.4% and 59.6%, respectively. The rates of chromosomally normal and abnormal embryos in the RIF group were 43.2% and 56.8%, respectively. The majority of abnormal embryos had aneuploidy (66.7%). Figures 17.7 and 17.8 show the distribution of the rate of chromosomally normal and abnormal embryos in the AMA and RIF groups.

Table 17.1. Results of chromosome analysis

Results	Rates of embryos analysed (%)
Normal	57.8
Aneuploidy	30.5
Trisomy	43.4
Monosomy	40.8
Double monosomy	3.9
Double trisomy	3.9
Trisomy-monosomy	3.9
Complex aneuploidy	5.6
Polyploidy	3.6
Haploidy	2.4

Although the number of embryos (n=21) evaluated chromosomally was low in cases with megalo-head sperm samples (n=6), a 76% aneuploidy rate was found, while 24% of embryos were chromosomally normal in this group (Fig. 17.9). High rates of aneuploidy (62.5%) and polyploidy (31.3%) were observed, probably due to a high incidence of diploidy in megalo-head sperm.

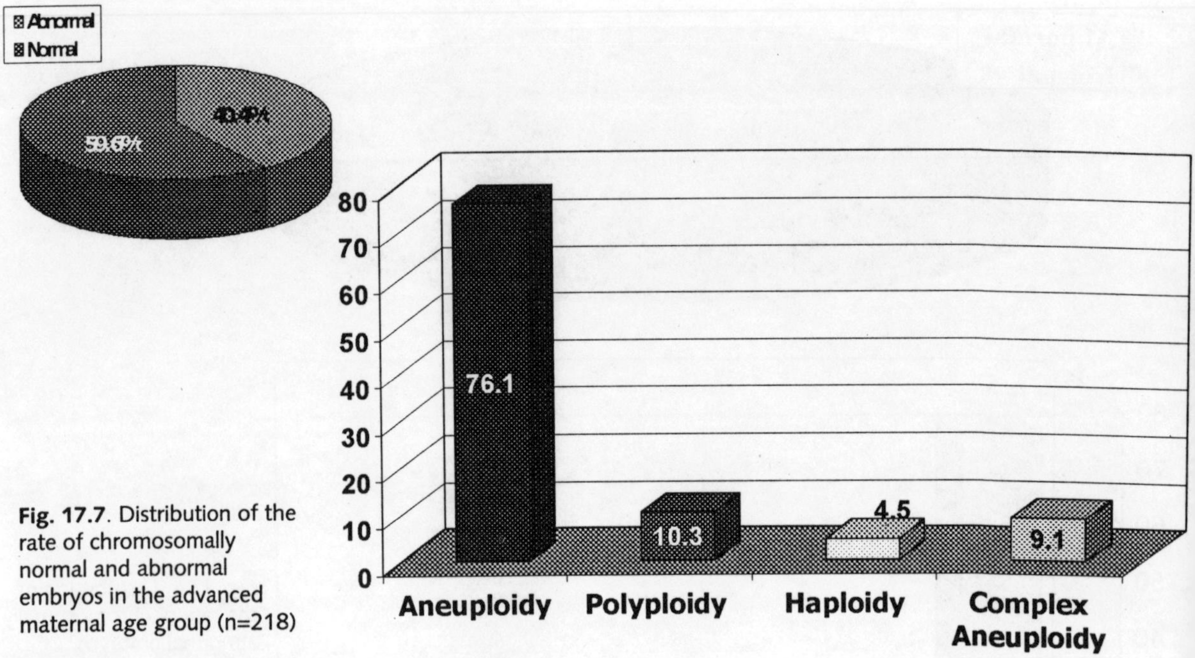

Fig. 17.7. Distribution of the rate of chromosomally normal and abnormal embryos in the advanced maternal age group (n=218)

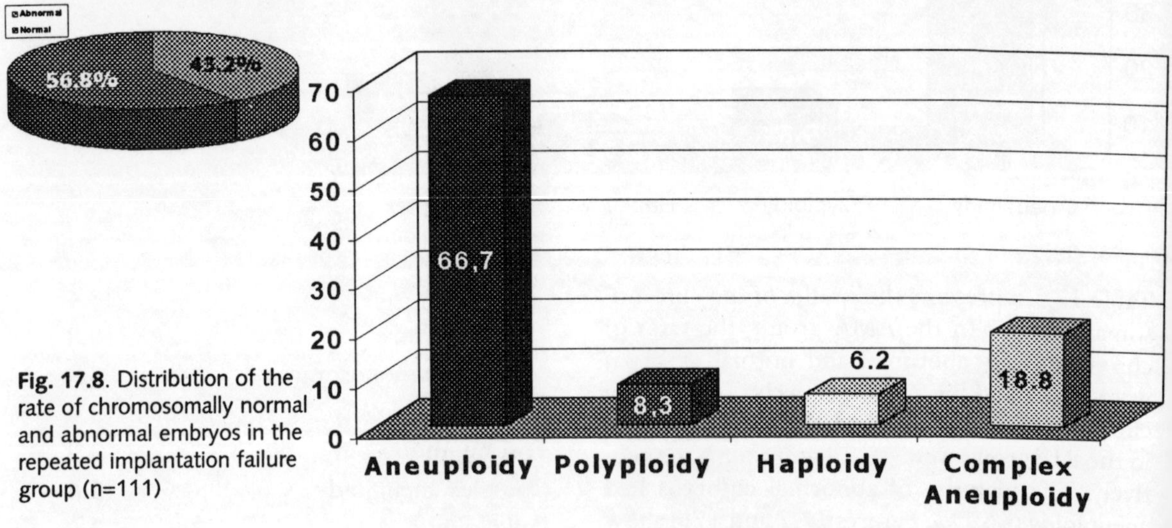

Fig. 17.8. Distribution of the rate of chromosomally normal and abnormal embryos in the repeated implantation failure group (n=111)

Eight patients had centrally located excessive granular oocytes in their previous and present cycles. As very low implantation and ongoing pregnancy rates (4.7%, unpublished data) were achieved, PGD was performed to evaluate a chromosomal complement of this group. Thirty-nine per cent of embryos were found to be chromosomally abnormal in the same group (Fig. 17.10). Of the 72 cases, 2 had no transfer due to the lack of chromosomally normal embryos. Out of the 110 chromosomally normal embryos transferred, a total of 22 pregnancies were achieved in 70 patients (31.4%). One pregnancy resulted in a spontaneous abortion at 8 weeks and one in a blighted ova at 6 weeks. The cytogenetic evaluation of both pregnancy material revealed 46, XY; 46, XX chromosomal complement by confirming the results of PGD. The rate of ongoing pregnancy

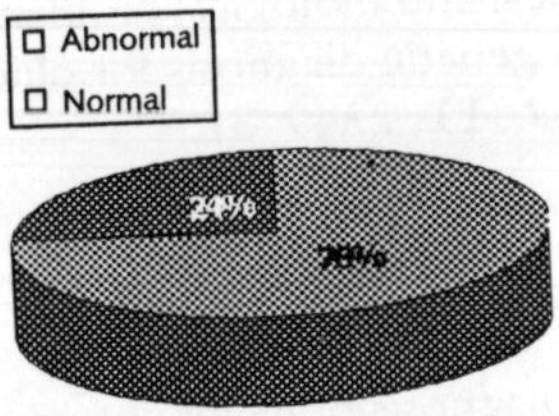

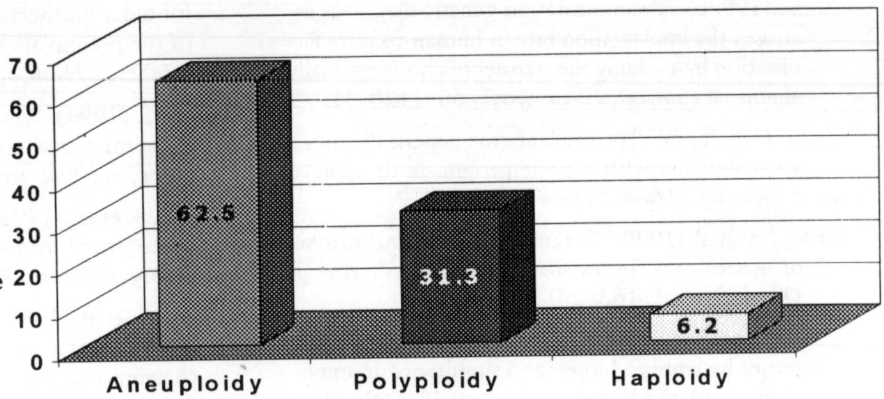

Fig. 17.9. Distribution of the rate of chromosomally normal and abnormal embryos in the megalo-head group (n=21)

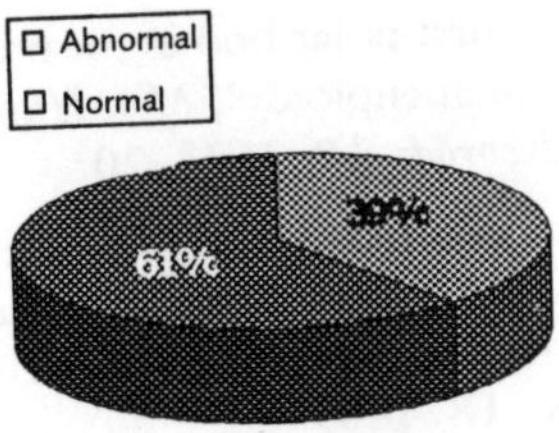

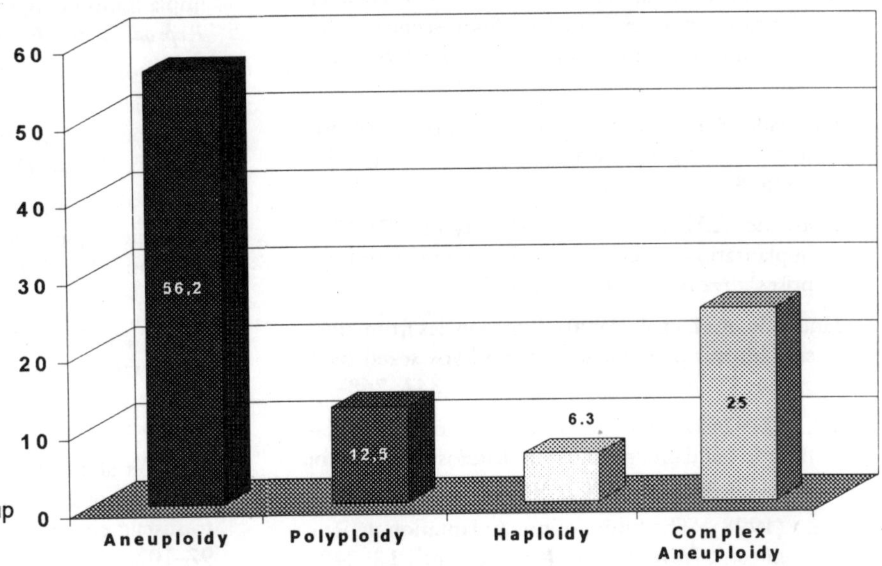

Fig. 17.10. Distribution of the rate of chromosomally normal and abnormal embryos in the centrally granular oocytes group (n=41)

was found to be 28.5% in total: a 25.5% ongoing pregnancy rate was achieved in the AMA group and 30.4% in the RIF group (p>0.05). Twelve healthy babies were born and other pregnancies are continuing into the third trimester.

REFERENCES

Angell, R.R. (1994). 'Polar body analysis: Possible pitfalls in preimplantation diagnosis of chromosomal disorders based on polar body analysis', *Hum. Reprod.*, **9**: 181–3.

Cieslak, J. et al. (1999). 'Three-dimensional partial zona dissection for preimplantation genetic diagnosis and assisted hatching', *Fertil. Steril.*, **71**: 308–13.

Ducibella, T. and E. Anderson (1979). 'The effect of calcium deficiency on the formation of the zona occludens and blastocoel in the mouse embryo', *Dev. Biol.*, **73**: 46–58

Dumoulin et al. (1998). 'Effect of Ca^{2+}/Mg^{2+}-free medium on the biopsy procedure for preimplantation genetic diagnosis and further development of human embryos', *Hum. Reprod.*, **13**: 2880–83.

Edwards, R.G., and R.L. Gardner (1967). 'Sexing of live rabbit blastocyst', *Nature*, **214**: 567–77

Gianaroli, L. et al. (1997a). 'Will preimplantation genetic diagnosis assist patient with a poor prognosis to achieve pregnancy', *Hum. Reprod.*, **12**: 1762–7.

______(1997b). 'Preimplantation genetic diagnosis increases the implantation rate in human *in vitro* fertilization by avoiding the transfer of chromosomally abnormal embyos', *Fertil. Steril.*, **68**: 1128–31.

______(1997c). 'Will preimplantation genetic diagnosis assist patients with a poor prognosis to achieve pregnancy', *Hum. Reprod.*, **12**: 1762–7.

Grifo, J.A. et al. (1990). 'Preembryo biopsy and analysis of blastomeres, by *in situ* hybridization', *Am. J. Obstet. Gynecol.*, **163**: 2013–9

______(1992). 'Ongoing pregnancy in a hemophilia carrier by embryo biopsy and simultaneous amplification of X and Y chromosome spesific DNA from single blastomeres', *JAMA.*, **6**: 727–9.

Grossmann, M. et al. (1998). 'Recurrent *in vitro* fertilization failure evaluated by fluorescence in situ hybridization: A case report', *Fertil. Steril.*, **69**: 558–60.

Handyside, A.H. (1998). 'Clinical evaluation of preimplantation genetic diagnosis', *Prenat. Diagn.* **18**: 1345–8.

Handyside, A.H. and J.D.A. Delhanty (1997). 'Preimplantation genetic diagnosis; strategies and surprises', *Trends Genet.*, **13**: 270–75.

Handyside, A.H. et al. (1990). 'Pregnancies from biopsied human preimplantation embryos sexed by Y spesific DNA amplification', *Nature*, **344**: 768–70

______(1992). 'Birth of a normal girl after *in vitro* fertilization and preimplantation diagnostic testing for cystic fibrosis', *N. Engl. J. Med.*, **327**: 594–8.

______(1998). 'The future of preimplantation genetic diagnosis', *Hum. Reprod.* (Supplement), **13**: 249–55.

Kahraman, S. et al. (1999). 'Fertility of ejaculated and testicular megalohead spermatozoa with intracytoplasmic sperm injection', *Hum. Reprod.*, **14**: 726–30

Lissens, W. and K. Sermon (1997). 'Preimplantation genetic diagnosis: Current status and new developments', *Hum. Reprod.*, **12**: 1756–61.

Liu, J. et al. (1994). 'Birth after preimplantation diagnosis of the cystic fibrosis delta F508 mutation by polymerase chain reaction in human embryos resulting from intracytoplasmic sperm injection with epididymal sperm', *J. Am. Med. Assoc.*, **272**: 1858–60.

Mancuso, S. et al. (1996). 'Preimplantation diagnosis for older mothers: Ethical and biological problems of the preimplantation genetic diagnosis for older mothers', *Hum. Reprod.*, **11**: 2349–51.

Munne S. (1994). 'Flow cytometry separation of X and Y spermatozoa could be detrimental for human embryos', *Biol. Reprod.*, **51**: 373–9.

Munne, S. et al. (1993). 'Diagnosis of major chromosome aneuploidies in human preimplantation embryos', *Hum. Reprod.*, **8**: 2185–91.

Munne, S. et al. (1995a). 'Embryo morphology developmental rates and maternal age are correlated with chromosome abnormalities', *Fertil. Steril.*, **64**: 382–91.

______(1995b). 'The use of first polar bodies for preimplantation diagnosis of aneuploidy', *Mol. Hum. Reprod.*, 1, see *Hum. Reprod.*, **10**: 1014–20.

______(1998). 'Preimplantation diagnosis of the aneuploidies most commonly found in spontaneous abortions and live births: XY, 13, 14, 15, 16, 18, 21, 22', *Prenat. Diagn.*, **18**: 1459–66.

______(1995). 'Enzymatic amplification of B-globin genomic sequences and restriction site analysis for diagnosis of sickle cell anemia', *Science*, **230**: 1350–54.

Munne, S. and H.U.G. Weier (1996). 'Simultaneous enumeration of chromosomes 13,18,21, X and Y in interphase cells for preimplantation genetic diagnosis', *Cytogenet. Cell Genet.*, **75**: 263–70.

Navot, D. et al. (1994). 'Age-related decline in female fertility is not due to diminished capacity of the uterus to sustain embryo implantation', *Fertil. Steril.*, **61**: 97–107.

Plachot, M. et al. (1988). 'Are clinical parameters and biological IVF parameters correlated with chromosomal disorders in early life: Multicentric study', *Hum. Reprod.*, **3**: 627–35

Reeve, W.J.D. (1981). 'The distribution of ingested horseadish peroxidase in the 16-cell mouse embryo', *J. Embryol. Exp. Morph.*, **66**: 191–207.

Santalo, J. et al. (1996). 'Does Ca^{2+}/Mg^{2+}-free medium have an effect on the survival of the preimplantation mouse embryo after biopsy', *Hum. Reprod. Update.*, **2**: 257–61

Staessen, C. et al. (1997). 'Preimplantation diagnosis by fluorescent in-situ hybridization in embryos from 47, XXY or 47, XXX patients', *J. Assist. Reprod. Genet.*, **14**: 468.

Strom, C. et al. (1997). 'Preimplantation diagnosis of single gene disorders by two-step oocyte genetic analysis', *J. Assist. Reprod. Genet.*, **14**: 469.

Verlinsky, Y. (1996). 'Preimplantation genetic diagnosis (Editorial)', *J. Assist. Reprod. Genet.*, **13**: 87–9.

Verlinsky, Y. et al. (1996). 'Polar body diagnosis of common aneuploidies by FISH', *J. Assist. Reprod. Genet.*, **13**: 157–62.

______(1995). 'Pregnancies following pre-conception diagnosis of common aneuploidies by fluorescent *in situ* hybridization', *Hum. Reprod.*, **10**: 1923–7

______(1996). 'Preimplantation genetic group: Birth of healthy children after preimplantation diagnosis of common aneuploidies by polar body fluorescent *in situ* hybridization analysis', *Fertil. Steril.*, **66**: 126–9.

______(1998). 'Polar Body Biopsy: Fertility and Reproductive Medicine', Proceedings of the XVI. World Congress on fertility and sterility, Elsevier Science, San Francisco, 4–9 October.

18

Ethical and Medico-legal Aspects of Assisted Reproductive Techniques

Pritam P. Phatnani

ASSISTED REPRODUCTIVE TECHNOLOGY (ART)

A certain element of risk is associated with ART procedures. It is, therefore, necessary to ascertain their therapeutic value in every case. An informed and written consent should be taken after duly counselling the couple/oocyte donor. They should be explained, in simple language, the various risk factors associated with the techniques, such as ovarian hyperstimulation, anaesthesia, laparoscopy, aspiration of ovum, etc. They should also be explained the possibility of multiple pregnancies, ectopic gestation, spontaneous abortion, premature births, higher perinatal and infant morality, growth and development problems, etc.

IVF-ET AND SURROGATE MOTHERHOOD

No medicolegal problems are posed by IVF-ET with an egg and a sperm of a married couple. With either egg or sperm donated, it is governed on the same lines as AID, with the married partner being the natural or biological mother. IVF-ET with a donated egg or sperm, or womb leasing, will create two to three sets of parents, genetic, biological and natural.

The doctor assumes the responsibility of selection of the suitable donor in terms of the following.

- Complete physical examination of the donor should be done to ascertain the good health of the donors of the semen, oocyte or embryo.
- The donor should be healthy, with good quality eggs or sperms and with a proven fertility record.
- The physical characteristics and mental make-up of the donor should match, as closely as possible, with that of the spouse of the recipient, specially with reference to colour of the skin, eyes and hair, height and built, religious and ethnic background, educational level and ABO blood type.
- The blood group of the proposed donor and donee should be tested with respect to Rh compatibility.
- No person suffering from any sexually transmitted disease (e.g., hepatitis -B, HIV) or genetically transmissible disease should be used as a donor.
- Sexually transmitted disease should be ruled out not more than one week before the seminal fluid is obtained. It is preferable that donated semen is cryopreserved and used only after 6 months as this would enable the centre to retest the donor after 3 months for HIV and eliminate the potential risk of HIV transmission in the 'window' period of HIV infection.
- The identities of the donor as well as the recipient should be protected from each other. However, all the records of the donor must be preserved in order to trace him/her in case of any eventuality.
- Confidentiality of the entire procedure and its outcome must be maintained and, therefore, no relative should be accepted as a donor, besides avoiding claims of parenthood and inheritance rights. (However, often the oocyte

donor is identified and brought by the couple, in which case the identity of the oocyte donor gets revealed.)

- Written consent of the donor should be taken towards unrestricted use of sperms or oocytes for AR, as well as an undertaking from him/her that he/she will not attempt to seek the identity of the recipient. In case the donor is married, taking the written consent of the spouse if possible.
- It is also desirable to restrict the use of semen from the same donor to 5–10 pregnancies to avoid the possibility of an incestuous relationship occurring among the offsprings at a later date.
- In case the oocyte donor incurs any health problems during the process of donation, the costs of the subsequent health care should be borne by the potential recipient couple, irrespective of whether they receive oocyte donation as planned or not.
- In case of unused surplus embryos, the consent of the couple concerned should be obtained to cryopreserve such embryos for donation to other needy couples. Such embryo donations should be kept anonymous.
- The doctor performing the AR procedure should avoid being the doctor who delivers the child as a precautionary measure to prevent falsification, on his part, of the birth records in terms of entering the names of the parents of the child.

It should be noted that AID in a married woman with the consent of the husband does not amount to adultery on the part of the wife or the donor, as there is no sexual intercourse involved. AID without the husband's consent can be a ground for divorce or judicial separation.

Surrogate Motherhood

The following consensus has emerged universally with respect to surrogate motherhood.

1. Surrogate motherhood should be legal only when it is coupled with authorized adoption.
2. It should be rebuttably presumed that the woman who carries the child and gives birth to it is its mother.
3. The intending parents should have a preferential right to adopt the child, subject to six weeks' postpartum delay for the necessary maternal consent.
4. It should be legal only if medically certified as the only solution to infertility, or any other bar on pregnancy, by the intending mother.
5. It should be supervised by a qualified consultant to enforce adequate genetic screening.
6. The contract for surrogacy, despite reasonable payment of compensation on the completion of adoption, would be valid subject to the surrogate's right to retain the baby if she so desires. The only remedy for the genetic father, then, would be to claim custody on the grounds of the best interest of the child.
7. Abortion under the Abortion Law, on medical grounds should be an inviolable right of the surrogate, and the adopting parents have no claim over the amounts already paid.
8. The physician will be held responsible for negligence in the selection of the donor or the surrogate, or for damage caused due to negligent surgical procedures.

Legitimacy Of The Child Born Through ART

A child born through ART is presumed to be the legitimate child of the couple, having been born within wedlock and with the consent of both spouses, with all the attendant rights of parentage, support and inheritance. The sperm/oocyte donor should have no parental right or duties in relation to the child and the donor's anonymity should be protected.

Rights Of An Unmarried Woman To ART/AID

There is no legal bar on an unmarried woman going for ART. However, it is universally recommended that AID should be performed only on married woman and, that too, with the written consent of her husband, a two-parent family always being better for the child, whose interests will always outweigh all other interests. Besides, a child born to a single woman through AID is deemed to be illegitimate.

Posthumous AIH Through Sperm Bank

The consensus of opinion is that artificial insemination by the husband's sperm, stored before his death, is to be treated on the lines of artificial insemination of a single woman; the children so born would definitely be considered illegitimate due to the marriage having come to an end with the death of the husband, and any child born thereafter would be out of wedlock.

Preservation, Utilization And Destruction Of Embryos

While passing The Human Fertilization and Embryology Act, 1990, the British Parliament accepted the Warnock Committee recommendations, prohibiting research on or keeping alive any live embryo over 14 days after fertilization, excluding the period during which the embryo was frozen, with a maximum storage period of 10 years and a 5-yearly review of semen and egg deposits. Under this law, early this month, nearly 3,000 frozen embryos were destroyed in the UK after the expiry of the 5-year statutory limit and with the absence of any consent coming forth from the parents to extend the limit by a further 5 years.

In a case of dispute arising between a couple following divorce, after the preservation of embryos, over the right of the woman to conceive the child and seek custody of the embryos, a recent judgement has gone in favour of the woman, the husband having consented to the conception at the time of fertilization. However, the child born in such a case would be deemed to be an illegitimate child.